Virology Methods Manual

VIROLOGY METHODS MANUAL

Edited by

Brian WJ Mahy

Director, Division of Viral and Rickettsial Diseases
National Center for Infectious Diseases
Center for Disease Control and Prevention
Atlanta, GA 30333
USA

and

Hillar O Kangro

Head of Clinical Immunology
SmithKlein Beecham Biologicals S.A.
Section for Biology/Immunology
Rue de l'Institut, 89
B-1330 Rixensart
Belgium

ACADEMIC PRESS
Harcourt Brace & Company, Publishers
London San Diego New York Boston Sydney Tokyo Toronto

ACADEMIC PRESS LIMITED
24–28 Oval Road
LONDON NW1 7DX

US Edition published by
ACADEMIC PRESS INC.
San Diego, CA 92101

This book is printed on acid free paper

A catalogue record for this book is available from the British Library

ISBN 0–12–465330–8

Typeset by J&L Composition Ltd, Filey, North Yorkshire
Printed and bound in Great Britain by Bath Press Colourbooks, Glasgow

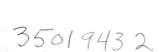

Preface

Viruses were first discovered and recognised as a separate class of microbes around the turn of the century. They were studied because they were found to be agents of some of the most important diseases of plants and animals, but because of their submicroscopic size and requirement to replicate within living cells it was not until the 1950s that virology became firmly established as a branch of science in its own right. At that time methods for cell culture and virus purification were developed, and the introduction of negative staining allowed electron microscopists to visualise the structures of viruses for the first time. The establishment of cell culture systems enabled studies of the replication of animal viruses and the development of attenuated live vaccines against important human pathogens such as measles, rubella and poliomyelitis. In the following twenty five years, virology made major contributions to the fields of cell and molecular biology and molecular genetics. Concepts arising directly from the study of animal virus replication include capping and polyadenylation of messenger RNAs, introns in cell DNA and splicing of RNA transcripts, interferons, reverse transcription, cellular oncogenes and the intracellular processing and presentation of antigens at the cell surface.

Our knowledge of virus structure and replication has increased in complexity, and so have the techniques required for virus detection, characterisation and diagnosis. The ability to sequence virus nucleic acids, whether DNA or RNA, by relatively simple technologies involving the polymerase chain reaction has led to our ability to trace virus movements in human or animal populations with great precision. A new field of molecular epidemiology has opened up and is providing the basis for World Health Organisation (WHO) campaigns to eradicate poliomyelitis and measles over the next five years. In addition, this genetic sequence information is being used as the basis for the rational design of new antiviral drugs as well as vaccines.

To help cope with the increased range and complexity of methods required for the study of viruses, we have assembled the present volume which aims to provide scientists working in clinical or research laboratories with clear descriptions and protocols of the most up-to-date, definitive techniques in virology. All the chapters are written by experts who have first-hand knowledge and experience of the methods they describe. We have divided the subject up into classical, molecular, and medical virology for convenience; these divisions are merely meant to guide the reader and are not intended to be exclusive. The chapters in Section 3 overlap somewhat in subject matter with those in Sections 1 and 2, but are written from the perspective of the medical virologist and provide additional insights that are important in the clinical setting when studying virus diseases.

We have included a number of appendices that may be used as a convenient information source on various aspects of virology. In each case reference to more substantial texts is made in the appendix, and these should be consulted if more detail is required.

The overall size and complexity of this volume was limited by our desire to create a useful methods book that would be affordable to most virologists. We would have achieved our aims if the book ends up in frequent use in the laboratory, not merely in the library.

We are grateful to Academic Press, especially to Tessa Picknett, for their patience and considerable professional input.

BRIAN WJ MAHY
HILLAR O KANGRO
JUNE 1995

Contents

Contributors

Dr Ali A Al-Jabri, Department of Academic Virology, The London Hospital Medical College, 64 Turner Street, London, E1 2AD, UK
Tel: + 171 375 2498
Fax: + 171 375 2597

Dr Eddie Ades, Division of Scientific Resources, National Center for Infectious Diseases, Centers for Disease Control and Prevention, 1600 Clifton Road N.E., Atlanta GA 30333, USA
Tel: + 1 404 639 3720
Fax: + 1 404 639 3129

Professor Max Chernesky, McMaster University Regional Virology Laboratory, St Joseph's Hospital, Hamilton, Ontario L8N 4A6, Canada
Tel: + 1 905 521 6021
Fax: + 1 905 521 6083

Dr Ian L Chrystie, Department of Virology, St Thomas' Hospital, London SE1 7EH, UK
Tel: + 171 928 9292 (Ext 3127)
Fax: + 171 928 0730

Dr Brian F Coles, National Center for Toxicological Research, Jefferson, Arkansas, AR 72079
Fax: + 1 501 5437136

Dr VG George, Scientific Resources Program, National Center for Infectious Diseases, Centers for Disease Control and Prevention, 1600 Clifton Road, NE, Atlanta, GA 30333, USA
Tel: + 1 404 639 3515
Fax: + 1 404 639 3129

Dr David Harper, Department of Virology, St Bartholomew's Hospital, Medical College, West Smithfield, London EC1A 7BE, UK
Tel: + 171 601 7351
Fax: + 171 726 4248

Dr John Hierholzer, Respiratory and Enteric Viruses Branch, DVRD, Centers for Disease Control and Prevention, 1600 Clifton Road N.E., Atlanta GA 30333, USA
Tel: + 1 404 639 3311
Fax: + 1 404 639

Dr TC Jarvis, Ribozyme Pharmaceuticals Inc., 2950 Wilderness Place, Boulder, Colorado 80301, USA

Professor Don Jeffries, Department of Virology, St Bartholomew's Hospital Medical College, University of London, 51–53 Bartholomew's Close, West Smithfield, London EC1A 7BE, UK
Tel: + 171 601 7351
Fax: + 171 726 4248

Dr Hillar Kangro, Head of Clinical Serology, Department of Immunology/Biology, SmithKline Beecham Biologicals SA, Section for Biology/Immunology, Rue de l'Institut, 89, B–1330, Rixensart, Belgium
Tel: + 32 2 656 9843
Fax: + 32 2 656 8113

Dr Richard Killington, Department of Microbiology, University of Leeds, Leeds LS2 9JT, UK
Tel: + 113 2431751
Fax: + 113 2834122

Dr Karla Kirkegaard, MCD Biology – HHMI, University of Colorado, Campus Box 347, Boulder, CO 80309–0347, USA
Tel: + 1 303 492 7882 (direct)/3600 (assistant)
Fax: + 1 303 492 7576

Contributors

Dr Keith Leppard, Department of Biological Sciences, University of Warwick, Coventry CV4 7AL, UK
Tel: + 1203 523579
Fax: + 1203 523701

Dr James Mahony, Head, Division of Virology, St Joseph's Hospital, 50 Charlton Avenue East, Hamilton, Ontario L8N 174, Canada
Tel: + 1 905 521 6021
Fax: + 1 905 521 6083

Dr Brian WJ Mahy, Director, Division of Viral and Rickettsial Diseases, National Center for Infectious Diseases, Centers for Disease Control and Prevention, Atlanta, GA 30333, USA
Tel: + 1 404 639 3574
Fax: + 1 404 639 3163

Dr Alison Mawle, Division of Viral and Rickettsial Diseases, National Center for Infectious Diseases, Centers for Disease Control and Prevention, 1600 Clifton Road, Atlanta, GA 30333, USA
Tel: + 1 404 639 1399
Fax: + 1 404 639 0049

Dr Dennis J McCance, Department of Microbiology and Immunology, University of Rochester, Box 672, Elmwood Avenue, Rochester, NY 14642, USA
Tel: + 1 716 275 0101
Fax: + 1 716 473 9573

Dr Malcolm McCrae, Department of Biological Sciences, University of Warwick, Coventry CV4 7AL, UK
Tel: + 1203 523524
Fax: + 1203 523568/523701

Dr JE Novak, Department of Molecular, Cellular, and Developmental Biology, Howard Hughes Medical Institute, University of Colorado, Boulder, Colorado 80309, USA
Tel: + 1 303 492 3600
Fax: + 1 303 492 7576

Dr John S Oxford, Department of Academic Virology, The London Hospital Medical College, 64 Turner Street, London E1 2AD, UK
Tel: + 171 375 2498
Fax: + 171 375 2597

Professor Craig Pringle, Department of Biological Sciences, University of Warwick, Coventry CV4 7AL, UK
Tel: + 1203 523565
Fax: + 1203 523701

Dr Steven Specter, Department of Medical Microbiology and Immunology, University of South Florida, College of Medicine, 12901 N Bruce B Downs Blvd, Tampa, FL 33612, USA
Tel: + 1 813 974 0897
Fax: + 1 813 974 4151

Dr A Stokes, Department of Microbiology, University of Leeds, LS2 9JT, UK
Tel: + 113 233 5614
Fax: + 113 233 5638

Dr Marcia D Wigg, Department of Academic Virology, The London Hospital Medical College, 64 Turner Street, London E1 2AD, UK
Tel: + 171 375 2498
Fax: + 171 375 2597

Section 1

Classical Techniques

Cell culture

V. G. George
J. C. Hierholzer
E. W. Ades

Cell culture is the art of growing cells *in vitro*. Although cells are probably influenced by the presence of each other, they have not become organized into a tissue. Cell culture allows one to look at cells in their entirety from the outside – that is, as a whole – before examining the intricacy of their component parts. In this chapter, we will provide the tools for using cell culture as an adjunct to the cell biology and molecular biology methods that break down the traditional borders between the disciplines of biology and virology.

As with any chapter on the methodology of cell culture, one must first determine the cell type of choice needed for a particular study. There are over 3200 characterized cell lines today, derived from over 75 species, including hybridomas and plant cultures. Several national and international cell banks, including the American Type Culture Collection (Rockville, Maryland, U.S.A.) and the European Collection of Animal Cell Cultures (Salisbury, Wiltshire, U.K.) are excellent resources for cells and specific cell information. Detailed information on media composition, plaque cultures, microcultures, and specialized techniques are also well documented (Freshney 1983; Schmidt 1989).

Once the cell type that exhibits some unique characteristic(s) has been selected, make certain that the life expectancy of these cells *in vitro* is sufficient to complete the project. It is preferable to use a cell line which can be propagated for at least 15–20 passages or subcultures beyond the seed stock while retaining its special characteristics.

Virology Methods Manual
ISBN 0–12–465330–8

Cell cultures

Primary cells

Primary cells are freshly isolated cells that are derived directly from the tissue of origin. The tissue source for the majority of primary cell cultures is either laboratory animals or human pathology specimens. Research institutions should have in place a review and approval process for procuring laboratory animals and human tissue. When a project utilizing laboratory animals, and particularly human tissue, is being developed, this approval process must be followed explicitly.

Healthy young or embryonic animals are preferable to adults. The younger the animal, the greater the potential for success in culturing the cells. Because there are numerous cell types, there are numerous methods of culturing these cells. The following is a general protocol for processing primary monkey kidney cells; it may need modification for use with other species or organs.

Removing the organ

1. The special skills of a veterinarian, or highly trained technician under the supervision of a veterinarian, are required for the successful removal of the monkey kidney. The kidney must be removed with a minimum of trauma to the animal and to the organ. The animal handlers and any technician involved in this process must be trained and certified by the supervising veterinarian.
2. To prevent drying and loss of viable cells, the kidney is placed in a flask containing an isotonic solution (balanced salt solution). Antibiotics are generally added to the medium to help prevent contamination.

Processing the organ

1. With sterile forceps, transfer the kidney to a beaker, and carefully remove the capsule with the forceps and surgical scissors. With surgical scissors, mince the kidney into small pieces (approximately 3 mm in diameter), add 100 ml of 0.22% trypsin–0.02% versene, and pour the contents of the beaker into a 250 ml indented Erlenmeyer flask (Melnick), which contains a magnetic stir bar.
2. Place the beaker on a magnetic mixer. Adjust the stirring speed to prevent foaming and stir for 2 min. Discard the first supernate-suspension as a wash, then add fresh enzyme and pour off every 20 min, repeating the interval harvest until the cortex tissue is exhausted. Collect the cell suspension by filtering through two layers of sterile gauze into 250 ml centrifuge bottles, and add 25–50 ml of cold growth medium.
3. Centrifuge the cell suspension immediately after each harvest at 65 g for 20 min at 4°C. Aspirate the trypsin–versene solution from the cells.
4. Add 50 ml of growth media to each bottle of packed cells and swirl vigorously until an even suspension is obtained.
5. After completing the cell harvest, filter the entire suspension through two layers of sterile gauze.
6. Determine the cell concentration (see page 13). Crystal violet is the dye of choice for primary cells, however, since cell fragments will also stain, count only the whole cells.
7. Seed the primary cells at 3×10^5 ml^{-1}

Continuous cell lines

Cell lines are continuously growing subcultures of the primary cells. Most cell lines may be propagated in an unaltered form for a limited number of cell generations, beyond which they either die out or give rise to continuous cell lines. The ability of a cell line to grow continuously probably reflects its capacity for genetic variation, which allows subsequent selection to occur (Freshney 1983).

Euploid cells

Normal human fibroblasts remain predominantly euploid (containing exact multiples of the normal chromosomal number) throughout their culture life-span, rarely give rise to continuous cell lines and at crisis (usually around 50 generations) will stop dividing (Hayflick and Moorhead 1961).

Aneuploid cells

Mouse fibroblasts and cell cultures from a variety of human and animal tumors, on the other hand, often become aneuploid (chromosome number is not an exact multiple of the normal number) in culture and give rise to continuous cultures with fairly high frequency. Continuous cell lines are usually aneuploid and have a chromosome complement between the diploid and tetraploid values. Nonfibroblast normal cells rarely give rise to continuous cell lines.

The alteration in a culture giving rise to a continuous cell line is commonly called 'in vitro transformation' and may occur spontaneously or be chemically or virally induced. The term 'transformation' has been applied to the process of formation of a continuous cell line partly because the culture undergoes morphological and kinetic alterations, but also because the formation of a continuous cell line is often accompanied by an increase in tumorigenicity (Freshney 1983). The condition that most predisposes primary cells to develop a continuous cell line is probably inherent genetic variation, so it is not surprising to find genetic instability perpetuated in continuous cell lines.

Insect cells

The most commonly utilized insect lines are the SF9 (ovary, fall armyworm, *Spodoptera frugiperda* (ATTC # CRL 1710) and mosquito cell lines such as *Aedes aegypti* (ATCC # CRL 125), and *Aedes albopictus* (ATCC # CRL 126).

The SF9 cell line culture medium consists of Graces' medium plus 3.3 g of lactalbumin hydrolysate and 3.3 g of yeastolate per liter with 10% heat-inactivated fetal bovine serum. This cell line is highly susceptible to infection with Baculoviruses and can be used to study recombinant genes in Baculovirus expression vectors and for other needs (Vaughn et al 1977; Smith et al 1985).

Mosquito lines are suitable for the replication of many mosquito-borne viruses (Singh 1968; Singh 1971; Yunker and Cory 1969; Buckley 1969). Mitsuhashi and Maramorosch Insect Medium supplemented with 5–20% fetal bovine serum is commonly used for the growth and maintenance of mosquito cell lines. Subcultures are prepared by scraping (see page 7) or by vigorous pipetting. A subcultivation ratio of 1:4 to 1:10 is recommended.

Propagation of cell cultures

All procedures involving cell lines should be performed in a Class II biological safety cabinet under strict aseptic conditions to minimize the risk of contaminating the cells with bacteria, yeasts, and mycoplasmas. All pipetting should be done using an automatic pipet-aid or manual propipetter, since **absolutely no** mouth pipetting should be allowed in the laboratory. Laboratory personnel should wear lab coats and surgical gloves while performing cell culture manipulations. All cell lines should be treated as potentially hazardous. Continuous cell lines are assumed to be free of infectious viruses, but in fact may harbor latent viruses that have the potential to infect the laboratory worker. Transformed cells may spontaneously produce a potentially oncogenic virus (Barkley 1979). Therefore, all cell lines should be treated as potentially hazardous, and all laboratory workers should become familiar with safe laboratory practices. Institution directors and laboratory supervisors should provide safety training and should enforce safety regulations. Laboratory workers should also share responsibility for their own safety.

Media and buffers

Most media in use today are chemically defined, but are supplemented with 5–20% serum. The medium used for any particular cells will be determined by the cell type and the procedures to be performed with these cells. Cells purchased from cell repositories will be accompanied by an instruction sheet which recommends the appropriate medium, subculture procedures, correct seeding concentrations, feeding schedule, and any safety concerns.

Generally, cells will grow well at pH 7.0–7.4. Phenol red is commonly used as an indicator in the culture medium. It is red at pH 7.4, becoming orange at pH 7.0 and yellow at pH 6.5, and in the alkaline direction, it becomes bluish at pH 7.6 and purple at pH 7.8 (Freshney 1983).

Culture media require buffering under two sets of conditions: (1) use of open dishes, in which exposure to oxygen causes the pH to rise, and (2) when CO_2 and lactic acid are overproduced in transformed cell lines at high cell concentrations, when the pH will fall. A buffer may be incorporated in the medium to stabilize the pH, but in open dishes, exogenous CO_2 may still be required by cell lines, particularly at low cell concentrations, to prevent the total loss of dissolved CO_2 and bicarbonate from the medium. In an overproduction scenario, it is usually preferable to leave the cap loose or to use a CO_2-permeable cap to promote the release of CO_2. Flasks with gas-permeable caps are available from Costar (Cambridge, MA), Corning (Corning, NY), and others. (**Use of trade names is for identification purposes only and does not imply endorsement by the Public Health Service or U.S. Department of Health and Human Services.**)

The CO_2 level is extremely important; a 1% increase can result in cell death in some cases. Therefore, even with a state-of-the-art incubator with digital read-outs, the CO_2 level must be monitored, since it can drift undetected by the read-out. In our laboratory, a Bacharach Fyrite Gas Analyzer (Bacharach, Inc., Pittsburgh, PA) is used once a week to monitor the CO_2 incubators.

The need for endotoxin-free water

Pyrogen-free water should be used to make any medium components made in-house. Small, inexpensive reagent grade water systems are available commercially (Culligan, Marietta, GA; Millipore, Bedford, MA). These units will produce Type I reagent grade water as described by NCCLS Document C3–A2: Preparation and Testing of Reagent Water in the Clinical Laboratory. We recommend that a reputable manufacturer of pure water equipment be contacted for guidance on the purchase of an appropriate system for laboratory applications. The manufacturer's recommendations will primarily depend on their analysis of the quality of the source water. The manufacturer will provide maintenance and sanitization on a contract basis or provide written procedures for laboratory maintenance.

Type I reagent grade water must be used as soon as it is produced because when it is stored, 'its resistivity will decrease, metals and/or organic contaminants will be leached from the storage container, and bacterial contamination will occur' (NCCLS Document C3–A2, 1991). Due to this degradation, purchased bottled water is not an acceptable alternative to an in-house pure water system.

Sterilization

Most reagents or media can be sterilized either by autoclaving if they are heat-stable (water, salt solutions, amino acid hydrolysates) or by membrane filtration if they are heat-labile. Filters appropriate for the sterilization of cell culture media are available from many sources such as Costar, Corning, Nalge, and Gelman. The type of filter membrane is important and care should be taken when selecting a filter system. Choose from cellulose acetate membranes for applications involving low protein binding. Cellulose nitrate membranes are appropriate for general purpose filtration in the cell culture laboratory. A membrane pore size of 0.22 μM should be used for sterilization. Thick cotton pads or membranes of larger pore size should be used for prefiltering.

Propagating cells by scraping

Removing anchorage dependent (adherent) cells from the cell culture flask requires a chemical or physical method. The enzymes used to detach cell monolayers may be toxic to some cells; therefore, disposable cell scrapers (Cat. # 3010, Costar Corp., Cambridge, MA) may be used. Cell scraping is a fairly simple method for cell harvesting. The growth medium is removed from the culture flask, and the cell sheet is then detached by physically scraping the cells from the flask surface. To disperse the cells, a growth medium is added to the flask and the medium is pipetted over the flask surface to obtain a single cell suspension. The cells are then counted and appropriately diluted (see page 13) for passage to new flasks or other types of cell culture containers.

Some laboratories depend on 'split ratios' rather than on cell counts to passage cells. These laboratories determine the optimum ratio at which a confluent flask may be divided to yield viable confluent monolayers within the

time frame necessary for their projects. This method is an option to be considered; however, dye exclusion cell counts are more reliable for consistent results because these counts provide the number of 'viable' cells, and the quantity of living cells that are actually being subcultured can be determined without guesswork.

Propagating cells by enzyme treatment

Advantages and disadvantages

For chemical detachment of adherent cells from tissue culture flasks, certain enzymes (trypsin, pronase and collagenase) and chelating agents (versene or ethylene-diamine-tetra-acetic acid (EDTA)) are routinely used. Utilizing a combination of trypsin and versene is a convenient and efficient method of detaching the majority of adherent cell lines with a minimum of cell damage; this method is detailed below. Note that some enzymes remove receptors or other important cell surface molecules; therefore, the effects of these enzymes on the characteristics of the cell line chosen must be determined.

Subculture protocol

1. Observe the cell monolayer under a microscope to determine the general condition of the cells and any obvious contamination. If the cells are healthy and appear to be free of contamination, proceed with trypsinization.
2. Decant or aspirate the spent medium and wash the cell layer with PBS that has been warmed to 37°C; the washing removes any remaining serum, which would inhibit the enzyme activity of the trypsin/versene.
3. Decant the wash solution and add trypsin/versene (0.05% trypsin, 0.53 mM EDTA; Cat. # 25300-047, GIBCO BRL, Grand Island, NY) to the

flask, approximately 3 ml per T-75 or 6 ml per T-150 flask. Place the flask at room temperature with the cell surface down until the cells detach. If trypsinizing a roller bottle, the bottle may be rotated at the work station during the wash, but should be placed on the roller drum while waiting for the cells to detach. Occasionally, a cell line will be difficult to remove from the flask; incubating at 37°C for a few minutes or gently tapping the flask against the heel of your hand will accelerate the process. Some cell lines such as MDCK may require two washes of trypsin–versene to accelerate detachment.

4. When cells detach, add growth medium to the flask and wash all flask surfaces by repeatedly pipetting up and down to suspend as many cells as possible in the medium and to break up any existing cell clumps.

5. Perform a cell count (see page 13) and seed new flasks or other vessels accordingly. Incubate the newly seeded vessels at 37°C.

Suspension cultures

Usefulness

Some cells will not adhere to a culture vessel but can be propagated in suspension. Many mouse and human leukemias and ascites tumors grow in suspension. These cells are incubated on shakers or on roller drums or allowed to settle to the bottom of a large culture flask such as a roller bottle. Alternatively, a mechanical method is available which forces normally adherent cells to grow in suspension. This is usually performed by using a spinner apparatus and medium formulated for suspension culture. Cells are available that are easily adapted to spinner culture, such as HeLa S3 (ATCC # CCL 2.2).

Subculture protocol

The subculture of suspension cells is a simple and fast procedure.

1. Allow the suspension to settle, and aspirate most of the spent medium before doing a cell count. Proceed with subculture by transferring the number of cells determined necessary to establish the new culture to the appropriate vessel containing fresh growth medium. If the cells do not settle well, centrifugation at a low speed may be necessary.

2. Suspension cells may also be cultured by dilution. A 1:10 dilution is usually sufficient to establish a new culture; one part cell suspension transferred to nine parts fresh growth medium will accomplish the subculture rapidly and efficiently. This procedure is less precise, however, and viability has not been assessed.

The pH of suspension cultures is critical. Observe cultures closely for the color changes described previously (page 6) and initiate appropriate procedures if the pH changes drastically. Culture vessels with vented caps are helpful in maintaining the pH in suspension cultures as well as in adherent cultures that require a CO_2 atmosphere.

Lymphocyte cultures

Fresh mononuclear cells can be isolated from whole blood by Ficoll-Hypaque gradient centrifugation (Boyum 1968) and cultured in suspension. These cells have multiple uses, including the following: after stimulation using lectins, such as phytohemagglutinin (PHA), they can be cocultivated with blood specimens to determine whether human immunodeficiency virus (HIV) is present. Other uses for these cells for diagnosis, evaluation of immunity, detection of disease or cellular networking are too numerous to discuss in this chapter.

Procedures for the isolation of particular subpopulations of cells (T cells, B cells, and macrophages) from peripheral blood or lymphoid tissues may be found in a National Institutes of Health publication (Coligan et al 1991).

Maintenance of adherent and suspension cells

The need for routine medium changes

Once a culture has been passaged, routine medium changes (feeding) (i.e. to replenish constituents in the medium, such as amino acids, vitamins, and glucose, which are essential for metabolism) are necessary to allow the cells to proliferate. The initial cell concentration and the metabolism rate will determine any feeding schedule instituted.

The need for subculturing

Close observation of color changes in the medium, which indicate an increase or decrease in pH level and the rate of metabolism, is necessary to determine if cells require feeding or subculturing. Epithelial cells such as HeLa and HEp2 metabolize rapidly and can be subcultured twice a week. Fibroblast cells such as MRC5 and WI-38 metabolize slowly and would probably be ready for subculture only once a week and would require feeding at least once during that week. Suspension cultures must be subcultured or the volume of medium increased as the cell population reaches 2×10^6 cells ml^{-1}, because, in general, the viability of suspension cells drops rapidly at higher concentrations.

Seeding concentrations of a rapidly proliferating cell line such as HeLa may be lowered to reduce subculturing to once a week. A seeding concentration as low as 20,000–30,000 cells cm^{-2} of surface area will result in a healthy monolayer. If cell viability begins to decrease, then the twice-a-week subculture schedule should be resumed.

A 'maintenance' medium, which is the regular medium with only 1 or 2% serum rather than 10–20%, may be used to hold some cell lines at a single cell layer for an extended period, even for 2–3 weeks if necessary. This holding or maintenance medium tends not to stimulate mitosis in most untransformed cells, which usually accompanies a medium change. This holding medium can also be used to maintain cell lines with a finite life-span without using up the limited number of cell generations available to them. Transformed cells, on the other hand, are unsuitable for this procedure because they may either continue to divide successfully or the culture may deteriorate.

Cell synchronization

The growth of cells in cultures can be divided into three stages: (1) a lag period, immediately after the inoculum; (2) a growth phase, during which the cell number increases rapidly and usually in an exponential fashion; and (3) a plateau or stationary phase, during which the cell number remains constant. In exponentially growing populations, the cells are distributed asynchronously throughout the cell cycle in its four phases – G_1, S, G_2 and M (Ashihara and Baserga 1979).

The M (mitosis) phase is the cell's reproductive cycle. The much longer phase between one cell division and the next is known as interphase, consisting of the G_1, S, and G_2 phases. The G_1 phase (G = gap) is the interval between the end of mitosis and the beginning of DNA synthesis or S phase. The G_2 phase is the interval between DNA synthesis and the beginning of mitosis.

Table 1.1. Cell synchronization.

A) Physical Methods of Synchronization
1. mitotic detachment*
2. gradient techniques*
3. centrifugal elutriation*

B) Chemical Methods of Synchronization
1. isoleucine deprivation*
2. serum deprivation and hydroxyurea*
3. double-thymidine block*
4. calcium deprivation*
5. FUdR and amethopterin[†]

* Ashihara and Baserga 1979.
[†] Nias and Fox 1971.

Any study of cellular events at specific times during the cell cycle is facilitated by culture synchronization, such that cells can be induced to proceed through the cell cycle together. Many ways to synchronize cultured cells have been described (Table 1.1); the method chosen depends on which cells are used and which events are to be studied. Synchrony of human diploid cells is short-lived, usually much less than the mean cell cycle time, and never complete. Human non-diploid established lines, such as HeLa cells, may respond to any of the methods generally applicable to mammalian cells, and synchrony may be more successful and lasting (Priest 1971).

Ideally, synchronized populations of cells in culture should meet the following criteria: (1) they should be perfectly synchronized at a specific point in the cell cycle; (2) the procedure used for synchronizing cells should have little or no effect on the metabolic processes of the cell; and (3) especially for the biochemist, the method should allow the harvesting of synchronized cells in large quantities (Ashihara and Baserga 1979).

Because mammalian cell populations have an intrinsic variability in cell doubling times, it is impossible to achieve perfect synchrony, i.e. all the cells passing through every point in the mitotic cycle simultaneously. The best that can be achieved is for all the cells to be at one single point in the cycle at a given time; thereafter they will lose synchronization as they progress through the mitotic cycle. Continued synchronization is only likely to be maintained by repeated treatment of the cell population, but the lack of synchronization at some time interval after a single treatment does not necessarily imply that the original synchronization procedure was ineffective (Nias and Fox 1971).

An example of synchronization is described by Held et al (1989). Their procedure is a simple, nontoxic protocol based on the selection of a rapidly attaching subpopulation of trypsinized cells. By limiting the time of attachment of trypsinized cells and the subsequent removal of unattached cells, a G_1 population of cells is isolated.

Quality assurance and contamination

Bacteria, yeasts, fungi

Many types of organisms may be found as contaminants of cell cultures. Some of them, such as bacteria, yeasts, and fungi may be detected by turbidity and pH change of the culture medium or, more definitively, by examining the cultures by microscope. Detailed protocols for the detection of most bacteria and fungi that would be expected to survive in cell cultures may be found elsewhere (ATCC 1985). These protocols should also be incorporated into the quality assurance of a cell culture media production laboratory to preclude the contamination of cells by the growth media.

Mycoplasmas and viruses

Organisms such as mycoplasmas and viruses usually do not cause turbidity or pH change and may or may not produce cytopathological effects (CPE) in the cells. They are thus difficult to detect and may be passaged with the cells indefinitely without detection, unless specific testing is performed. Primary rhesus monkey kidney cells (MK), primary African green monkey kidney cells (AGMK), and primary bovine kidney cells (PBEK) are particularly notorious for adventitious virus contamination (Crandell et al 1978; Hsiung 1969; Schmidt 1989). Commercial testing services are available for mycoplasmas and viruses. Test kits are commercially available for mycoplasma, such as the MycoTect test (GIBCO #189–5672). Two of the most common methods for mycoplasma detection in the cell culture laboratory are culture and fluorescent staining. These methods may be incorporated into the quality assurance procedures of a laboratory relatively easily. The DNA specific fluorescent stain (Chen 1977) may be used as the presumptive test, and the culture method (Hayflick 1973) as the confirmatory test.

Other cell lines

Cross-contamination between cell lines has occurred often, the most problematic being the intrusion of HeLa cells into many other lines. Therefore, it is extremely important to take the following precautions. **Never** work with more than one cell line at a time. Do not use a bottle of medium, trypsin/versene etc on more than one cell line. Allow a 'resting' period of approximately 30 min between cell lines in a biological safety cabinet, and decontaminate cabinet surfaces before introducing another cell line to the work area.

Determining species of origin

Species of origin can be determined for cell lines by a variety of immunological tests, by isoenzymology and/or by cytogenetics (ATCC 1985). This testing requires expertise that is not available in most cell culture laboratories; however, testing services are available for these procedures (e.g. Childrens' Hospital, Detroit, MI).

If a laboratory routinely receives cell lines from other research institutions, an area should be established to isolate these cell lines until the quality assurance testing can be performed on them and they are declared to be free of contamination and the correct species is identified. This may seem extreme, but our laboratory has on several occasions received cells that were contaminated with mycoplasma or with another cell line. Also, quality testing information from the sending laboratory should be reviewed by the receiving laboratory before culturing the cells.

We cannot emphasize strongly enough that these quality assurance tests must be performed *routinely* in any laboratory in which cell cultures are used. Contaminants may cause irreversible changes in cell cultures, and they can completely confound the interpretation of a diagnostic test. Therefore, results from diagnostic tests or any research in which cells were used would be suspect unless these quality assurance tests were performed with satisfactory results.

Quantifying by cell counts

Purpose and choice of method

Cells are counted in order to seed stock cultures with a known number of viable cells, to determine cell propagation rates, and to determine viability in a cell culture. Cells are usually counted in the presence of a vital stain, a dye which is only incorporated into a cell if it is no longer alive. Hence dyes such as trypan blue, which stain only the dead cells, can be used to determine cell viability. Since the cell membrane of living cells prevents the cells from taking up the dye, procedures in which these vital stains are used are known as dye exclusion tests.

Trypan blue vital stain procedure

A cell suspension sample which has been combined with a dye is placed in the counting chamber of a hemocytometer, and the cells are counted with a low-power microscope. The count is then mathematically converted to the number of cells per milliliter. The stained (dead) cells and the unstained (living) cells are counted separately to determine the percentage that are viable. Trypan blue and erythrosine B are the most common dyes used for viability dye exclusion tests. Other dyes, such as methylene blue, acridine orange, eosin, nigrosin, and safranin, have been used as 'exclusion' dyes but are no longer preferred (Tolnai 1975). Dyes such as crystal violet stain both living and dead cells and are best used to clarify morphology (Bird and Forrester, 1981).

A working solution of trypan blue (0.4% in physiological saline) that has been filtered through membrane (and can be stored at room temperature) may be purchased through several suppliers, including GIBCO BRL (Cat. # 15250-012).

1. Gather the cell suspension sample, trypan blue dye, counting chamber (Improved Neubauer 0.1 mm deep, conversion factor = 10,000), coverslip, and hand tally counter (the counting chamber, coverslips, and tally counter may be purchased through a scientific supply catalog such as Fisher or Thomas).
2. Prepare the chamber and coverslip. Clean the counting chamber and coverslip with 70% alcohol. Dry both thoroughly, being careful not to scratch either. Moisten the edges of the coverslip slightly and apply to the supporting edges of the counting chamber.
3. Mix the cell sample thoroughly and add 1 ml of dye to 1 ml of the cell sample. Allow mixture to stand for at least 5 min, but not more than 15 min, before performing the cell count.
4. Using a Pasteur pipette, gently fill one side of the counting chamber. For an accurate count, the chamber should not be underfilled or overfilled.
5. Examine the cells through a microscope at about 100× magnification by first focusing on the grid of the chamber and then on the cells themselves. Count the cells in the four large corner squares. Each corner square is made up of sixteen small squares. Count cells within each small square, and to avoid counting some cells twice, count overlapping cells using the line method (i.e. count

the left and top lines of each small square or the right and bottom lines, but not both). Count each cell in a clump of cells.

6. Determine the number of viable cells per milliliter in the original suspension, using the following formula:

[(no. of cells counted) ÷ (no. of squares counted)] × [counting chamber conversion factor] × [dilution factor] = cells per ml

(For counting chamber conversion factor see package insert.)

Example: 1 ml of dye added to a ml of cell suspension = 1:2 dilution, therefore the dilution factor = 2. The conversion factor of the hemocytometer = 10,000. Therefore, 356 (cells) ÷ 4 (large sqs.) × 10,000 (conversion) × 2 (dilution) = 1.78×10^6 (cells/ml)

We recommend that at least 100 cells be counted for routine subcultures. It may be necessary to concentrate the cell suspension by centrifugation for more accurate results. If the cell suspension is heavily concentrated and results in too many cells to count, the sample may be diluted in growth medium before the dye is added.

Example: 1 ml cell suspension added to 4 ml of medium = 1:5 dilution. 1 ml of the 1:5 dilution added to 1 ml of dye = 1:2 dilution, and thus the dilution factor used in the formula is the product of both factors: 5 × 2 = 10 (the total dilution factor).

Viability determination

For viability determination, use the cell counting procedur described above to count viable and nonviable cells.

Using the following formula, determine the percentage of viable cells.

$$\frac{\text{Viable cells (Unstained)}}{\text{Viable Cells + Dead Cells (Stained)}} \times 100$$
$$= \text{\% Viable cells}$$

Example: 254 ÷ (254 + 5) × 100 = 98% Viable cells

Stock cell culture seeding

The volume of the initial cell suspension needed to seed subsequent cultures is determined by the standard volume/concentration equation:

Initial Concentration × Volume of Initial Concentrate = Final Concentration × Final Volume

For example: To determine what volume of a cell suspension containing 5×10^6 cells ml^{-1} should be diluted to 1 ml to yield 2×10^6 cells ml^{-1}

5×10^6 cells ml^{-1} X (X ml) = 2×10^6 cells ml^{-1} X (1 ml)

$$Xml = \frac{2 \times 10^6 \text{ cells } ml^{-1}}{5 \times 10^6 \text{ cells } ml^{-1}}$$

X   = 0.4 ml

Therefore: 0.4 ml of original suspension diluted with 0.6 ml of medium will yield 1 ml of suspension at 2×10^6 cells ml^{-1}.

Cell preservation and storage

Cryopreservation procedure

Cells may be preserved by freezing or 'cryopreserved'. This provides a ready stock of cells if cells are lost due to contamination, malfunction of the incubator, natural senescence, or a genetic drift that may affect their ability to exhibit the expected response characteristics to a routine procedure or assay.

As most laboratories are not equipped with a controlled rate freezing apparatus, we find the following procedure yields successful cryopreservation results. First and foremost, only cells that are healthy, free from contamination, and in active logarithmic growth phase should be selected for preservation. In general, cells should be frozen at a minimum of 1×10^6 cells ml^{-1}; a routine number of $2-4 \times 10^6$ cells ml^{-1} is used as the standard in our laboratory.

After enumeration by trypan blue cell counting technique (page 13), the cells are centrifuged at 80–100 g and resuspended in the preservation or freeze medium that has been warmed to room temperature. The preservation medium consists of the culture medium containing 5–20% serum plus 5% dimethylsulfoxide (DMSO) or glycerol, preferably DMSO (Lovelock and Bishop 1959; Freshney 1983; Schmidt 1989). The cells are then dispensed into cryovials, 1 ml per vial. Cryovials, which are recommended for −70°C or nitrogen storage, may be purchased from numerous commercial sources, such as the Nalgene Cryovial (Nalge Company, Rochester, NY).

The cell suspension should be frozen slowly at 1°C min^{-1} (Leibo and Mazur 1971; Harris and Griffiths 1977). If a controlled rate freezing apparatus is not available, the cells may be cooled gradually by placing at 4°C for 1 h, then at −20°C for at least 1 h and transferred to −70°C or a liquid or gas phase nitrogen freezer. The much lower temperature (−165°C) obtained in nitrogen is preferable for long-term storage.

An inexpensive and extremely efficient controlled rate freezing apparatus is now available (9001 BTRL Cell Freezer, Biotech Research Laboratories, Inc., Rockville, MD). The 9001 BTRL Cell Freezer consists of a can with a foam grid support and vial grid that will hold 24 vials. The can is filled with methanol, ethanol, or isopropanol as a refrigerant to a level that will be slightly higher than the level of the cell suspension in the freezing vials. After the vials are placed in the vial grid, the 9001 freezer can is sealed and placed in a −70°C to −90°C freezer. The 9001 unit should be left undisturbed for at least 5 h, after which the vials can be transferred to a liquid nitrogen freezer.

Recovery of frozen cells

A vial of cells is thawed rapidly by agitating the vial in a water bath at 37°C. The cells are then diluted, but not washed, with the appropriate culture medium and placed in a cell culture flask. The dilution should be determined by the concentration of viable cells present at the time of freezing. A vial containing 2×10^6 cells ml^{-1} may be diluted successfully to 1:10 or 1:20.

During the initial growth period, the pH should be carefully controlled. Therefore, it is standard procedure in our laboratory to place these cultures in a 5% CO_2 atmosphere. The medium must be replaced after 24 h to remove all traces of DMSO or glycerol. The medium

exchange on a suspension culture would necessitate centrifugation and resuspension in the new culture medium.

During all phases of this procedure, precautions should be taken to prevent inhalation of DMSO fumes and contact of DMSO with the skin. A face shield or safety glasses should be worn while removing the vial from the freezer and during the thawing process.

Transformation and transfection

Most vertebrate cell lines die after a finite number of divisions in cell culture, although rare 'immortal' variant cells can arise spontaneously in culture and can be maintained indefinitely as cell lines. DNA cloning and genetic engineering have given us techniques that enable us to isolate specific genes, redesign them, and insert them back into cells. This technology has revolutionized the study of living cells. Eukaryotic cell lines are being developed with indefinite replication ability to express at least some of the differentiated properties of their cell of origin, and to not necessarily cause tumors if injected into animals.

The procedures for generation of transformed cell lines are well documented (Freshney 1983). Genetic engineering procedures are too numerous and involved for this chapter; an excellent source of detailed procedures is Ausubel et al (1991).

Cytopathologic effects in cell cultures due to viruses

The general principles of collection, shipment, and processing of specimens, choice of viral isolation systems, and choice of diagnostic tests can be found in the next chapter and in other reference works (Fields et al 1990; Hierholzer 1993; Leland and French 1988; Mandell et al 1990; Schmidt and Emmons 1989). Information surrounding viral CPE is given here because cell culture is so vital to the laboratory diagnosis of viral infections.

Viral growth is usually evidenced by the CPE that occur in the infected cell monolayer. CPE are scanned under light microscopy at 40–100× and observed in greater detail at 200–400×. The exact nature of the CPE and the time required for it to appear in a particular cell type are often indicative of the virus group present there. Thus, careful observation of the monolayers is important so that the proper identification test can be expediently applied. CPE caused by different viruses in various cells are summarized below.

Types of CPE in standard cell cultures

Enlarged, round, refractile cells in clusters

Grape-like clusters of round, refractile, enlarged cells in cultures of HEK, HEp2, A549, NCI-H292, HeLa, and many other cells indicate adenovirus or herpes simplex virus. For adenovirus, the same CPE may develop, but more slowly, in fibroblast cells. At complete (4+) CPE, all cells become lysed and detached from the glass surface. Generally, both viruses grow in the same cells, but adenovirus grows more slowly (3–14 days) depending on serotype, and makes more discrete, irregularly-shaped cell clusters, whereas herpes type 1 grows very fast (1–2 days), makes fewer clusters, and may produce ballooned, multinucleate giant cells with granulated cytoplasm.

Multinucleate giant cell CPE

Measles virus produces classic giant cell CPE in AGMK, Vero, and HEK cells after 7–14 days of roller culture. This CPE is characterized by fusion of the cells, with the nuclei of the fused cells surrounding a granular area in the cytoplasm. Cytomegalovirus produces giant cells resembling elongated foci of refractile, swollen cells, but more slowly (12–30 days) and only in diploid fibroblast cells, also on a roller apparatus.

Syncytial CPE

The classic example of this CPE is respiratory syncytial virus (RSV), which produces patches of multicell syncytia in HEp2, HeLa, and NCI-H292 cells in 5–12 days in roller cultures. The balled-up syncytia usually become detached from the glass surface and float freely in the medium. Some strains of RSV, particularly of type B, produce more cellular degeneration than syncytia both in HEp2 and NCI-H292 cells.

The influenza, parainfluenza, and mumps viruses cause a combination of syncytia, rounding, and degeneration in roller cultures of NCI-H292 and MK cells. In addition, chick embryo and MDCK cells for influenza virus isolation and NCI-H292 cells for parainfluenza virus isolation require a fortified medium containing trypsin for optimal sensitivity (Castells et al 1990; Frank et al 1979; Klenk et al 1975; Meguro et al 1979). The syncytia may be accompanied by vacuolation with influenza, especially type B; by a granular degeneration with parainfluenza virus types 1–4; and is often noted as large syncytia with mumps virus. The CPE induced by these viruses may develop in 4–7 days, but the cultures must generally be blind-passaged and held an additional week to ensure viral growth. The cells rarely become detached.

Enlarged, round, glassy cells in small foci

Varicella-zoster (VZ) virus exhibits this CPE in 2–10 days; it is distinct from that caused by CMV, although both grow in diploid fibroblast cells in roller culture. VZ can produce large foci of multinucleate giant cells when the individual foci coalesce.

Cell fusion CPE with plaques

The cell fusion/plaque type of CPE is caused by vaccinia virus and certain other poxviruses growing in MK, Vero, NCI-H292, and diploid fibroblast cells. Plaques ranging from 1 mm to 6 mm in diameter, depending on the virus, are formed in 2–4 days, during which the infected cells fuse, form cytoplasmic bridging, and then disintegrate.

Shrunken cell degeneration CPE

The enteroviruses and rhinoviruses typify this CPE in NCI-H292, MK, RD, and diploid fibroblast cells, preferably in roller cultures. The CPE is often observed as tadpole shaped, shrunken cells with pycnotic nuclei, beginning in patches at the edges of the monolayer and progressing inward. CPE for polioviruses and some coxsackie B viruses is very rapid, becoming 4^+ in 1–3 days with all cells detached from the glass. CPE for the remain-

ing enteroviruses and the rhinoviruses generally requires 4–7 days or longer, is often accompanied by individual small, rounded, and sometimes refractile cells or by a degenerative appearance across the monolayer, and may not ever progress to 4^+ or general cell lysis.

Granular, degenerative, slowly-lytic CPE

Reoviruses cause a nondescript, gradual degeneration with granulation of the cytoplasm in NCI-H292, MK, and HeLa cells under stationary or roller conditions after 5–14 days of culture. MK cultures must be rolled. Polyoma BK virus in HEK, NCI-H292, and diploid fibroblast cells, and the polyoma JC virus in primary human fetal glial cells cause a similar, slowly-developing CPE.

Certain arboviruses belonging to the *Togaviridae*, *Flaviviridae*, *Filoviridae*, *Bunyaviridae*, and *Arenaviridae* families can be isolated in primary hamster kidney, chick or duck embryo cells, or derivative cell lines such as BHK-21, Vero, and LLC-MK2, after 2–10 days of culture. The CPE may be nonexistent at first, but become a generalized degeneration in subpassages or form plaques under agarose. Other arboviruses grow best in mosquito suspension cultures (see pages 5 & 8), whereas others can only be recovered in whole animal systems such as embryonated chicken eggs, suckling mice or hamsters, or mosquitoes (these systems not discussed here).

The gastroenteritis viruses also belong to diverse virus families and have unique requirements for culture. Rotaviruses, after treatment with trypsin, will replicate in BSC–1, MA104, and primary AGMK cells under roller conditions (Babiuk et al 1977). Caliciviruses and astroviruses may replicate in primary HEK under a fortified medium with trypsin. Enteric adenoviruses (see Chapter 2) and enteric coronaviruses (discussed below) round out this difficult group of viruses.

New or specialized culture systems

Organ cultures

Laboratory cultures of pieces of human embryonic lung, kidney, intestine, and other organs have proven essential to the discovery of many viruses, such as the respiratory coronaviruses and rhinoviruses. Organ cultures are tiny explants of whole tissue, so that many cell types are present in their natural form, and feeding medium has to be perfused through the explants to maintain viability. The human enteric coronaviruses – although their existence is still in dispute – may replicate in primary human fetal intestinal organ cultures containing trypsin. Once the tissue culture is inoculated with a suspected virus specimen, the presence of virus may be detected by cessation of ciliary movement (in lung and intestine) or by specific tests for the viral products accumulated in the medium (Caul and Clarke 1975; Caul and Egglestone 1977; McIntosh et al 1967; Tyrrell and Blamire 1967).

Microcultures

Early attempts to reduce the size of cell cultures and to manipulate cultures into 4-, 6-, 8- and 96-well formats were met with severe problems of external contamination, cross-contamination between wells, overoxygenation, and toxic plastics. All of these problems have now been overcome. Today, microcultures of most cell types are commonplace in the 4- to 8-well format in plastic plates with sealable lids (or snug lids for CO_2 incubators) for plaque assays. Microculture plates in the 96-well microtiter plate configuration, but with flat well bottoms, made of nontoxic plastic, and sterilized without toxic residues, are also a standard laboratory item today. Microcultures are especially useful for large volume neutralization tests, tissue culture EIA tests, monoclonal antibody testing, and most screening assays requiring cell cultures

(Anderson et al 1985; Hierholzer and Bingham 1978; Hierholzer et al 1990, 1993; Schmidt and Emmons 1989). Macrocultures in standard glass tubes, however, are still preferred for primary virus isolation because of the ease of setting up stationary or roller cultures in ordinary incubators, of reading the monolayers for CPE, and of obtaining sufficient volume of virus culture to use in identification tests and for subpassaging and storage.

Shell vial cultures

These cultures utilize the Leighton tube concept, in which the cell monolayer is established on one side of a glass coverslip inside a glass tube. The tube is then inoculated as usual and is subjected to a low-speed centrifugation, which apparently distorts the cell surface and renders it more susceptible to viral attachment. After just 1–3 days of incubation, regardless of the presence of any CPE, the coverslip is brought out, washed briefly, and tested by IFA or immunoperoxidase tests for suspected viruses. Shell vials have been particularly useful as a rapid culture test for adenoviruses, myxoviruses, herpes simplex, and cytomegalovirus, to name a few (Espy et al 1987; Gleaves et al 1985; Leland and French 1988; Matthey et al 1992).

Other specialized systems

Suspension cultures of human peripheral blood lymphocytes are sensitive to the Epstein-Barr herpes virus, where it is detected by a transformation assay, and, under cocultivation procedures, to the HTLV and HIV retroviruses; these highly specialized techniques are described elsewhere (Fields et al 1990; Leland and French 1988; Schmidt and Emmons 1989; Warfield and Feorino 1992). Immortalized human microvascular endothelial cell cultures derived from foreskin are sensitive to a wide variety of viruses under special culture conditions, and potential for use as a model to study the biology of these important cells (Ades et al 1992).

Extracellular matrix systems have recently been introduced for the three-dimensional growth of cells, as opposed to monolayer cultures. The Matrigel Invasion Chamber (Collaborative Biomedical Products, Bedford, MA), for instance, can support the growth of many fastidious cell types, and is currently being explored for its use in viral culture and alterations in cell physiology following viral infection (Bissell et al 1990; Thompson et al 1991).

Acknowledgement

We wish to thank Lynda Royer for excellent secretarial assistance.

References

Ades EW, Hierholzer JC, George V, Black J, Candal F (1992) J Virol Meth 39: 83–90.

Anderson LJ, Hierholzer JC, Bingham PG, Stone YO (1985) J Clin Microbiol 22: 1050–1052.

Ashihara T, Baserga R (1979) In: Methods in Enzymology, Vol. LVIII (Cell Culture) Jakoby WB, Pastan IH (Eds.), Academic Press, New York, pp. 248–262.

ATCC (1985) In: ATCC Quality Control Methods for Cell Lines. American Type Culture Collection, Rockville, MD, pp. 11–12.

Ausubel FM, Brent R, Kingston RE, Moore DD, Seidman JG, Smith JA, Struhl K (Eds.) (1991) Current Protocols in Molecular Biology. Green Publishing Associates and Wiley–Interscience, New York.

Babiuk LA, Mohammed K, Spence L, Fauvel M, Petro R (1977) J Clin Microbiol 6: 610–617.

Barkley WE (1979) In: Methods in Enzymology, Vol. LVIII Jakoby WB, Pastan IH (Eds.) Academic Press, New York, pp. 36–43.

Bird RB, Forrester FT (1981) Basic Laboratory Techniques in Cell Culture. Centers for Disease Control, Atlanta: U.S. Dept. of Health and Human Services.

Bissell DM, Caron JM, Babiss LE, Friedman JM (1990) Mol Biol Med 7: 187–197.

Boyum A (1968) Scand J Clin Lab Invest Suppl 21: 77–89.

Buckley S (1969) Proc Soc Exp Biol Med 131: 625–630.

Castells E, George VG, Hierholzer JC (1990) Arch Virol 115: 277–288.

Caul EO, Clarke SK (1975) Lancet 2: 953–954.

Caul EO, Egglestone SI (1977) Arch Virol 54: 107–117.

Chen TR (1977) Exp Cell Res 104: 255–262.

Coligan JE, Kruisbeek AM, Margulies DH, Shevach EM, Strober W (Eds.) (1991) Current Protocols in Immunology, Vol. 1. Green Publishing Associates and Wiley-Interscience, New York.

Crandell RA, Hierholzer JC, Krebs JW, Drysdale SS (1978) J Clin Microbiol 7: 214–218.

Espy MJ, Hierholzer JC, Smith TF (1987) Am J Clin Pathol 88: 358–360.

Fields BN, Knipe DM, Chanock RM, Hirsch MS, Melnick JL, Monath TP, Roizman B (Eds.) (1990) Virology, Vols. 1 and 2, 2nd edn. Raven Press, New York.

Frank AL, Couch RB, Griffis CA, Baxter BD (1979) J Clin Microbiol 10: 32–36.

Freshney RI (1983) Culture of Animal Cells: A Manual of Basic Technique. Alan R. Liss, New York.

Gleaves CA, Smith TF, Shuster EA, Pearson GR (1985) J Clin Microbiol 21: 217–221.

Harris LW, Griffiths JB (1977) Cryobiology 14: 662–669.

Hayflick L (1973) In: Tissue Culture Methods and Applications, (Kruse PF, Patterson MK, Eds.) Academic Press, New York, pp. 43–45.

Hayflick L, Moorhead PS (1961) Exp Cell Res 25: 585–621.

Held PG, Doyle JW, Sell C, Janakidevi K (1989) In Vitro Cell Dev Biol 25: 1025–1030.

Hierholzer JC (1993) Immunol Allergy Clin N Amer 13: 27–42.

Hierholzer JC, Anderson LJ, Halonen PE (1990) Med Virol 9: 17–45.

Hierholzer JC, Bingham PG (1978) J Clin Microbiol 7: 499–506.

Hierholzer JC, Bingham PG, Castells E, Coombs RA (1993) Arch Virol 130: 335–352.

Hsiung GD (1969) Ann NY Acad Sci 162: 483–498.

Klenk HD, Rott R, Orlich M, Blodorn J (1975) Virology 68: 426–439.

Leibo SP, Mazur P (1971) Cryobiology 8: 447–452.

Leland DS, French MLV (1988) In: Laboratory Diagnosis of Infectious Diseases: Principles and Practice, Vol. II, Viral, Rickettsial, and Chlamydial Diseases, Lennette EH, Halonen P, Murphy FA (Eds.) Springer-Verlag, New York, pp. 39–59.

Lovelock JE, Bishop MWH (1959) Nature 183: 1394–1395.

Mandell GL, Douglas RG, Bennett JE (Eds.) (1990) Principles and Practice of Infectious Diseases, Churchill Livingstone, New York.

Matthey S, Nicholson D, Ruhs S, Alden B, Knock M, Schultz K, Schmuecker A (1992) J Clin Microbiol 30: 540–544.

McIntosh K, Dees JH, Becker WB, Kapikian AZ, Chanock RM (1967) Proc Natl Acad Sci 57: 933–940.

Meguro H, Bryant JD, Torrence AE, Wright PF (1979) J Clin Microbiol 9: 175–179.

Nias AHW, Fox M (1971) Cell Tissue Kinet 4: 375–398.

Priest JH (1971) In: Human Cell Culture in Diagnosis of Disease, Newton IN (Ed.) Charles C. Thomas, Springfield, IL, pp. 44–45.

Schmidt NJ (1989) In: Diagnostic Procedures for Viral, Rickettsial and Chlamydial Infections, 6th edn. Schmidt NJ, Emmons RW (Eds.) American Public Health Assn., Washington, D.C., pp. 51–100.

Schmidt NJ, Emmons RW (1989) In: Diagnostic Procedures for Viral, Rickettsial and Chlamydial Infections, 6th edn. Schmidt NJ, Emmons RW

(Eds.) American Public Health Assn., Washington, D.C., pp. 1–35.

Singh KRP (1968) Curr Sci (Bangalore) 37: 65–67.

Singh KRP (1971) Curr Top Microbiol Immunol 55: 127–133.

Smith GE, Ju G, Ericson BL, Moschera J, Lahm HW, Chizzonite R, Summers MD (1985) Proc Natl Acad Sci U.S.A. 82: 8404–8408.

Thompson EW, Nakamura S, Shima TB, Melchiori A, Martin GR, Salahuddin SZ, Gallo RC, Albini A (1991) Cancer Res 51: 2670–2676.

Tolnai S (1975) In: TCA Manual, Vol. 1, Evans VJ,

Perry VP, Vincent MM (Eds.) Tissue Culture Association, Rockville, MD, pp. 37–38.

Tyrrell DAJ, Blamire CJ (1967) Brit J Exp Path 48: 217–227.

Warfield DT, Feorino PM (1992) In: Clinical Microbiology Procedures Handbook, Isenberg HD (Ed.) American Society for Microbiology, Washington, D.C., pp. 8.15.1–8.15.11.

Vaughn JL, Goodwin RH, Tompkins GJ, McCauley P (1977) In Vitro 13: 213–217.

Yunker CE, Cory J (1969) J Virol 3: 631–632.

Virus isolation and quantitation

2

J. C. Hierholzer
R. A. Killington

This chapter outlines the two most commonly used methods of virus isolation, namely tissue cultures and embryonated eggs. We have chosen to present the first section by describing the methodology involved for the predominant virus groups, which cover the majority of viruses encountered in the clinical situation. Virus isolation is a prelude to the diagnostic methodology described in a later chapter. We also describe selected methods of virus assay and the calculation of virus titers.

Virology Methods Manual
ISBN 0–12–465330–8

Primary isolation of viruses

For clinical samples, the type of specimen and the manner of collection are dependent on the laboratory methods anticipated (see Chapter 15). Ideally specimens should be collected within two days of onset of symptoms, because most viruses are shed only in the initial stages of illness. (Exceptions are adenovirus types 8, 19, and 37 in keratoconjunctivitis in which the virus is shed from the eye for 14 days; mumps virus, which is shed from the parotid gland and saliva for up to 12 days; and various adenoviruses and picornaviruses which are shed in the stool for weeks or months after onset, particularly in children). Nasal swabs are the easiest specimens to collect for respiratory viruses and are also the best specimens (i.e., they contain the most virus) for the majority of the respiratory viruses described here. For nasal swabs, urogenital calginate swabs are inserted into the nasal passages, gently rotated to absorb mucus and cells, and then vigorously twirled into 2 ml of transport medium (such as tryptose phosphate broth with 0.5% gelatin, veal heart infusion broth, or trypticase soy broth), preferably without antibiotics. Throat swabs can be obtained with cotton-tipped wooden applicator sticks that are rubbed against the posterior nasopharynx and then placed in the transport medium. The stick can easily be broken off to leave the cotton tip in the medium. Nasopharyngeal aspirates are collected with a neonatal mucus extractor and mucus trap to which transport medium is added. Swabs or scrapings of vesicular lesions are likewise carefully obtained and placed in transport medium. Urine and stool specimens are collected as for any pathogen. For more unusual viruses, the preferred specimen may be a lesion scraping, cerebrospinal fluid, biopsy or autopsy specimens, or serum or blood cells. Which specimen to collect is often determined by the sites exhibiting clinical symptoms (see Chapter 15).

Specimens should be placed on wet ice and transported to the laboratory for immediate testing. This is particularly critical for specimens for fluorescent antibody tests, because the epithelial cells must remain intact for a reliable test result. If testing is not possible within 5 days after collection, the specimens should be frozen on dry ice and stored at −70°C until processed, although this may decrease the amount of viable virus.

When processing for viral isolation, the specimens are treated with antibiotics, vigorously mixed, clarified at 1000 g for 3 min at 4°C to remove cell debris and bacteria, and inoculated onto appropriate cell culture monolayers in glass tubes. The cultures should include a continuous human epithelial line (e.g., HEp2, A549, HeLa), a human embryonic lung diploid fibroblast cell strain (e.g., HLF, HELF, MRC5, WI38), human lung mucoepidermoid cells (NCI-H292) to replace MK cells for most applications (Castells et al 1990; Hierholzer et al 1993b), and human rhabdomyosarcoma cells (RD) for the broadest coverage of viruses within practical limitations (Hierholzer 1993; Hierholzer and Hatch 1985; Matthey et al 1992; Meguro et al 1979; Smith et al 1986; Woods and Young 1988). The Epstein-Barr virus (EBV)-transformed marmoset cell line is particularly useful for isolation of measles virus. The inoculum (0.5 ml tube^{-1}) is adsorbed to the cell monolayers (whose growth medium has been decanted) for 1 h at ambient temperature, and the cultures are then fed with maintenance medium and incubated at 35–36°C for several weeks, with subpassaging as required.

Some cell types and certain viruses require roller cultures, while others do best with stationary cultures during their incubation period. In general, all tube cultures of primary monkey kidney cells (MK, AGMK) and their derivative cell lines (Vero, BSC-1, LLC-MK2, etc.), all diploid fibroblast cell cultures, and NCI-H292 cells should be rolled in roller drums or agitated on rocker platforms to remove toxic by-products from the cell surface and to replenish critical nutrients to the cells more quickly. Cultures of HEK, HEp2, KB, A549, and HeLa do not need to be rolled except for measles virus isolation in HEK and RSV isolation in HEp2.

Small variations in media composition and incubation temperature are also important for the successful isolation of certain viruses. For instance, some viruses require prior treatment with trypsin for successful cultivation, and some cells require the presence of trypsin in the maintenance medium for them to be sensitive to certain viruses. Cooler temperatures (33–35°C) are required for certain, less-invasive viruses, such as coronaviruses, rhinoviruses, and those enteroviruses causing hemorrhagic conjunctivitis (Hierholzer 1976; Hierholzer and Hatch 1985; Lennette et al 1995). These details are best found in current reference works concentrating on the virus families and their diagnostic tests (Fields et al 1990; Hierholzer 1993; Lennette et al 1988, 1995; Mandell et al 1990). One other caution is that any time primary monkey kidney cells are used, such as for influenza, measles or rubella, the laboratory worker must be acutely aware of the probable presence of simian adventitious agents which will confound the isolation and identification of human viruses (Arya 1975; Hsiung 1968, 1969; Hull 1968). Details of these and of the media required for different cells and viruses can be obtained elsewhere (Murray et al 1995; Rose et al 1992; Lennette et al 1995). Viral growth is seen as CPE in the cell monolayer visible under light microscopy (see Chapter 1) or by other means (see page 33).

Primary isolation of viruses in cell cultures

Herpesviridae

As a Family, the herpesviruses are spread by aerosolized droplets, fomites, and direct contact, and cause a wide variety of ocular, oropharyngeal, genital and generalized diseases in man. Herpes simplex viruses types 1 and 2 grow well in many cell types, notably primary rabbit kidney, HEK, HEp2, HeLa, A549, HLF

and NCI-H292 cells; type 2, usually a genital isolate, grows more slowly than type 1. Roller cultures are not necessary. Cytomegalovirus (CMV), a notably labile virus, is the only herpes virus that is shed in great amounts in the urine, and replicates slowly in roller cultures of diploid fibroblast cells, producing giant cells in 12–30 days. Varicella-zoster (VZV), the cause of chickenpox and shingles, also grows slowly in fibroblast cells on roller culture.

EBV, associated with infectious mononucleosis, Burkitt's lymphoma and nasopharyngeal carcinoma; human herpesvirus type 6 (HHV-6), the cause of roseola infantum (exanthema subitum or fourth disease) in children; and HHV-7, the probable cause of some roseola cases, require special conditions and cells for successful cultivation in the laboratory. In culture, EBV infects both B-lymphocytes and epithelial cells with the CD21 receptor (Fields et al 1990; Lennette et al 1995), HHV-6 grows best in primary CD4[+] T-lymphocytes rendered more susceptible by the presence of antibody to CD3 (Hall et al 1994; Inoue et al 1994; Pellett et al 1992), and HHV-7 also replicates in CD4[+] T-lymphocytes (Black and Pellett 1993; Black et al 1993; Tanaka et al 1994; Yasukawa et al 1993).

The herpes virus group is readily visualized by electron microscopy (EM), with the cubic icosahedral shape of the capsid being prominent (Palmer and Martin, 1988). The viruses are commonly speciated by indirect fluorescent antibody (IFA), enzyme immunoassay (EIA), DNA probes, and polymerase chain reaction (PCR) (Fields et al 1990; Hall et al 1994; Inoue et al 1994; Hierholzer 1991; Lennette et al 1988, 1995; Mandell et al 1990; Pellett et al 1992).

Adenoviridae

Adenoviruses are another group of viruses associated with diverse clinical syndromes. They are spread by droplets, fomites and the fecal–oral route; some serotypes are also spread venereally. Most serotypes replicate readily in HEK, HEp2, A549 and NC1-H292 cells, with or without rolling. Types 40 and 41, associated with infantile gastroenteritis grow best in an Ad5-transformed HEK line (Graham-293 cells) or in HEp2 under a fortified Opti-MEM medium (Gibco BRL) containing low serum (0.4% fetal calf serum) and 0.1% 2-mercaptoethanol. The adenoviruses are among the easiest viruses to identify because they are unique in producing prodigious quantities of soluble antigens as they grow in cell culture, and these antigens possess many type- and group-specific properties that lend themselves to a wide variety of diagnostic tests. Adenoviruses are differentiated from other viruses which may grow in the same cells and with similar cytopathic effects (CPE) by EM, complement fixation (CF), latex agglutination (LA), IFA, EIA, time-resolved fluoroimmunoassays (TR-FIA), DNA probes, restriction enzymes, PCR with suitable primers and cytological and inclusion-body staining methods; they are then serotyped by hemagglutination (HA)/hemagglutination-inhibition (HI) and neutralization (SN) tests (Adrian et al 1986; Hierholzer 1991, 1993; Hierholzer et al 1990; Lennette et al 1988, 1995; Murray et al 1995).

Papovaviridae

The papovaviruses consist of two genera, but only members of one can be isolated in cell culture. Polyoma BK virus can be recovered in HEK, NCI-H292, and diploid fibroblast cells, and the polyoma JC virus replicates in primary human fetal glial cells, but both viruses may be missed because their CPE develops slowly and is vague. BK virus is identified by HA/HI tests at 4°C with human 'O' erythrocytes and specific antiserum; BK and JC virus are identified by EIA, SN, and probes. The papillomaviruses, forming the other genus, cannot be propagated in cell culture or identified serologically, so are only identified in biopsied tissues by various DNA hybridization techniques (Fields et al 1990; Lennette et al 1988, 1995).

Poxviridae

Vaccinia virus and certain other pox viruses can be isolated in MK, Vero, NCI-H292, and diploid fibroblast cells, and identified by the type of plaques formed and by EM, HI, EIA and various DNA tests (Murray et al 1995; Ropp et al 1995).

Reoviridae

Reovirus 1, 2 and 3 are frequently isolated from throat and rectal specimens in NCI-H292, MK and HeLa cells under stationary or roller conditions after 5–14 days of culture, but they have never been clearly associated with human disease. They are easily visualized by EM and serotyped by HA/HI tests with human 'O' erythrocytes and antisera and by SN tests.

Paramyxoviridae

The Family Paramyxoviridae comprises the genera *Paramyxovirus* (parainfluenza virus types 1, 2, 3, 4A, 4B and mumps virus), *Morbillivirus* (measles virus or rubeola), and *Pneumovirus* (respiratory syncytial virus [RSV]). The parainfluenza and mumps viruses replicate well in roller cultures of NCI-H292 cells under a fortified medium containing trypsin for optimal sensitivity, and in MK cells without trypsin (Castells et al 1990; Meguro et al 1979). The CPE induced by these viruses may develop in 4–7 days but the cultures must generally be blind-passaged and held an additional week to ensure viral growth. The cells rarely become detached, and may not show obvious CPE at all, so that NCI-H292 or MK cultures for these viruses must be hemadsorbed with guinea pig, human, or monkey erythrocytes at the end of the culture period, and the viruses then typed by HI, IFA, EIA, or TR-FIA tests (Hierholzer et al 1993a; Lennette et al 1995).

Measles virus is most easily isolated using the marmoset cell line, B95/8 (Bellini and Rota 1995). The virus also causes CPE in primary African green monkey kidney (AGMK), Vero and HEK cells after 7–14 days of roller culture. But because the CPE usually develops slowly and may not be recognized, the monolayers should be hemadsorbed with vervet monkey erythrocytes to ensure detection of the virus. The virus is then further identified by HI tests with vervet erythrocytes, IFA, EIA and SN tests, or by probe or PCR tests (Fields et al 1990; Hummel et al 1992; Lennette et al 1995; Mandell et al 1990; Murray et al 1995).

RSV produces distinct syncytia in HEp2, HeLa and NCI-H292 cells in 5–12 days in roller cultures. Group A and B strains of RSV are readily identified by IFA, EIA and TR-FIA tests (Anderson et al 1985; Hierholzer et al 1990, 1994b; Lennette et al 1995; Murray et al 1995).

Orthomyxoviridae

Influenza A, B and C viruses are spread by aerosol droplets and fomites and are best recovered in roller cultures of MK and MDCK cells and in embryonated eggs. Chick embryo, MDCK and other cells require a fortified medium containing trypsin for optimal sensitivity (Frank et al 1979, Klenk et al 1975; Lazarowitz and Choppin 1975; Meguro et al 1979). The viruses are detected in MK cells by hemadsorption and in MDCK cells by HA, and are then identified by IFA, EIA, HI or SN tests (Grandien et al 1985; Lennette et al 1988, 1995; Mandell et al 1990; Murray et al 1995).

Picornaviridae

This very large Family includes the genus *Enterovirus* (polio virus 1, 2, 3; 23 Coxsackie A viruses; 6 Coxsackie B viruses; 31 echoviruses; and 5 more recent enteroviruses), and the genus *Rhinovirus* (125 serotypes). The enteroviruses are spread by aerosolized droplets, fomites and the fecal–oral route, whereas the rhinoviruses are spread by aerosols and fomites only (Dick et al 1987; Mandell et al 1990). These viruses produce CPE in NCI-H292, MK, RD, trypsin-treated MA-104 and diploid fibroblast cells, preferably in roller cultures, although some Coxsackie A viruses grow only in suckling mouse brain. Enteroviruses are distinguished from rhinoviruses by acid- and chloroform-lability tests in which both genera are chloroform-stable but only enteroviruses are acid-stable; the viruses are identifiable to serotype only by type-specific SN tests (Agbalika et al 1984; Hierholzer and Hatch 1985; Hyypia and Stanway 1993; Lennette et al 1995; Murray et al 1995).

Viruses difficult to isolate

Togaviridae, Flaviviridae, Rhabdoviridae, Filoviridae, Bunyaviridae and Arenaviridae families contain the formerly-known arboviruses, so named because they are spread by insect and/or rodent vectors, plus many rare and unusual viruses that cause disease in geographically distinct parts of the world. These viruses are numerous and have too many specialized isolation requirements to enumerate here. Certain arboviruses can be isolated in primary cells or derivative cell lines like BHK-21, Vero and LLC-MK2, after 2–10 days of culture. The CPE may be difficult to detect, particularly in mosquito suspension cultures (see Chapter 1). Many arboviruses can only be recovered in whole animal systems such as embryonated chicken eggs, suckling mice or hamsters, or mosquitoes. Fortunately, most diagnostic laboratories will not encounter these viruses, either because of their rarity in most parts of the world or their requirement for Biosafety Level 3 or 4 containment facilities. Other works detail the isolation requirements and systems, the specific identification tests and the laboratory precautions for these viruses (Fields et al 1990; Lennette et al 1988, 1995).

Of particular interest is the isolation in deer mice of the causative agent of the newly-described Hantavirus Pulmonary Syndrome. The virus, named Sin Nombre virus, is a member of the Bunyaviridae and can be propagated in the Vero-E6 cell line after growth in deer mouse lungs (Elliott et al 1994).

The gastroenteritis viruses also belong to diverse virus families and have unique requirements for culture. Rotaviruses, after treatment with trypsin, will replicate in BSC-1, MA104 and primary AGMK cells under roller conditions

(Babiuk et al 1977). Caliciviruses and astroviruses may replicate in primary HEK or LLC-MK2 cells under a fortified medium with trypsin (Sanchez-Fauquier et al 1994). The human enteric coronaviruses and toroviruses cannot be isolated in the laboratory (Koopmans and Horzinek, 1994; Lennette et al 1988, 1995), and the enteric adenoviruses were discussed above.

The human parvovirus B19 causes fifth disease (erythema infectiosum) and is easily spread by aerosolized droplets and fomites in schools, and vertically to the fetus during the first trimester of pregnancy. The virus has been reported to grow in specialized erythropoietic stem cell cultures, but will not be recovered in standard culture systems. Thus, B19 infection is documented by EIA testing of the patient's acute-phase serum sample, where both virus and antibodies are sought; EM, Western blots, DNA hybridization probes and PCR have also been used extensively (Anderson 1987; Durigon et al 1993; Fields et al 1990; Mandell et al 1990; Murray et al 1995).

The human coronaviruses cause a significant proportion of 'common colds' and are spread by droplets, but are best identified directly in nasal and throat specimens by IFA, EIA and TR-FIA because the viruses are extremely labile and difficult to recover in the laboratory. The peplomers constitute the primary antigen detected in all tests, including the HI test for strain OC43 (Hierholzer et al 1994a; Lennette et al 1988, 1995; Schmidt et al 1979).

The HIV and HTLV viruses (family Retroviridae) also require specialized systems for isolation and identification, and will not be recovered by standard culture methods (Lennette et al 1995; Warfield and Feorino 1992).

The interpretation of any cell culture isolation result or of any test used to identify the isolate is dependent on the methods used. An isolate's association with human disease is dependent on the patient data obtained with the specimen and on the known epidemiology of the virus. All of these interpretive elements are reviewed elsewhere (Fields et al 1990; Hierholzer 1993; Lennette et al 1988, 1995; Mandell et al 1990; Murray et al 1995; Rose et al 1992).

Primary isolation of viruses in embryonated eggs

In most cases the advent of tissue culture techniques has superseded the need to isolate viruses in embryonated hen eggs. However, for some viruses, e.g., influenza and avian species, the embryonated egg is still

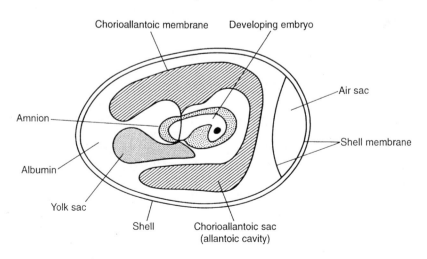

Chorioallantoic membrane Developing embryo

Air sac

Amnion

Shell membrane

Albumin

Yolk sac

Shell Chorioallantoic sac
(allantoic cavity)

Figure 2.1. The embryonated egg

often used for virus isolation. As will be determined later, the embryonated egg is also used for infectivity (pock) assays. The embryonated egg provides an ideal 'receptacle' in which to grow viruses, as it is sterile and has a range of tissue types and cavity fluids which both support the replication and allow the concentration of infectious virus. The anatomy of the egg is shown in Fig. 2.1.

Fertile hens' eggs are acquired from a suitable hatchery and incubated at 37°C in an atmosphere of about 62% humidity with a forced (usually fan driven) air circulation. This prevents drying out of the egg and allows for good air exchange in the developing embryo. More elaborate incubators also have a mechanism for gently rocking the egg at frequent time intervals. The embryo and developing membranes and cavities go through a variety of anatomical changes up to hatching. Particular sites of injection are therefore optimal at various times in the development of the embryo, e.g., infectious bronchitis virus is propagated in the yolk sac of a 5–6 day old embryo, whereas Newcastle Disease and Influenza viruses are inoculated into the chorioallantoic sac of a 9–11 day embryo.

The procedure of egg inoculation can be divided up into a series of steps.

1. Eggs are 'candled' to check for viability and to determine the positions of the embryo, membranes and blood vessels. Dead eggs will have little or no vasculature and have a characteristic translucent appearance. Darkly stained eggs are usually heavily contaminated. Candling is carried out in a darkened room using a light box which has one small egg-shaped hole surrounded by a piece of foam on which the egg is placed. Rotating the egg immediately reveals its anatomical make-up.

2. Eggs are disinfected with alcohol and marked on the shell in preparation for the drilling of holes, care being taken to avoid areas rich in blood vessels.
3. The virus is injected via the appropriate route, and the hole is covered with tape, glue or wax.
4. Contaminated eggs (which appear 24 h post inoculation) are discarded – such eggs can often be detected by their smell!
5. Eggs are chilled and harvested 2–5 days post infection

Procedure

We have chosen to describe the procedure for chorioallantoic sac inoculation, a common method of isolating influenza virus. Inoculation onto the chorioallantoic membrane for pock formation is described on page 40. In addition, Fig. 2.2 shows diagrammatically

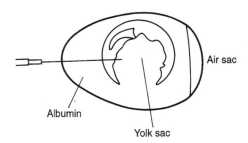

(A) Yolk sac route

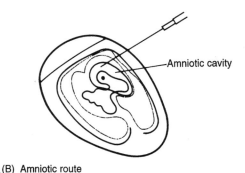

(B) Amniotic route

Figure 2.2. Yolk sac and amniotic routes of inoculation.

the routes for amniotic and yolk sac inoculations

1. Candle 9–11 day old eggs to determine viability and sterilize with alcohol. Place the egg pointed end down and drill a small groove in the blunt end of the egg.
2. Mark, with a pencil, an area towards the pointed end of the egg above the embryo and free of blood vessels. Carefully drill a groove in the shell, without damaging the chorioallantoic membrane, at the point of the mark.
3. Inject 0.1 ml virus suspension using a tuberculin syringe fitted with a 26G-$\frac{3}{8}$ needle into the chorioallantoic sac through the groove created in step 2 above.
4. Seal both grooves with adhesive tape.
5. Incubate the egg with the blunt end uppermost in a humidified incubator at 33°C.
6. Collect fluids 2–4 days after inoculation.
7. Place the eggs at 4°C overnight in order to kill the embryo.
8. With the blunt end uppermost, insert scissors into the groove and cut away the area of shell above the air sac taking care not to puncture membranes.
9. This reveals the secondary shell membrane which should be carefully removed with forceps.
10. Gently lift the chorioallantoic membrane to the top of the egg and introduce a pasteur pipette into the sac by piercing the membrane. Remove the allantoic fluid, taking care not to puncture the yolk sac.
11. The fluid should be clear. If the fluid contains erythrocytes centrifuge at 500 g for 10 min and collect the supernatant.
12. The fluid can be assayed using the haemagglutination test (see page 41). Store at −70°C.

Detection of viruses in cell cultures in the absence of CPE

Hemadsorption tests

Hemadsorption is a fast and convenient method of detecting orthomyxoviruses (influenza A, B, C) and non RSV paramyxoviruses (parainfluenza 1, 2, 3, 4A, 4B; mumps; measles) in cell cultures in which the CPE can vary from obvious to minimal. It is even used in the presence of CPE to obtain a quick delineation from other virus groups which may cause similar CPE in the same types of cultures. The method conserves the virus and viral antigens, because the supernatant fluid is decanted from the cell culture into a sterile tube at the end of the incubation period (7–10 days); the monolayer is washed twice with 2–3 ml of plain Hanks Balanced Salt Solution (HBSS) at room temperature; 1 ml of fresh HBSS followed by 0.2 ml of 0.4% mammalian erythrocyte suspension from the appropriate species is added to the monolayer; the tube is incubated stationary with the fluid covering the monolayer; and the test is read 3 times at 20-min intervals by agitating the tube in a sideways motion and then observing the monolayer at 40–100× magnification to see if the erythrocytes are firmly attached to the cultured cells or are floating free in the fluid (see Fig. 15.4). The hemadsorbed monolayer should be regarded as contaminated at this point because the erythrocyte suspension would more than likely not be sterile; subpassaging and virus-specific identification tests should be carried out with the decanted and saved supernatant fluid.

Viral interference tests

Rubella virus was originally detected only by its ability to prevent another virus from infecting the same cells it was replicating in. Current diagnostic testing for rubella may employ specialized cultures in which CPE may become evident; rubella can, under certain culture conditions, cause a vague and variable CPE in rabbit cornea, rabbit kidney and Vero cells. Most commonly, however, rubella specimens are inoculated onto Vero, BHK-21, or primary vervet monkey kidney cell cultures for recovery of the virus, under roller conditions for 4–10 days. Virus is detected by the viral interference test, in which a known quantity of another virus (such as echovirus-11 or coxsackievirus-A9, both enteroviruses) is added to the culture fluid at the end of the culture period allowed for rubella, and the culture is then reincubated for 3 days and observed for enterovirus CPE. The challenge virus is chosen and standardized to give 3+ CPE in 3 days in that particular cell line. In the test, cultures containing rubella are refractory to the enterovirus infection while control cultures (not containing rubella) are sensitive and exhibit the expected degree of CPE within 3 days.

Cellular toxicity by viral autolysis

The human respiratory coronaviruses growing in diploid fibroblast cells (229E virus) or in RD cells (OC43 virus) do not cause any visible CPE during their replication phases. Only when viral replication is complete and the virus titer has peaked (at about 10^7 Tissue Culture Infective Doses (TCID$_{50}$) per 0.1 ml), after 26–30 hours of roller incubation, do changes begin to be evident in the monolayer. For the next several days, CPE is seen as a degeneration evenly across the monolayer. The CPE increases to 4+ concomitant with autolysis of the newly-formed virions; by the time complete CPE is achieved, there is very little infectious virus left in the culture (Hierholzer, 1976; Schmidt et al., 1979).

Standard tests for viral antigens and nucleic acids

Arboviruses replicating in mosquito suspension cell cultures at 20–30°C may be detected by subpassaging to monolayer cultures in which CPE may be evident or by HA/HI, EIA, complement-fixation, or nucleic acid tests for the specific viruses suspected. Hepatitis A virus replicates in primary rhesus MK cultures in 1–4 weeks but is non-cytolytic; it is detected by EIA or hybridization tests. The standard tests for viral antigens and viral RNA or DNA, such as these, can of course be applied to any culture of any suspected virus, regardless of the type and degree of CPE observed. CPE by itself should never be considered pathognomonic.

Quantitation of virus

For most virology experiments it is essential to know the concentration of the total or infectious virus particles present in any given virus suspension. Such quantitation forms the basis for example of determining one-step growth curves, examining the neutralization of virus infectivity, assessing the activity of chemotherapeutic agents, monitoring the stages of virus purification, and assessing virus pathogenicity. Animal viruses are quantified by either an infectivity assay (e.g., $TCID_{50}$, Egg Infective Dose$_{50}$ (EID$_{50}$), Lethal Dose$_{50}$ (LD$_{50}$), pock assay), other biological/chemical assays (e.g., haemadsorption, haemagglutination, total protein), or by direct total virus particle counting using the electron microscope. Most virologists however, would consider the plaque assay to be the easiest, most accurate and sensitive form of assaying virus infectivity. The plaquing efficiency of some viruses however is often poor and hence other methods are needed (e.g., haemagglutination by influenza).

Those readers who teach virology at a practical level may find the comparative titration methods of e.g., herpes simplex virus, a useful class experiment. This virus can be titrated by plaque, pock, $TCID_{50}$, LD_{50} and total particle counting methods, thus allowing the accuracy, sensitivity and practicality of each method to be demonstrated.

This section of the chapter highlights the essential features of these methods drawing upon specific virus assays as examples. The reader should be aware however, that this book is not a manual for all viruses but serves to outline the basic techniques. Specific details for individual viruses can be obtained from the published literature.

Infectivity assays

Probably the most important attribute of a virus is its ability to infect and replicate within a cell. The virus replicative cycle is accompanied by a number of biochemical and morphological changes within the cell which usually culminates with cell death. These morphological changes, which are often readily visualized with the naked eye, but may require light microscopy are, as stated earlier, referred to as the virus cytopathic effect (CPE) and may take several forms e.g., cell rounding, cell fusion (syncytia formation) or total cell lysis. A few viruses (e.g., selected Retroviruses) do not kill infected cells or cause cytopathic effect but instead transform the cells into rapidly growing foci, capable in many cases of forming tumors in animals. Such foci of infection can be observed in infected monolayers in a similar way to the detection of virus CPE.

Infectivity assays, like other forms of assay, are designed so as to allow the calculation of a virus 'titer' (the number of infectious units per unit volume, e.g., plaque forming units per milliliter). Infectious units are usually thought of as being the smallest amount of virus that will produce a detectable biological effect in the assay, e.g., a plaque forming unit, a pock forming unit). Infectivity assays are of either the quantal or focal type. Quantal assays detect the presence of infectious virus by use of an 'all or none' approach. Does a tissue culture monolayer show CPE? Is an egg infected? Has an animal died? Focal assays rely on the detection and counting of foci of infection, e.g. a focus of CPE (plaque) or a focus of inflammatory response (pock) which allows for the quantitative determination of the number of infectious units as opposed to the qualitative approach of the quantal assay.

Virus dilution

Virus titers are determined by making accurate serial dilutions of virus suspensions, the diluent usually being either tissue culture maintenance or growth medium. Such serial dilutions are usually done using factors of 2, 5 or 10, the former obviously giving a more precise titer. For routine use 10-fold dilutions are usually carried out.

When setting up such a dilution series consideration should be given to the final volume of diluent needed for the assay and thus aliquots of 0.9, 4.5, 9.0 ml are usually made in a series of sterile tubes or bottles. In order to conserve virus stocks it is usual for the first (lowest) dilution in the series to be achieved by the use of 0.1 ml stock suspension. With subsequent dilutions it is very important to use a new sterile pipette for each transfer and to thoroughly mix each virus dilution before further transfer. Use of the same pipette will transfer millions of virus particles along the series, resulting in a very large dilution error. Once diluted, virus should be assayed as soon as possible although, if necessary, some viruses will withstand storing at 4°C for a few hours before assay. The use of such a storage procedure should obviously be checked to determine if it is suitable for the virus under assay.

TCID$_{50}$

The TCID$_{50}$ is defined as that dilution of a virus required to infect 50% of a given batch of inoculated cell cultures. The assay relies on the presence and detection of cytocidal virus particles (i.e., those capable of causing CPE).

Host cells are grown in confluent healthy monolayers, usually in tubes or 96-well tissue culture grade plastic plates, to which aliquots of virus dilutions are added. The method becomes more accurate with increasing numbers of tubes or wells per dilution, but it is usual to use either 5 or 10 repetitions per dilution.

On incubation the virus replicates and progeny virions are released into the supernatant, these infecting healthy cells in the monolayer. The CPE is allowed to develop over a period of days (depending on the virus and cell type) at which time the cell monolayers are observed microscopically (they can be fixed and stained

if necessary). Tubes are scored for the presence or absence of CPE.

It is thus a quantal assay in that each tube provides only one piece of information, i.e., is there CPE or not? The data is used to calculate the TCID$_{50}$ of the initial virus suspension by one of two ways – the Reed-Muench and the Spearman-Kärber methods (see below). The calculation does not tell us how many infectious units are present in the original virus suspension but what dilution of virus will give CPE in 50% of the cells inoculated.

Procedure

1. Seed tissue culture tubes/wells at a density of cells which will be confluent on the day of virus assay.
2. Make serial dilutions of virus suspension in appropriate diluent.
3. Remove tissue culture growth medium from healthy confluent monolayer and replace with appropriate dilution of virus. This would usually be 1 ml of virus dilution in a tissue culture tube and 0.1 ml in the well of a 96-well plate. Set up at least 5 tubes/wells per virus dilution.
4. Also include at least 5 control tubes/wells which contain diluent alone, i.e. no virus.
5. Incubate at appropriate temperature in either a closed or open incubator system and monitor the development of CPE. Record CPE after a designated time, having observed the cell control tubes/wells first.
6. CPE is usually graded on a 0–4 system; 0 (no CPE) 1 (less than 50% of cells showing CPE) 2 (about 50% of cells showing CPE) 3 (about 75% of cells showing CPE) 4 (the monolayer is totally destroyed or shows 100% CPE).
7. Calculate the TCID$_{50}$ counting all the tubes/wells with 1–4 CPE as being positive.

Table 2.1. Data used to calculate $TCID_{50}$ using Reed-Muench or Spearman-Kärber method

Log of virus dilution	Infected test units	Cumulative infected (A)	Cumulative non-infected (B)	Ratio of A/(A + B)	Percent infected
−5	5/5	9	0	9/9	100.0
−6	3/5	4	2	4/6	66.7
−7	1/5	1	6	1/7	14.3
−8	0/5	0	11	0/11	00.0

Calculation of $TCID_{50}$

The data shown in Table 2.1 will be used to demonstrate the calculation by either the Reed-Muench or Spearman-Kärber methods.

Reed-Muench method (Burleson et al 1992, Reed and Muench 1938)

The dilution in Table 2.1 that corresponds to the 50% end point obviously lies somewhere between the 10^{-6} (66.7% infected) and 10^{-7} (14.3% infected) dilutions. The proportionate distance between these two dilutions is calculated in the following manner:

$$\frac{(\% \text{ positive above } 50\%) - 50\%}{(\% \text{ positive above } 50\%) - (\% \text{ positive below } 50\%)}$$
$$= \text{Proportionate distance}$$

i.e., $\dfrac{66.7\% - 50\%}{66.7\% - 14.3\%} = 0.3$

Given that the log of the dilution above 50% is −6, the proportionate distance is 0.3 and the log of the dilution factor is −1 (i.e., serial 10 fold dilutions were used) the 50% end point is now calculated in the following way:

(log dilution above 50%) + (proportionate distance × log dilution factor) = log ID_{50}

$$(-6) + (0.3 \times -1.0) = -6.3$$

Therefore $ID_{50} = 10^{-6.3}$

This is the end point dilution, i.e., the dilution that will infect 50% of the test units inoculated.

The reciprocal of this number gives rise to the virus titer in terms of infectious doses per unit volume. If the inoculation of virus dilution was 0.1 ml the titer of the virus suspension would therefore be:

$$10^{6.3} \ TCID_{50} \ 0.1 \ ml^{-1}$$
$$= 10 \times 10^{6.3} \ TCID \ ml^{-1}$$
$$= 10^{7.3} \ TCID_{50} \ ml^{-1}$$

Spearman Kärber method (Spearman, 1908; Kärber, 1931)

Again using the data from Table 2.1 the following formula is used to directly estimate the 50% end point:

Highest dilution giving 100% CPE $+ \frac{1}{2} -$

$$\frac{\text{total number of test units showing CPE}}{\text{number of test units per dilution}}$$
$$= TCID_{50}$$

$$-5 + \tfrac{1}{2} - \tfrac{9}{5} = -6.3 \ TCID_{50}$$
or $10^{-6.3} \ TCID_{50}$ unit volume^{-1}

The titer, given a volume of 0.1 ml, is therefore:

$$10^{6.3} \ TCID_{50} \ 0.1 \ ml^{-1}$$
$$= 10 \times 10^{6.3} \ TCID \ ml^{-1}$$
$$= 10^{7.3} \ TCID_{50} \ ml^{-1}$$

The principle involved in the $TCID_{50}$ experiment is the same for either animal deaths (LD_{50}) or infection of a developing fertile hen's egg (EID_{50}).

Plaque assay

The plaque assay is an infectivity assay that quantifies the number of infectious units in a given virus suspension. Plaques are localized discrete foci of infection denoted by zones of cell lysis or CPE within a monolayer of otherwise healthy tissue culture cells. Each plaque originates from a single infectious virion thus allowing a very precise calculation of the virus titer.

Plaque assays are essentially of two types, suspension assays and monolayer assays. In suspension assays a high concentration of healthy tissue culture cells, in a small volume, are shaken with a suitably diluted aliquot of virus to allow virus adsorption to take place; cells are seeded onto a tissue culture grade vented petri dish. The monolayer assay on the other hand requires a small volume of virus diluent to be added to a previously seeded confluent tissue culture cell monolayer for virus adsorption to take place. In both assays, prior to incubation, an overlay medium is added to the cell suspension or cell monolayer. Overlay media, composed of either agar/agarose or methylcellulose solution prevent the formation of secondary plaques by forcing those virus particles released from the initial infected cell to invade adjacent cells as opposed to spreading to other areas of the cell monolayer.

Following the addition of overlay medium the assay dishes are incubated at an appropriate temperature until plaques are readily discernible. At this point petri plates or microplates are 'fixed' with formol saline solution and stained with crystal violet solution. Plaques are observed either macro- or microscopically.

For statistical reasons 20–100 plaques per monolayer are ideal to count, although the actual number is often dependent on the size of the plaque and the size of the vessel used for the assay.

The infectivity titer is expressed as the number of plaque forming units per ml (pfu ml^{-1}) and is obtained in the following way:

plaque number $\times$ reciprocal of dilution $\times$ reciprocal of volume in ml

e.g. if there is a mean number of 50 plaques from monolayers infected with 0.1 ml of a 10^{-6} dilution there are:

$$50 \times 10^6 \times 10 = 5 \times 10^8 \text{ pfu ml}^{-1}$$

It is essential that the reader experiments to determine the most sensitive and suitable plaque assay for their own virus/cell system as the methods vary in relation to detail. Such details include:

a) sensitivity of the cell to virus infection – plaquing efficiencies varying from cell to cell
b) the time required for virus adsorption to cells
c) the type of agar used in the overlay medium, i.e. some can be inhibitory for virus replication
d) the time of incubation, i.e. plaques must be visible but discrete
e) the constituents of the medium in which the overlay is dissolved, i.e. some viruses require high Mg^{2+} concentrations for plaque formation
f) the ability of the virus to cause a detectable CPE in tissue culture
g) the ability of the cells to form a confluent monolayer
h) the need to add a protease (e.g. trypsin) to the overlay medium for plaque formation.

Monolayer assay procedure

This method, modified from Burleson et al 1992, is for the assay of EMC virus in BHK cells.

1. Seed an appropriate number of tissue culture grade vented petri dishes with a sufficient concentration of tissue culture cells to reach confluence on the day of assay.
2. On the day of assay observe the cell monolayers, which must be healthy and confluent. Thin monolayers are not suitable for assay purposes.

3. Prepare an overlay medium using Difco agar:
Eagle's minimal essential medium (8.3 ml)
FBS (1.7 ml) ⎤(Solution A)
TPB (1.7 ml) ⎦
Agar (30% in Hanks Basal Salt Solution and autoclaved) (5.0 ml) (Solution B)
adjust pH with sterile $NaHCO_3$ solution
   a) melt the agar and maintain in the 48°C water bath
   b) prepare solution A and equilibrate at 48°C in the water bath
   c) combine solutions A and B in a sterile bottle and adjust the pH
   d) keep in the water bath until needed
   e) do not use the overlay medium if it is 'clumpy'
4. Prepare appropriate virus dilutions.
5. Discard the medium from the previously seeded petri dishes.
6. Carefully add 0.2 ml virus dilution to each of duplicate tissue culture monolayers and gently rock the dish to achieve an even distribution of virus.
7. Allow the virus to adsorb for 30 min at 37°C in a CO_2 incubator or atmosphere of CO_2. The monolayers may be tilted after 15 min to avoid the cells drying up, although this step may not be necessary.
8. Remove unadsorbed virus – if many assays are to be done use a suction apparatus. Many virologists wash the monolayer at this stage with sterile PBS but others consider this step optional.
9. During the last five minutes of virus adsorption remove the agar overlays from the water bath, thus permitting them to cool. Beware of solidification – trial and error will give experience of how long this takes. The agar should be warm but not uncomfortable to the touch.
10. Add 5 ml of appropriate overlay/plate and allow to solidify. Incubate at 37°C for 48 h.
11. Fix plates in formol saline (10%) for at least 60 min. Plates can be left in this solution until they can be conveniently stained.
12. Remove agar overlay using something similar to a 'bent pin' and stain the monolayer with crystal violet solution (10%) for 10 min.
13. Invert and drain the plates and count using, if necessary, a stereomicroscope.

Suspension assay method

The method outlined below was devised by Russell (1962) for herpes simplex virus assayed in BHK cells.

1. Dilute virus to the appropriate dilution in Eagle's medium containing tryptose phosphate broth (10%) and calf serum (10%) (ETC).
2. Remove 2 ml virus dilution to a fresh Universal or McCartney bottle to which are added a total of 8×10^6 BHK cells.
3. Shake the cell-virus suspension at 37°C for 30 min. This is normally achieved by using a Luckhams Shaker or something similar.
4. Following adsorption add 8 ml overlay medium (ETC containing 0.8% carboxymethyl cellulose solution) and thoroughly mix with the infected cell suspension.
5. Remove 5 ml of the resulting suspension to each of two 60 mm vented tissue culture plastic petri plates and incubate in a CO_2 atmosphere at 37°C.
6. Plates may be observed microscopically after 1 day to observe the development of plaques.
7. After 2 days incubation the medium is decanted into a disinfectant solution

and the cell sheet fixed in formol saline solution (10%). If time does not permit this, plates can be fixed with formol saline solution prior to decanting the overlay medium.

8. Wash the cell sheet gently with water from a beaker and stain for 10 min with crystal violet solution (10%).

9. Decant the stain into a beaker, invert the plates to dry them and count the plaques with the aid of a stereomicroscope.

Pock assays

As discussed earlier the fertile hen's egg is routinely used in virology for both virus growth and virus assay. It has also been used in the diagnostic laboratory for the typing of virus strains, often using the criterion of pock size or pock type. A pock is essentially an area of inflammatory response which results from the virus invasion of an epithelial cell on the chorioallantoic membrane (CAM) of a fertile hen's egg. Like the plaque assay the method is quantitative and each pock results from the infection caused by an infectious unit of virus (pock forming unit). The method is considered by some to be very messy and time consuming and recent animal licencing reforms have restricted the use of the fertile hen's egg (particularly in the UK) to animal licence holders.

As a result the egg is no longer used to the same degree as it was several years ago.

The method requires the creation, in the egg, of a false air sac, onto which is inoculated an aliquot of diluted virus. Following incubation the membrane is observed and the pocks counted. Fig. 2.3 shows a diagram of the egg before and after the creation of the false air sac.

The infectivity titer is obtained in the following way:

pock number $\times$ reciprocal of dilution $\times$ reciprocal of volume in ml

e.g. if there is a mean number of 50 pocks from eggs inoculated with 0.1 ml of a 10^{-6} dilution there are:

$$50 \times 10^6 \times 10 = 5 \times 10^8 \text{ pkfu ml}^{-1}$$

Pock assay procedure

The procedure outlined below is used routinely in our laboratory for demonstrations of the herpes simplex virus pock assay:

1. Candle 9–11 day old embryonated hen eggs to determine viability (described earlier).
2. Mark the air sac and an area for inoculation over the centre of the chorioallantoic membrane free from blood vessels.

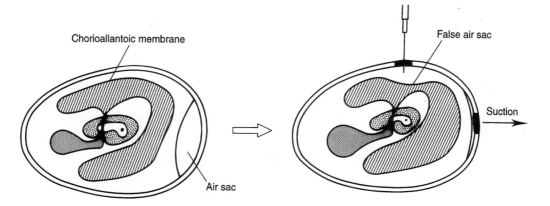

Figure 2.3. Creation of false air sac in embryonated egg.

3. Swab both areas of the egg with alcohol and drill a 3–4 mm groove in the shell at centre of the air sac and also over the CAM (position already marked). Avoid damage to the shell membrane.

4. Using a sterile mounting needle puncture the shell membrane over the air sac.

5. Place a small drop of sterile saline on the exposed shell membrane over the CAM.

6. Place the tip of a mounting needle or hypodermic syringe, through the drop of saline, on the exposed shell membrane, vertically to the long axis of the egg, and press gently but firmly to split the fibres of the shell membrane. *Avoid puncturing the CAM which lies directly beneath.*

7. Using a rubber teat apply suction to the air sac hole. The chorioallantoic membrane should detach and drop away from the shell membrane, the drop of saline acting as a 'wet wedge'.

8. The contents of the egg become transposed and an artificial air sac forms beneath the hole over the CAM. Check this by candling.

9. Using a 1 ml syringe filled with an appropriate virus dilution, inoculate the eggs (by inserting the needle into the artificial air sac through the hole over CAM to depth of about 4–5 mm) with 0.1 ml of virus suspension. Inoculate two eggs with each dilution of the virus.

10. Rock the eggs gently to distribute the inoculum.

11. Seal the holes in the shell with adhesive tape or wax.

12. Incubate the eggs at 37°C for two days in a humidified environment with the false air sac uppermost.

13. Chill eggs at 4°C overnight prior to harvesting.

14. Place each egg in a petri dish with the inoculated area uppermost.

15. Cut the egg into two halves around the long axis using sterile scissors.

16. The chorioallantoic membrane should remain in the top half of the shell and can be removed with forceps. Discard the rest of the egg contents.

17. Place the harvested membrane in a fresh petri dish containing saline.

18. Wash the membrane free of yolk, shell, etc., and transfer to a further petri dish containing 10% formol saline.

19. Examine the membranes for presence of pocks. This is easier if they are placed over a black background. Count the pocks and calculate pock forming units per millilitre of original virus suspension.

Haemagglutination

The ability of some viruses to aggregate various species of red blood cells (RBCs) is referred to as haemagglutination. This effect is brought about by the interaction of specific virus glycoproteins with surface receptors present on the plasma membrane of RBCs. Not all viruses are capable of causing this reaction and those that do may only react with RBCs of particular species and may do so only under stringent conditions of pH and ionic strength. Other viruses, however, may react with a whole range of RBCs in a basic saline solution.

For the reaction to occur, the virus should be in sufficient concentration to form cross-bridges between RBCs, causing their agglutination. Thus, RBCs left in a hemispherical well unagglutinated will fall to the bottom of the well and form a well-defined RBC pellet. Agglutinated RBCs on the other hand will form a lattice-work structure which coats the sides of the well. The two morphological appearances (pellet and lattice) are easily discernible with the naked eye.

The assay, one of the most common indirect methods of determining virus titer, is not a measure of infectivity. Indeed, virus replication does not take place during this assay. Instead it measures those particles of virus in

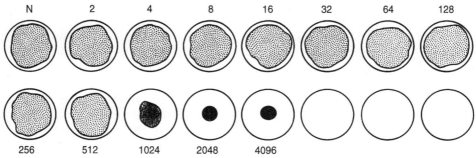

Figure 2.4. Diagram of a sample haemagglutination assay. Serial doubling dilutions of virus shows complete agglutination end point at 1:512 and 50% end point at 1:1024.

a given suspension capable of causing haemagglutination and as such the assay is not at all sensitive, as a very large number of particles are needed to produce the effect.

The haemagglutination assay is done by end point titration. Serial two fold dilutions of virus suspension are mixed with an equal volume of RBCs of known concentration and wells are observed for the presence or absence of a lattice. RBCs are routinely used at 0.3% or 0.5%. The end point of the titration can be interpreted in two ways: (a) the last dilution showing complete agglutination or (b) the dilution which shows 50% agglutination. Most laboratories use the former and by definition such a dilution is said to contain 1 HA unit. The HA titer of a virus suspension is therefore defined as being the reciprocal of the highest dilution which causes complete agglutination and is expressed as the number of HA units per unit volume for a given concentration of RBCs. An example upon which a calculation of the HA titer can be made is shown in Fig. 2.4. The end point in this figure, assuming this to be the highest dilution capable of complete agglutination, is $\frac{1}{512}$. If 0.2 ml of virus were added per well the HA titer would be 512 HA units 0.2 ml^{-1} or 2560 HA units ml^{-1}. Using the 50% end point calculation the titer would be 1024 HA units 0.2 ml^{-1} or 5120 HA units ml^{-1}.

Burleson et al (1992) document a method whereby the number of haemagglutinating virus particles can be obtained, given the HA titer and the fact that the number of RBCs in the well approximates the number of HA particles. In the above example, knowing that a 0.3% RBC suspension gave rise to a titer of 512 HA units 0.2 ml^{-1}, the number of haemagglutinating virus particles in the original suspension can be calculated. A 10% solution of RBCs is defined as having 8×10^8 RBCs ml^{-1}. A 0.3% solution therefore contains 2.3×10^7 RBCs ml^{-1}. As 0.2 ml of RBC were added to each well this represents 4.8×10^6 RBCs per well. At a 1:512 dilution there were 4.8×10^6 haemagglutinating virus particles in the well. As 0.2 ml of virus was used this represents 2.4×10^7 virus particles ml^{-1}. When multiplied by the dilution factor (512) this means that 1.2×10^{10} haemagglutinating virus particles ml^{-1} are present in the original virus suspension.

Procedure

The procedure outlined below is routinely used in our laboratories to assay influenza virus using chicken RBCs.

1. Chicken RBCs are 'brought in' in preservative solution. Alternatively, acquire by bleeding the wing vein of a chicken.
2. Prepare a stock solution of RBCs (10%) in phosphate buffered saline. Once washed away from preservative these cells will last for 1–2 weeks only at 4°C. The 10% solution can be achieved by a haemocytometer count, i.e. a suspension of 8×10^8 cells ml^{-1}, or by use of a haematocrit tube.
3. Carry out the assay in a large 80 well

WHO plate or in a 96 well plate. For the former 0.2 ml volumes are used, for the latter 0.1 ml. We will assume a WHO 80 well plate is being used.

4. Add 0.2 ml saline to all wells in the two rows of the plate (apart from well 1).
5. Add 0.2 ml virus suspension to well 1. This represents neat virus.
6. Add 0.2 ml virus suspension to well 2 and mix by pipetting up and down into the pipette tip. Transfer 0.2 ml to well 3 and repeat the mixing step. Carry out the serial two fold dilutions along the row and transfer 0.2 ml to row 1 of column 2. Again dilute along the row, this time discarding the tip (+0.2 ml) into disinfectant after the last well.
7. Add 0.2 ml RBCs (0.3% or 0.5%) to each well. Gently tap the plate to ensure good mixing of RBCs and virus.
8. Leave for 1 h at ambient temperature and read the end point

As will be seen in later chapters virus haemagglutination can be inhibited by specific antisera, this forming the basis of the haemagglutination-inhibition test.

Particle counting

A later chapter of this book discusses and elaborates upon the electron microscope and its uses in virology. In this chapter we highlight the basic methodology of virus particle counting using the technique of negative staining. This procedure was excellently described by Watson et al (1963).

The counting procedure relies on the use of a 'reference particle'. The principle is that if viruses can be mixed with reference particles of known concentration (i.e. number per unit volume) a simple determination of the ratio of virus to reference particles will yield the virus count. The Dow Corning Company, many years ago, made this possible by producing suspensions of spherical polystyrene latex particles of uniform diameter, with physical properties allowing calculation of their count. However, early problems in virus particle counting arose because of the inability to differentiate, in some cases, between the latex beads and the virus particles when observed in the electron microscope!

The problem of identification was easily overcome by the incorporation in the reference particles/virus mixture of a negative stain, phosphotungstate (PTA), which reveals the characteristic structures on virus particles (Watson 1962).

The mixture of virus, negative stain and latex beads is deposited, in droplet form using a bacteriological loop, onto a specimen grid. Upon observation in the electron microscope a virus/latex ratio can be derived by examination of substantial parts of the grid.

Procedure

The loop drop procedure, described below, may be used for any virus suspension containing approximately 10^9 particles ml^{-1}, and was developed for herpes simplex virus.

1. Portions of latex and virus suspensions (0.1 ml) each diluted to contain about 10^9 particles ml^{-1} are mixed with 0.1 ml of 0.5% PTA and 0.1 ml of 0.5% bovine serum albumin. The dilution of virus if no infectivity titer is known, will be by trial and error.
2. Introduce a drop of the above mixture, using a platinum loop onto a carbon Formvar grid held carefully with fine tweezers.
3. Wait for 1–2 minutes and then dry the grid by touching it with blotting paper.
4. Scan the grid in the electron microscope at a screen magnification of ×40,000.
5. Virus particles and latex beads are clearly visible and counts are made of the number encountered using five groups of 20 latex beads.
6. The number of particles is calculated by the method outlined below:

Table 2.2.

	Latex	Virus ($\frac{1}{50}$ dilution)
	20	9
	20	8
	20	8
	20	9
	20	6
mean	20	8

Assuming the latex to have been used at a concentration of (for example) 2.84×10^9 beads ml^{-1}, the total number of virus particles per millilitre is given by:

$$\frac{8}{20} \times 2.84 \times 10^9 \times 50$$
$$= 5.7 \times 10^{10} \text{ particles ml}^{-1}$$

If the infectivity titer, e.g. pfu ml^{-1}, is known it is possible from the above to calculate the particle:infectivity ratio of the virus. Assuming the titer of the above virus suspension to be 5.0×10^8 pfu ml^{-1} the particle: infectivity ratio would be:

$$\frac{5.7 \times 10^{10}}{5.0 \times 10^8} = 114$$

Determination of this ratio is important for many areas of virology, e.g. monitoring virus purification regimes, looking for defective interfering particles, determining the state or age of a virus suspension.

References

Adrian T, Wadell G, Hierholzer JC, Wigand R (1986) Arch Virol 91: 277–290.

Agbalika F, Hartemann P, Foliguet JM (1984) Appl Environ Microbiol 47: 378–380.

Anderson LJ (1987) Ped Infect Dis J 6: 711–718.

Anderson LJ, Hierholzer JC, Bingham PG, Stone YO (1985) J Clin Microbiol 22: 1050–1052.

Arya SC (1975) Indian J Med Res 63: 1238–1241.

Babiuk LA, Mohammed K, Spence L, Fauvel M, Petro R (1977) J Clin Microbiol 6: 610–617.

Bellini WJ and Rota PA (1995) In Diagnostic Procedures for Viral, Rickettsial and Chlamydial Infections. Lennette EH, Lennette DA, Lennette ET (Eds.) 7th edn. American Public Health Assn, Washington DC pp. 447–454.

Black JB, Inoue N, Kite-Powell K, Zaki S, Pellett PE (1993) Virus Res 29: 91–98.

Black JB, Pellett PE (1993) Rev Med Virol 3: 217–223.

Burleson FG, Chambers TM, Wiedbrauk DL (1992) Virology, A Laboratory Manual, Academic Press.

Castells E, George VG, Hierholzer JC (1990) Arch Virol 115: 277–288.

Dick EC, Jennings LC, Mink KA, Wartgow CD, Inhorn SL (1987) J Infect Dis 156: 442–448.

Durigon EL, Erdman DD, Gary GW, Pallansch MA, Torok TJ, Anderson LJ (1993) J Virol Meth 44: 155–165.

Elliott LH, Ksiazek TG, Rollin PE, Spiropoulou CF, Morzunov S, Monroe M, Goldsmith CS, Humphrey CD, Zaki SR, Krebs JW, Maupin G, Gage K, Childs JE, Nichol ST, Peters CJ (1994) Am J Trop Med Hyg 51: 102–108.

Fields BN, Knipe DM, Chanock RM, Hirsch MS, Melnick JL, Monath TP, Roizman B (Eds.) (1990) Virology Vols 1 and 2, 2nd Edn. Raven Press, New York.

Frank AL, Couch RB, Griffis CA, Baxter BD (1979) J Clin Microbiol 10: 32–36.

Grandien M, Pettersson CA, Gardner PS, Linde A, Stanton A (1985) J Clin Microbiol 22: 757–760.

Hall CB, Long CE, Schnabel KC, Caserta MT, McIntyre KM, Costanzo MA, Knott A, Dewhurst S, Insel RA, Epstein LG (1994) New Engl J Med 331: 432–438.

Hierholzer JC (1976) Virology 75: 155–165.

Hierholzer JC (1991) In Rapid Methods and Automation in Microbiology and Immunology. Vaheri A, Tilton RC, Balows A (Eds.) Springer-Verlag Berlin, pp. 556–573.

Hierholzer JC (1993) Immunol Allergy Clin North Amer 13: 27–42.

Hierholzer JC, Anderson LJ, Halonen PE (1990) Med Virol 9: 17–45.

Hierholzer JC, Bingham PG, Castells E, Coombs RA (1993a) Arch Virol 130: 335–352.

Hierholzer JC, Castells E, Banks GG, Bryan JA, McEwen CT (1993b) J Clin Microbiol 31: 1504–1510.

Hierholzer JC, Halonen PE, Bingham PG, Coombs RA, Stone YO (1994a) Clin Diag Virol 2: 165–179.

Hierholzer JC, Hatch MH (1985) In Viral Diseases of the Eye. Darrell RW (Ed.), pp. 165–196. Lea and Febiger, Philadelphia.

Hierholzer JC, Tannock GA, Hierholzer CM, Coombs RA, Kennett ML, Phillips PA, Gust ID (1994b) Arch Virol 136: 133–147.

Hsiung GD (1968) Bacteriol Rev 32: 185–205.

Hsiung GD (1969) Ann NY Acad Sci 162: 483–498.

Hull RN (1968) Virol Monogr 2: 1–66.

Hummel KB, Erdman DD, Heath J, Bellini WJ (1992) J Clin Microbiol 30: 2874–2880.

Hyypia T, Stanway G (1993) Adv Virus Res 42: 343–373.

Inoue N, Dambaugh TR, Pellett PE (1994) Infect Agents Dis 2: 343–360.

Kärber G (1931) Arch exp Path Pharmak 162: 480–487.

Klenk HD, Rott R, Orlich M, Blodorn J (1975) Virology 68: 426–439.

Koopmans M, Horzinek MC (1994) Adv Vir Res 43: 233–273.

Lazarowitz SG, Choppin PW (1975) Virology 68: 440–454.

Lennette EH, Halonen P, Murphy FA (Eds.) (1988) Laboratory Diagnosis of Infectious Diseases: Principles and Practice, Vol. II, Viral Rickettsial, and Chlamydial Diseases. Springer-Verlag, NY.

Lennette EH, Lennette DA, Lennette ET (Eds.) (1995) Diagnostic Procedures for Viral, Rickettsial and Chlamydial Infections. 7th edn. American Public Health Assn, Washington D.C.

Mandell GL, Douglas RG, Bennett JE (Eds.) (1990) Principles and Practice of Infectious Diseases. Churchill Livingstone, NY.

Matthey S, Nicholson D, Ruhs S, Alden B, Knock M, Schultz K, Schmuecker A (1992) J Clin Microbiol 30: 540–544.

Meguro H, Bryant JD, Torrence AE, Wright PF (1979) J Clin Microbiol 9: 175–179.

Murray PR, Baron EJ, Pfaller MA, Tenover FC, Yolken RH (Eds.) (1995) Manual of Clinical Microbiology. 6th edn. American Society for Microbiology Press, Washington D.C.

Palmer EL, Martin ML (1988) Electron Microscopy in Viral Diagnosis. CRC Press, Boca Raton, FL.

Pellett PE, Black JB, Yamamoto M (1992) Adv Virus Res 41: 1–52.

Reed LJ, Muench H (1938) Amer J Hyg 27: 493–497.

Ropp SL, Jin Q, Knight JC, Massung RF, Esposito J (1995) J Clin Microbiol 33: 2069–2076.

Rose NR, deMacario EC, Fahey JL, Friedman H, Penn GM (Ed.) (1992) Manual of Clinical Laboratory Immunology. 4th ed, American Society for Microbiology, Washington, D.C.

Russell WC (1962) Nature 195: 1028–1029.

Sanchez-Fauquier A, Carrascosa AL, Carrascosa JL, Otero A, Glass RI, Lopez JA, San Martin C, Melero JA (1994) Virology 201: 312–320.

Schmidt OW, Cooney MK, Kenny GE (1979) J Clin Microbiol 9: 722–728.

Smith CD, Craft DW, Shiromoto RS, Yan PO (1986) J Clin Microbiol 24: 265–268.

Spearman C (1908) Brit J Psychol 2: 227–242.

Tanaka K, Kondo T, Torigoe S, Okada S, Mukai T, Yamanishi K (1994) J Pediatr 125: 1–5.

Warfield DT, Feorino PM (1992) In Clinical Microbiology Procedures Handbook. (Ed.) Isenberg HD, pp. 8.15.1–8.15.11; American Society for Microbiology, Washington, D.C.

Watson DH (1962) Biochim Biophys Acta 61: 321–331.

Watson DH, Russell WC, Wildy P (1963) Virology 19: 250–260.

Woods GL, Young A (1988) J Clin Microbiol 26: 1026–1028.

Yasukawa M, Yakushijin Y, Furukawa M, Fujita S (1993) J Virol 67: 6259–6264.

Preparation of antigens

3

J. C. Hierholzer
R. A. Killington
A. Stokes

Virtually every diagnostic and research-oriented test in virology begins with an antigen that has been specially prepared for that test. For some tests, the antigen can simply be the supernatant fluid from the cell culture the virus was propagated in, with no regard to the maintenance medium used in culture or the storage conditions for the final product. For others, intact virus is required at the highest titers achievable, so that several freeze–thaw or sonication cycles are applied to the virus culture at complete (4^+) CPE to thoroughly disrupt all remaining cells containing virus; or, a particular viral product needs to be enriched in proportion to other products, but not purified in the biochemical sense. For still others, only a specific viral protein can be used in the test, so that it has to be purified, concentrated, and preserved while all other interfering viral products and medium components are removed. The procedures described in this chapter will accomplish all of these tasks.

The most general concept to begin with is also the most important – viz, the microbiological purity of the starting viral culture. Wherever possible, laboratories should be equipped with recirculating laminar-flow safety cabinets; all operations likely to produce aerosols of infectious materials should be carried out in the cabinet. Minimum requirements for protective clothing include a lab coat or gown and, for more hazardous operations, gloves and masks. During operations involving infectious materials, the workbench would be covered with disposable plastic-lined table soakers to prevent contamination. All work areas should be decontaminated with 0.5% hypochlorite solution. All discarded materials must be placed in discard pans and sterilised by standard procedures. One product should be worked with at a time in a very clean environment. All virus products should be certified to be free of viable bacterial, fungal, and mycoplasmal contamination by appropriate culturing in thioglycollate broth, trypticase soy broth, 5% sheep blood agar pour/streak plates, Sabouraud dextrose slants for yeasts, and mycoplasma biphasic medium. While these concepts may seem basic, many a lengthy piece of work has been erroneously interpreted or had to be discarded because the starting culture was contaminated and the test results were obfuscated by the contaminant.

In most cases, infected cell antigens are derived from cells previously infected at a high moi, i.e. 2–10 pfu cell^{-1}. For every virus antigen there should be a parallel 'normal antigen' to serve as the negative control in the test. Normal antigens are prepared by sham-inoculating cell cultures with negative culture material (without virus), and following these cultures through the entire virus culture and antigen preparation steps in exact parallel fashion.

Depending on the test and the day-to-day usage, many antigens can be preserved by adding thimerosal to the final product to a

Virology Methods Manual
ISBN 0–12–465330–8

final concentration of 1:10,000, or sodium azide to a final concentraton of 0.1%.

Conditions for storing virus antigens must be monitored carefully. For some 4°C is adequate, others require storage at −20°C or −70°C. The potency of antigen batches should be regularly tested following thawing, usually by means of a serological test.

Special preparation of antigens is required for many diagnostic tests, for monoclonal or polyclonal antibody production, for many EIA and LA tests, etc. Many viruses and antigens have their own peculiarities based on the specific properties of each virus group; these can be found elsewhere in this book and in other reference works (Fields et al 1990; Hierholzer 1993; Hierholzer et al 1990; Lennette et al 1988; Schmidt and Emmons 1989).

Particular subsets of antigens can be prepared in similar ways to those outlined below; in some cases with previous treatment of infected cells with inhibitory drugs, e.g. inhibitors of DNA synthesis. This allows early and late antigens to be selected. Time of cell harvest also allows for a predominant antigen type to be selected. Non-glycosylated virus proteins can be prepared from cells treated with glycosylation inhibitors (e.g. tunicamycin and monensin). For the preparation of structural antigens the starting material may be purified virus, prepared as outlined in chapter 4.

Whole-cell antigen preparations

Total extracts of infected cells have a wide range of uses in virology. The simplest and most often used techniques for liberating virus from the host cells, for dislodging the host cells from the cell culture surface, and sometimes for disrupting virions to liberate particular antigens, are outlined below.

Freeze–thawing

1. At the appropriate time during the culture period, usually at 4+ CPE, lay the flasks or tubes in a −70°C or −80°C freezer such that the maintenance medium is covering all the cells.
2. Alternatively, wash the cell monolayer with phosphate buffered saline to remove maintenance medium and replenish with a similar volume of buffer before freezing.
3. Allow to freeze solid (the time will depend on the temperature and the volume).
4. Thaw under warm (but not hot) water or at room temperature. When enough ice has thawed to form a slush, use the slush to further dislodge the cells by striking the flask several times against the palm of the hand.
5. Repeat the freeze–thaw cycle at least twice more. For labile viruses, stop at two freeze–thaw cycles.
6. Clarify the final material by low-speed centrifugation (e.g. 1000 g, 30 min, 4°C). The supernatant is the antigen product, and can be further treated by any of the following procedures if necessary.

Sonication

1. At the appropriate time during culture, usually at 4+ CPE, the cultures may be either freeze–thawed as above but not clarified by centrifugation, or the cells scraped off the glass or plastic surface with a rubber policeman.
2. For some viruses (e.g. herpes viruses) the majority of antigens may remain intracellularly bound and a centrifugation step is necessary in order to remove infected cells from the supernatant. Low speed centrifugation is used to pellet the cells which are washed in PBS before resuspending in an appropriate volume of buffer.

   The cells/medium/virus mixture is then sonicated at sufficient energy to disrupt all the cells and release the virus, or with additional energy to disrupt the virions to release particular antigens. The energy level must be determined by pilot trials for the test procedure in use. Usually, 30–70 watts for 1–3 min with multiple pulses per minute will break the cells. For labile viruses such as CMV and RSV, a 60-second sonication at 60 watts output is sufficient to produce an enhanced antigen. **Note**: The manufacturer's instructions for the sonicator must be followed carefully, and all sonication steps must be done in an ice bath and in vessels which will not shatter. It is absolutely essential that the antigen does not become heated.

   For many viruses, sufficient energy can be created from the small ultrasonic baths that are used to clean jewelry. These are usually cheap and easily obtainable. For all procedures, aerosols must be avoided.

3. Sonicated material is usually clarified by low speed centrifugation (as above). For some purposes a batch of 'soluble' antigen may be necessary and therefore virions will need to be removed. In this case the sonicated material is ultracentrifugated and the pellet discarded, the supernatant being a preparation of 'soluble' antigen which is particularly useful for immunodiffusion purposes.

Solubilization of infected cell antigen can also be achieved by chemical treatment. This procedure is particularly useful for the preparation of antigens for PAGE/Western blotting techniques. Washed pelleted cells are solubilized by resuspending in RIPA buffer (1% NP-40, 0.1% SDS, 0.1 M NaCl, 50 mM Tris-HCl, pH 7.4) then protein solubilizing buffer (0.125 M Tris-HCl pH 6.8; 4% (w/v) glycerol and, if required, a drop of bromophenol blue).

Alkaline glycine treatment, and others

High-titered intracellular antigens for CF, IHA, and RIA tests, such as for CMV, can be pre-pared by alkaline glycine extraction. In this procedure, the infected cell monolayer is scraped and the cells packed by centrifugation; then the cell pellet is mixed with 0.1 M glycine-buffered saline, pH 9.5, for 6 h at 37°C, followed by clarification at 600 g for 20 min (Cremer et al 1975; Schmidt and Emmons 1989). Alternatively, the infected cell monolayer is rinsed with 0.01 M PBS (1.096 g Na_2HPO_4 + 0.315 g $NaH_2PO_4.H_2O$ + 8.5 g NaCl + 1000 ml distilled water; pH 7.2; filter sterilized) before 4+ CPE, and is overlayered with a small amount of 0.05 M glycine-buffered saline (3.75 g glycine + 0.35 g NaOH + 8.5 g NaCl + 1000 ml distilled water; pH 9.0; 0.22 μ filter-sterilized). The cells are scraped thoroughly into this buffer, and the slurry is sonicated (70 watts, 1 min, 0°C), gamma-irradiated (0.5 MRads, 0°C), stabilized with 10% sorbitol (final concentration), preserved with 0.01% thimerosal, packaged, and tested (Chappell et al 1984).

Another simple antigen preparation, usually made for EIA tests, involves washing an infected cell monolayer with cold PBS, treating with 0.25% trypsin or trypsin/versene (see chapter 1), further washing of the dislodged cells with cold PBS to remove the trypsin, suspension of the cells in a buffer suitable for the test, sonication in an ice bath, and finally centrifugation at 1500 g for 15 min at 4°C to remove the cellular debris. This procedure has worked well for EIA antigens for CMV and VZV and for HA antigens for certain arboviruses (Ardoin et al 1969; Schmidt and Emmons 1989). IFA antigens can also be prepared with trypsin, utilizing the washed, suspended cells as the test antigen.

Fractionation of antigens by various extraction procedures (sub-unit preparations)

Tween-80/ether extraction

1. Obtain a virus culture as above, at 4+ CPE or maximum hemadsorption in companion flasks. Treat the cultures by freeze–thaw cycles, sonication, or scraping the cells from the flasks, and pool.
2. Clarify by centrifugation (1000 g, 30 min, 4°C).
3. Add Tween-80 slowly to 0.125% final concentration to disrupt the virus.
4. Add an equal volume of diethyl ether (reagent grade) to extract lipids, with constant mixing on a magnetic stirrer. Mix for about 1 h at ambient temperature or in the cold, depending on the virus. **Note:** Good ventilation and the absence of fire are mandatory!
5. Centrifuge to form a distinct ether layer (on top), which is aspirated away. Residual ether in the lower, aqueous layer is removed by slowly bubbling filtered nitrogen gas through the layer until no odor of ether can be detected.
6. The product may need to be clarified again by light centrifugation. This procedure makes excellent HA antigens for rubella, influenza, parainfluenza, mumps, and measles viruses, and CF antigens for influenza and parainfluenza viruses (Chappell et

al 1984; Norrby 1962; Schmidt and Emmons 1989).

β-Propiolactone (BPL) extraction

1. Clarify culture by centrifugation (1000 g, 30 min, 4°C).
2. Add 1 M Tris in PBS [12.11 g Tris(hydroxymethyl)amino-methane + 100 ml PBS, pH 7.2 (see page 50); 0.22 μ filter-sterilized] to the virus supernatant in a 1:10 ratio (i.e., 1 ml Tris per 9 ml supernatant).
3. Add cold reagent-grade BPL, dropwise and with constant mixing at room temperature, to a final concentration ranging from 0.05% to 0.3%, depending on the virus and the antigen test system. Final concentration must be determined in pilot trials, but 0.3% is suitable to inactivate and extract CF antigens for herpesvirus 1 and 2, rotavirus, RSV, rabies, parainfluenza, measles, and echoviruses, polioviruses, and some other enteroviruses; 0.2% is sufficient for coronavirus CF antigens; 0.1% treats HA antigens of NDV and CF antigens of mumps virus, Coxsackie A

and B viruses, and some other enteroviruses; and 0.05% inactivates and extracts HA antigens of influenza, mumps, and parainfluenza viruses (Chappell et al 1984; Schmidt and Emmons 1989; Sever et al 1964). **Note:** Use gloves, and avoid eye and skin contact with BPL.

4. Let stand 4–18 h at 4°C, or place in a 37°C water bath for 2 h, with occasional mixing. Time and temperature must be determined in pilot trials.
5. Adjust to pH 7.3–7.4 as necessary.
6. Clarify by light centrifugation as above, and add preservative if desired. Thimerosal at 0.01% is generally preferred for CF antigens, while sodium azide at 0.1% usually has least interference in HA tests, but there is no solid rule for this. Test for potency.
7. The BPL extraction of CF and HA antigens from many Togaviridae (EEE, Ross River, Sindbis, VEE, WEE, and other formerly Group A arboviruses), Rhabdoviridae (VSV), Reoviridae (Colorado tick fever), Flaviviridae (Powassan), Bunyaviridae (California encephalitis virus, Trivitattus), and some other arboviruses, is done slightly differently. Included here, because of the need for the borate-saline buffer, is the CF antigen for the Arenavirus LCM and the HA antigen for the Poxvirus vaccinia. For these antigens, prepare 10% mouse brain suspensions or infected cell cultures in borate-saline [100 ml of 0.5 M H_3BO_3 + 80 ml of 1.5 M NaCl + 24 ml of 1.0 N NaOH, QS to 1000 ml with distilled water; pH 9.0; 0.22 μ filter-sterilized]. Homogenize the mixture for 1–3 min in a tightly-capped container in an ice bath, and allow to sit for 30 min. Then, add 1 M Tris in borate-saline [12.11 g Tris + 100 ml borate-saline, pH 9.0; 0.22 μ filtered] to 1/10 the volume of the original suspension. Slowly add cold BPL to achieve the desired final concentration, usually 0.3%, in the cold and with constant mixing. Hold the suspension at 4°C for 18–24 h, clarify by centrifugation at 1000–9000 g for 1 h at 4°C, and save the supernatant. If desired, wash the pellet with additional borate-saline one or more times and combine the supernatants. Thimerosal may be added to a final concentration of 0.01% for a preservative. Aliquot and store at −70°C or colder; then safety-test the antigen for complete loss of infectivity in appropriate host systems, and test the antigen for homologous CF and HA titers. **Note:** Hemagglutination by Togaviruses and Flaviviruses is often pH-dependent (e.g. Powassan at pH 6.1), so the HA antigen and the HA test may have to be prepared in buffers with the required pH.

For Tween-80/ether and sucrose/acetone/BPL extractions of certain arbovirus HA and CF antigens, see Chappell et al (1984) and Schmidt and Emmons (1989).

Nonionic detergent extraction

A rapid means of separating, for example, virus envelope proteins from capsid and surrounding tegument is to treat with detergent. Such a treatment will also serve for the preparation of plasma membranes from infected cells. Nonidet P-40 (NP-40) is usually the non-ionic detergent of choice and may be used with or without sodium deoxycholate. The infected cell pellet or purified virus is resuspended in NP-40 at a final concentration of 1%, sodium deoxycholate being the same concentration. The suspension is left at 4°C for 20 min and a further 20 min at 25°C before centrifuging at 38,000 rpm in an ultracentrifuge. Depending on the size of virus and other characteristics, the detergent treated suspension may be centrifuged in an 'Eppendorf' microfuge. The supernatant is retained as the detergent extract.

Excreted protein fraction

Many viruses selectively release specific proteins into the extracellular medium and this may be a useful means of making preparations of antigens of restricted specificity (Randall et al, 1980). Extracellular medium from infected cell monolayers is centrifuged to remove debris – if possible at 16,000 rpm for 1.5 h. The supernatant is concentrated, initially by polyethylene glycol dialysis (see chapter 4), followed by either vacuum dialysis or ultrafiltration (e.g. Amicon concentration). The concentrated suspension is ultracentrifuged to remove virion particles and dialyzed against either PBS or 0.05 M Tris/HCl buffer pH 7.0, resulting in an infected cell released protein fraction (Randall et al, 1980).

High-salt extraction

A high-salt extract of antigens from infected cells often forms the starting point for a series of further fractionation steps. An example is the purification of virus-specific DNA binding proteins which, following high salt extraction, are exposed to DEAE cellulose, phosphocellulose or DNA cellulose chromatography (Alberts et al 1968; Purifoy and Powell 1976; Powell and Purifoy 1977).

Washed and pelletted infected cells are resuspended in buffer containing 20 mM Tris HCl pH 7.5, 2 mM β-mercaptoethanol, and bovine serum albumin (4000 μg ml^{-1}). Following ultrasonic cellular disruption, the cells are suspended in an equal volume of high-salt buffer containing 5 mM EDTA and 1.7 M KCl and incubated at 0°C for 60'. Insoluble protein and free DNA are removed by centrifugaton at 16,000 rpm for 1 h and the supernatant dialyzed against several changes of low-salt buffer containing 50 mM KCl, 20 mM Tris HCl pH 7.5, 1 mM EDTA, 2 mM β-mercaptoethanol, and 10% glycerol. The dialysate is centrifuged at 20,000 rpm for 32 h to yield a high-salt extract.

Partial purification by adsorption/elution techniques

Adsorption and elution from erythrocytes

This simple technique is based on the hemagglutinability of certain viruses. Viruses which agglutinate red blood cells can be partially purified by adsorbing them to the appropriate erythrocytes at low temperatures, thoroughly washing the cells to remove all non-virion and non-HA antigen components, and then eluting the virus into a simple buffer at higher temperatures. The method has been used effectively for partial purification of intact, infectious influenza, parainfluenza, mumps, measles, and coronaviruses, for removing hemagglutinins from CF antigens, and for obtaining reagents enriched in hemagglutinins (Chappell et al 1984; Hierholzer and Dowdle 1970; Hierholzer et al 1972; Schmidt and Emmons 1989). Because of the number of washes the cells must undergo, the success of the procedure depends on being able to use one of the 'tougher' species of erythrocytes, such as human, monkey, or chicken, rather than rat, mouse, or guinea pig red blood cells which tend to disintegrate from the physical trauma incurred by the procedure.

1. Begin with a large-volume harvest of virus from cell culture, 20% suckling mouse brain suspension in PBS, amniotic or allantoic fluids from embryonated eggs, or any other system. Multiple freeze–thaw cycles may be indicated to release maximum virus from the cells, if the virus is stable under this treatment. Clarify the harvest at abut 5000 g for 20–40 min at 4°C to remove gross cellular debris. At this point, the supernatant will contain maximum amounts of whole virus and soluble antigens (if produced).

2. If a hemagglutinin preparation free of infectious virus is desired, treat the supernatant with SLS in distilled water to a final concentration of up to 5% for 1 h at ambient temperature, or with some other ionic or nonionic detergent, followed by dialysis against PBS to remove the detergent.

3. Select erythrocyte species that gives high HA titers with virus being purified, choosing a more durable cell if possible. Obtain sufficient volume of red blood cells to carry out the procedure; the blood must be obtained in Alsever's solution [20.5 g glucose + 8.0 g sodium citrate ($Na_3C_6H_5O_7.2H_2O$) + 0.55 g citric acid ($C_6H_8O_7.H_2O$) + 4.2 g NaCl + 1000 ml distilled water; final pH 6.1; filter-sterilized] as gently as possible, and used fresh to minimize trauma to the cells.

4. Gently wash the cells three times with a large excess of cold PBS, being sure to aspirate off the leukocytes which layer on top of the erythrocytes. Use a suitably large centrifuge bottle so that the reaction to follow can be carried out in the bottle. Do all wash steps at 4°C.

5. Placing the bottle with packed, washed cells in an ice bath, slowly add ice-cold virus supernatant (from

steps 1 or 2) to the cells at the final ratio of 60 ml of virus to 40 ml of packed erythrocytes. [**Note:** For influenza and mumps viruses grown in embryonated eggs, 95 ml of cold fluid harvest per 10 ml of packed chicken red cells is generally sufficient.] Mix gently and frequently over a 2 h adsorption period.

6. Pack the red cells by centrifugation at 1000 g for 15 min at 0°C. If removing hemagglutinins from a CF, EIA, or other antigen preparation, *save* the supernatant and stop here. If preparing an HA antigen, *discard* the supernatant and proceed as follows.

7. Wash the cells three times under the same centrifugation conditions, always discarding the supernatant. It is critical to re-suspend the cells as gently as possible at each wash step, preferably using a wooden applicator stick.

8. Elute the virus or hemagglutinins from the red cells by two successive incubations, each with 10 ml of PBS for 40–60 min at 38°C, with frequent gentle agitation, followed by centrifugation as above but at ambient temperature. Collect the supernatant, now containing the virus or hemagglutinins.

9. Pool the two eluates and test for virus or antigen titer, as appropriate. Thimerosal may be added to 0.01% final concentration as a preservative. Assuming a starting volume of 60 ml of virus, this yields a 3× concentration of virus that is free of all cell and medium components and all non-intact virus, non-HA antigen viral components. Some erythrocyte membranes and proteins, however, may be picked up in the elutions by disintegration of some red blood cells.

Adsorption and elution from calcium phosphate gel

The freshly-prepared brushite form of calcium phosphate ($CaHPO_4.2H_2O$) is one of the oldest but still most useful ways to purify viruses, proteins, and antigens (Taverne et al 1958). In hydroxyapatite form [$Ca_{10}(PO_4)_6(OH)_2$] calcium phosphate is used to separate the various forms of DNA and RNA, nucleohistones, and polynucleotides (Alberts et al 1989; Bernardi 1971). The brushite procedure, with little modification, has been used to partially purify many viruses and antigens, including adenovirus capsid components, influenza virus and hemagglutinins; Group A arboviruses belonging to Togaviridae and Group B arboviruses belonging to Flaviviridae, along with their CF and HA antigens; vaccinia virus; coronaviruses; and enteroviruses (Dowdle et al 1971; Hierholzer 1976; Hierholzer and Dowdle 1970; Hierholzer et al 1972; Simon 1962; Smith and Holt 1961; Taverne et al 1958). The method works best for virus cultures grown under maintenance medium without calf serum or other added proteins; and the final culture must be clarified by low-speed centrifugation and dialyzed thoroughly against 0.001 M phosphate buffer, pH 7.3, for 24 h at 4°C.

1. Prepare the brushite form of $CaHPO_4$ by adding equal volumes of 0.5 M $CaCl_2.2H_2O$ and 0.5 M $Na_2HPO_4.2H_2O$, both in distilled water, dropwise into a beaker, with constant mixing at ambient temperature, at a drop rate of about 60 drops min^{-1} for each salt. The precipitate $CaHPO_4.2H_2O$ + 2NaCl is formed.

2. Allow the precipitate to settle for about 1 h, decant or aspirate off the supernatant, and wash the precipitate six times in distilled water by

low-speed centrifugation, such as 700 g for 5–10 min. The final wash may be tested for chloride content, but this is usually not necessary.

3. Resuspend the final packed gel in 0.001 M phosphate buffer, pH 7.3, at which point the gel may be stored in the refrigerator for up to two weeks. Degas the gel under vacuum before using for column chromatography.

4. To continue with column chromatography, fill a chromatographic column with 0.001 M phosphate buffer, begin dripping out the buffer, and pour in the gel slurry (slowly to avoid bubbles and channels) until the column has the desired height of gel. The column should have a length : diameter ratio of 5:1 to 10:1, and must have a series of mesh filters at the bottom of the column to prevent blockage by the fine gel particles. The top of the gel bed should be covered with a nylon or filter paper 'float' to effect even loading of the surface. The virus sample can then be loaded, the column rinsed with one void volume of distilled water, and the desired components eluted by a gradient of increasing molarities of phosphate buffer at pH 7.3.

5. To continue with batch chromatography, which is preferable for $CaHPO_4$ work, transfer the gel slurry to a 50 ml conical centrifuge tube to obtain about 15 ml of packed gel. Centrifuge and discard the supernatant buffer. Add about 30 ml of clarified virus supernatant that has already been dialyzed against the 0.001 M phosphate buffer.

6. Gently but constantly mix the gel (now at about 33% v/v) with the virus for 2 h at ambient temperature. (This step may be done in an ice bath to protect a labile virus. Likewise, mixing may be accomplished by periodically inverting the tube rather than using a magnetic mixer, to prevent physical destruction of the virus.)

7. Centrifuge the mixture at 4°C; discard the supernatant.

8. Wash the gel once with distilled water and once with 0.001 M buffer to remove nonadsorbed components.

9. Elute with 0.005, 0.01, 0.05, 0.1, 0.15, 0.2, 0.25, 0.3, 0.35, 0.4, and 0.5 M phosphate buffers, all at pH 7.3, in stepwise fashion to release different proteins and whole virus from the gel. (Whole virus usually elutes between 0.2 and 0.4 M.) Each elution step is done with 10–40 ml of buffer, depending on whether any concentration is desired, by incubating the buffer–gel mixture for 30–60 min in a 30–37°C water bath (as dictated by experience) with occasional mixing, and then packing the gel by centrifugation as above. All supernatants should be tested for the desired components or whole virus, as appropriate, before discarding them.

Partial purification/ purification by chromatographic procedures

Chromatography is considered by many to be the most effective means of producing purified preparations of virus proteins, this being achieved by gel filtration, ion exchange or affinity chromatography. Antigens are separated by the process of selective retention, when a 'mobile' phase (liquid) moves through a liquid or solid 'stationary' phase, the retention being based on the size and chemical or immunological attributes of the individual antigens. Gel filtration separates molecules according to their size and the choice of pore size selected in the stationery gel. Small molecules enter the pores and are retained, whereas larger molecules elute through the gel very quickly thus giving rise to a differential elution of antigens, collected in small volume fractions from the gel column. Ion exchange chromatography utilizes the intrinsic ionic charge of a molecule as the differentiating property. In this case the stationary phase of a column contains groups of chemicals with various anionic or cationic charges, these retaining ions from the mobile phase of virus antigens as they pass through the column. Ions that react strongly with the exchange are retained and eluted much later than those with weaker attachment kinetics. Elution is achieved by slowly increasing, with time, the salt concentration of the eluting buffer. More recently this technique has been refined by the introduction of high-performance liquid chromatography (Chicz and Regnier 1990).

For the purpose of antigen separation in this chapter we have chosen to describe, in detail, the method of affinity chromatography, using a monoclonal antibody as the ligand which is immobilized onto the stationary matrix.

Affinity chromatography

The reader is referred to Harlow and Lane (1988) or to Wilchek et al (1984) for excellent review manuals.

The production of columns or slurries which consist of a monoclonal antibody attached to a solid matrix allows the purification of single proteins from mixtures of antigens which are passed through the column, the selected protein being specifically retained by the antibody for later elution. The procedure is more efficient if the starting mixture of viral antigens is in a 'semi-pure' state. Purification of single virus proteins of 1000–10,000 fold are common practice with such procedures. The efficiency of the procedure depends on three criteria: (a) the purity of the starting antigen, (b) the affinity of the antibody for the antigen, and (c) the relative ease with which the bond can be split and the protein eluted.

Preparation of the antibody–matrix

This first step in the procedure requires the attachment of antibody to the solid matrix. A number of matrices exist, e.g. agarose beads, cross-linked agarose beads, polyacrylamide beads, copolymer of polyacrylamide and agarose, and polyacrylic beads. The authors commonly use Sepharose (Pharmacia). There are also a number of procedures for achieving attachment of antibody. Essentially, however, there are three methods of coupling antibodies: (a) directly to Protein A beads; (b) to chemically activated beads; or (c) by activating the antibody before coupling. Matrices modified so as to contain secondary reagents are the most commonly used.

Preparation of a Protein A Bead–Antibody column

The method described is suitable for binding mouse monoclonal antibodies of sub class IgG2a, IgG2b and IgG3.

1. 2 mg purified antibodies/ml of wet beads are mixed in a slurry by incubating at room temperature for 60 min with gentle rocking.
2. The beads are washed twice with 10 volumes of 0.2 M sodium borate (pH 9.0), being centrifuged at 3000 g for 5 min or 10,000 g for 30 s.
3. Resuspend the beads in 10 volumes of 0.2 M sodium borate buffer (pH 9.0) and add dimethylpimelimidate (solid) to bring to a final concentration of 20 mM.
4. Mix for 30 min at room temperature with shaking.
5. Stop the reaction by washing the beads in 0.2 M ethanolamine (pH 8.0) and incubating for 2 h at room temperature in 0.2 M ethanolamine with gentle mixing.
6. After the final wash, the beads are resuspended in PBS with 0.01% merthiolate.

    The beads at this stage are ready for binding to antigen.

Preparation of chemically activated beads

This procedure requires the matrix to be activated using one of a number of chemical reagents prior to interaction with antibody. The chemicals most widely used include cyanogen bromide, carbonyldiimidazole, gluteraldehyde, hydroxysuccinimide, and tosyl chloride. Procedures for activating the beads with either of these are well documented in Harlow and Lane (1988).

Many laboratories, however, purchase pre-activated beads for use in antibody binding from commercial companies. These include Reacti-Gel (Pierce), CNBr-activated Sepharose (Pharmacia), Act-Ultragel ACA 22(IBF), Affigel 10 (Bio Rad), and Activated Microspheres (KPL). The authors have used Affigel 10 (Bio Rad) with success. This comes as an immunoaffinity kit.

Cyanogen-bromide activated beads

This procedure has been selected for description as it is the most commonly used. It is suitable for agarose, cross-linked agarose, and polyacrylic beads. The method is based on that of Harlow and Lane (1988), Axen et al (1967), March et al (1974), and Kohn and Wilchek (1984).

1. Transfer 10 ml of wet beads to a sintered glass filter. Wash with distilled water. Wash with 1 M sodium carbonate buffer (pH 11.0).
2. Add 10 ml of 1 M sodium bicarbonate (pH 11.0) and transfer the beads to a suitable beaker.
3. Move to a fume hood. Weigh out 1 g of cyanogen bromide (CNBr) and dissolve in 1 ml of acetonitrile. Add the CNBr to the beads. Cyanogen bromide is extremely toxic; use only in a fume hood.

4. Incubate at room temperature for 10 min with constant agitation. Monitor the pH. Adjust as necessary to keep between 10.5 and 11.0 by adding 4 N NaOH.
5. Transfer the beads to a sintered glass filter. Use suction to draw the CNBr buffer into a vacuum flask containing 100 mM ferrous sulfate to inactivate the CNBr.
6. Sequentially wash the beads with water, several milliliters of 95% acetone, and several changes of 100 mM sodium phosphate (pH 7.5) (or an alternative binding buffer).

The beads are ready for coupling to antibody.

Coupling of antibody to activated beads
(Harlow and Lane 1988)

1. The antibody preparations must not contain extraneous compounds with amino groups, and, if these compounds have been used during the purification, the antibody preparation should be extensively dialyzed against the binding buffer of 0.5 M sodium phosphate (pH 7.5).
2. Prepare a solution of antibody at the desired concentration in 0.5 M sodium phosphate (pH 7.5). 5–10 mg of antibody per milliliter of beads should yield a high capacity column.
3. Add the activated beads and mix gently overnight at room temperature on a rocker.
4. Wash the beads twice with 0.5 M sodium phosphate (pH 7.5) and once with 1 M NaCl/0.05 M sodium phosphate (pH 7.5).
5. Add 10 volumes of 100 mM ethanolamine (pH 7.5). Incubate at room temperature for 4 h to overnight, with gentle mixing.
6. Wash twice with PBS. Add merthiolate

to 0.01%. The beads can be stored at 4°C where they should be stable for several months.

The beads are now ready for binding of the antigen.

Note

A check for binding can be made by testing the protein concentration in a sample taken from step 2 and comparing it to the wash in step 4. Should antibody activity be drastically reduced through coupling, a different approach should be tried (see Harlow and Lane 1988).

Binding of antigens to antibody
(Harlow and Lane 1988)

Antigen can be bound to antibody-coated beads either by mixing in a slurry or by passing the antigen down a column of antibody bound beads.

Binding in suspension

1. Mix the antigen solution with the antibody beads.
2. Rock for 1 h to overnight at 4°C, ensuring that beads are maintained in suspension.
3. Stop agitation, transfer the beads to a suitable column and wash with 20 bed volumes of binding buffer.

The antigen is now ready for elution.

Binding in a column

Antigen samples added to columns should be free of particulate matter and need centrifugation at 100,000 g for 30 min prior to use.

1. Transfer antibody beads to a suitable column and wash with 20 bed volumes of PBS.
2. Apply the antigen solution to the column and allow to pass through by

gravity (three times) or with a fixed flow rate of approximately 2 ml h^{-1}.

3. Wash the column with 20 bed volumes of binding buffer.

Elution of antigens from immunoaffinity columns
(Harlow and Lane 1988)

Elution of antigen from columns requires a series of optimal conditions to be determined in order that the process is quick and efficient. Conditions vary from harsh to mild, depending on the antibody used; strategies for testing elution conditions are described in Harlow and Lane (1988). In essence, the procedure is as outlined below.

1. Use a pre-elution buffer and pass 10 bed volumes through the column.
2. Using a stepwise elution, sequentially pass samples of elution buffer (0.5 bed volumes/step) through the column. Collect each fraction in separate tubes. If either high or low pH is used to elute the column, the collection tubes should contain a neutralizing buffer. When using a gradient elution, pass the gradient of increasingly harsher elution buffer through the column.
3. Check each tube for the presence of the antigen. Combine tubes with high concentrations.
4. Return the column to the starting buffer by passing 20 column volumes through the matrix. Add 0.01% merthiolate for long-term storage (4°C).

Note

After the elution of the antigen, the eluant will often need to be changed by dialysis or by chromatography on a desalting column.

The above procedures have been used successfully in many laboratories to produce batches of purified viral antigens. It should be noted, however, that they are generalized procedures and may need specific refinements for the antibody and antigen of choice. Commercially available purification 'kits' come with excellent step-by-step protocols. The reader is also referred to Deutscher (1990) for a guide to purifying antigens.

Preparation of antigens for immunization

Formol saline inactivation

Many antigen preparations, particularly those containing virions, need inactivating before immunization protocols can commence; for most preparations this can be achieved by incubation with 0.015% formaldehyde.

Production of solid matrix antigen/antibody complexes

Binding antigens to antibodies is thought to induce a much better immune response than antigen alone (Harlow and Lane 1988). The immunogenicity can be enhanced further by binding the complex to a solid matrix such as *Staphylococcus aureus* (Randall and Souberbielk 1990). The procedure below describes the preparation of *S. aureus* (Staph A Protein), and attachment to a monoclonal antibody and an antigen resulting in a solid matrix antigen antibody (SMAA)

Preparation of formalin fixed *S. aureus*

1. Grow *S. aureus* Cowan I strain in tryptone soya broth for approximately 8 h. Centrifuge 9000 rpm for 10 min.
2. Resuspend in PBS (pH 6.95) containing 0.1% (w/v) sodium azide (PBS/azide) to give a 10% (w/v) cell suspension.
3. Wash cells twice in PBS/azide and resuspend in 10% (w/v) PBS/azide containing 1.5% (v/v) formalin. Leave stirring overnight at room temperature.
4. Wash cells in PBS/azide to remove formalin and transfer to a large flask such that the depth of liquid is ⩽ 1–2 cm.
5. Heat at 80°C for 5 min and cool rapidly in ice bath.
6. Wash cells twice in PBS/azide, resuspend in 10% w/v PBS/azide and store in aliquots at −70°C.

Preparation of a SMAA complex

The procedure is essentially that of Randall & Young (1988) and Randall et al (1988).

1. A 10% (w/v) suspension of formalin fixed *S. aureus* is saturated with antibody by mixing with an excess of monoclonal antibody (concentrated tissue culture supernatant or ascitic fluid) at 4°C for 4 h.
2. Centrifuge at 13,000 rpm for 1–1.5 min in an Eppendorf microcentrifuge and wash twice in PBS. Resuspend in PBS to give a 10% (w/v) suspension of *S. aureus*.
3. The antibody-bound *S. aureus* is shaken overnight at 4°C with an excess of solubilized virus antigen prepared by any of the procedures outlined above.
4. The SMAA complex produced is washed three times in ice cold RIPA buffer (20 mM Tris-HCl pH 7.2, 5 mM EDTA, 0.5% (v/v) NP40, 0.1% (w/v) SDS, 0.65 M NaCl and 1 mM PMSF) followed by three washes with PBS. The complex is resuspended at 10% (w/v) or 0.5 (w/v) in PBS. The 0.5% suspension is used for immunization purposes.

Expression of antigens *in vitro*

The advent of advanced techniques in molecular biology and biotechnology has lent itself to the production of more refined systems for both the *in vitro* expression and purification of viral antigens. These may comprise several amino acids or a larger sequence complete with the post-translational modifications of the authentic protein. The nature of the desired end-product determines the system of choice (i.e. prokaryotic or eukaryotic). Whilst prokaryotic systems are convenient, with the availability of inexpensive scale-up reagents, there are distinct disadvantages in their use for protein expression. This is due to differences in processing pathways which lead to the absence of both amino terminal modifications and di-sulphide bond formation, a lack of glycosylation, and an inability to facilitate the proteolytic cleavage of signal sequence from mature polypeptide chains. In addition, because vertebrate viruses replicate in cells of eukaryotic origin, in some instances it is more feasible to produce the relevant antigen in one of the many eukaryotic systems available where any post-translational modifications can be ensured.

Ultimately, the choice of the expression system will be dependent on the role the antigen is to play. Thus it may be required for either diagnostic or therapeutic purposes. Diagnostic tests often involve the detection of anti-viral antibodies in body fluids such as serum, saliva, cerebrospinal fluid or synovial fluid which indicate prior exposure to an agent. The diagnostic tests which are used extensively include the ELISA, Western blotting, radioimmunoprecipitation, indirect immunofluorescence, single radial haemolysis-in-gel, and radio-immunoassay. For each of these systems, a different form of the antigen may be required. For therapeutic purposes, the antigen may be required as a subunit vaccine and extensive purification steps may have to be carried out before the antigen can be of use.

The initial steps in obtaining antigen expression, including the isolation of the gene or a small nucleotide sequence and its cloning into a suitable expression plasmid, are common to most systems. These and further steps are summarized below.

(i) The selection of a suitable expression plasmid;
(ii) The isolation of the whole of the gene of interest or a truncated form of it;
(iii) The cloning of the gene into the expression plasmid;
(iv) the expression and detection of the protein product.

Eukaryotic gene expression

Many references are available which describe the successful production of viral antigens in eukaryotic systems. Several types of virus have been engineered as vectors for this purpose, including adenoviruses, herpesviruses, poxviruses, baculoviruses and adeno-associated viruses. The baculovirus and poxvirus systems are here described in detail.

Baculovirus expression systems

The prototype baculovirus *Autographa california* nuclear polyhedrosis virus (AcMNPV) is commonly used for the production of recombinant baculoviruses which are engineered for high-level protein expression. The production of the recombinant first involves the cloning of the gene into one of the many baculovirus expression vectors available. The most commonly used vectors employ one of two very late baculovirus gene promoters, although studies have been carried out to stably transfect insect cells with plasmids containing genes under the control of one of the immediate early promoters (Jarvis 1991). The former include the polyhedrin or the p10 promoters. The polyhedrin gene encodes the polyhedrin protein which surrounds newly synthesized virus particles in the nucleus of the cell. The p10 promoter is thought to be involved in the assembly of occlusion bodies. Such promoters are flanked by sequences which allow recombination into the baculovirus genome to occur, and unique restriction endonuclease sites are incorporated downstream of them for the insertion of coding sequences. Further modifications to baculovirus vectors include the insertion of the beta-galactosidase gene which is of use for the screening of recombinant viruses by blue colour selection (Vialard et al 1990) or the addition of a histidine tag (i.e. pBlue Bac His ABC) which can be used for the purification of the expressed protein on nickel columns. Vectors are also commercially available which allow for the insertion of multiple coding sequences (i.e. p2Bac).

Careful consideration must be given when selecting the vector and designing the insert. The vector may be such that the insert is fused to the polyhedrin gene, in which case the translation initiation codon of the novel gene is not required but subsequent amino acids are inserted in-frame (i.e. pAC360). In non-fusion vectors (i.e. pVL1392 and pVL1393) there is a mutation (ATG to ATT) in the initiation codon of the polyhedrin gene, resulting in a requirement for an ATG codon in the inserted gene. The baculovirus transfer vector pVT-bac (Tessier et al 1991) contains the honeybee mellitin signal sequence under the control of the polyhedrin promoter; this construct has been used successfully by Sisk et al (1994) to substitute for the signal sequence of HSV-1 gD, enabling up to 25 mg of protein to be purified from one litre of culture medium.

Procedure

The propagation of baculoviruses and tissue culture maintenance is carried out at 27°C. Baculoviruses are routinely stored at 4°C.

Types of insect cell in which baculoviruses can be propagated

A number of cell lines of insect origin have been used in the propagation of baculoviruses and are commercially available. These include Sf 9 cells, Sf 21 cells, High 5 cells and MG1 cells. Sf 9 cells are derived from *Spodoptera frugiperda* ovarian cells. Sf 21 cells are of a similar origin but are larger in size and allow for elevated levels of protein production. High 5 cells are adherent cells and are derived from *Trichoplusia ni* egg cell homogenates. These cells also give 25 fold higher levels of protein expression than Sf9 cells. Cells are routinely cultured at 27°C in commercially available 'Grace's' insect medium which is supplemented with foetal calf serum. Serum-free preparations of insect medium are available for the production of recombinant proteins free from serum contaminants.

Plasmid preparation

1. 1 µg of 100 µg ml^{-1} of the baculovirus expression plasmid is added to 100 µl of competent cells which are left on ice for 30 min.
2. Cells are heat shocked at 42°C for 45 s.
3. 400 µl SOC medium is added.
4. Cells are shaken at 37°C for 1 h.
5. Cells are plated out on LB agar plates containing antibiotics (ampicillin at 100 µg ml^{-1}).
6. Plates are inverted and incubated at 37°C overnight.
7. 250 ml LB broth containing ampicillin at 100 µg ml^{-1} is inoculated with a

single colony from the plate and shaken overnight.

8. Plasmid DNA is purified from the bacteria using caesium chloride gradient centrifugation or one of the commercially available DNA purification kits.

9. The plasmid is digested with a suitable restriction enzyme, treated with calf intestinal, alkaline phosphatase and purified following agarose gel electrophoresis.

10. The gene of interest is either excised from an existing plasmid or amplified from viral nucleic acid by the polymerase chain reaction (PCR). Suitable restriction endonuclease sites are incorporated into synthetic oligonucleotide primers for cloning purposes.

11. The PCR product is phenol/chloroform extracted.

12. 100 µl chloroform is added, the sample vortexed and centrifuged at 14,000 rpm.

13. The upper phase is removed and 100 µl Tris-saturated phenol plus 100 µl chloroform is added. The upper phase is again removed and the DNA is precipitated with 1/10 volume 3 M sodium acetate pH 7.0 and 2.5 volumes ethanol at $-70°C$ for 1 h.

14. The sample is centrifuged at 14,000 rpm, dried and digested with a compatible restriction enzyme.

15. The DNA is purified by PAGE and electroelution.

16. The DNA is quantitated and ligated into the baculovirus vector.

17. Competent cells are transformed as described above and the baculovirus expression plasmid and insert purified. This material is then co-transfected with linear AcMNPV DNA into Sf 9 insect cells.

Production of the recombinant virus

1. Sf 9 cells are seeded into 60 mm tissue culture dishes at a density of 2×10^6 and allowed to adhere for 30 min.

2. 1 µg AcMNPV DNA is mixed with 2 µg circularized plasmid DNA containing the gene of interest in 1 ml of Grace's medium containing no supplements.

3. 20 µl cationic liposome solution is added and the solution vortexed.

4. The solution is incubated at room temperature for 15 min.

5. The medium is aspirated from the Sf 9 cells and replaced with 2 ml Grace's medium without supplements and cells are allowed to remain in this medium for 10 min.

6. The medium is removed from the plates; the transfection mix is then added dropwise and the plates are placed on a rocking platform for 4 h. An additional 1 ml of complete medium is then added to the plates and the plates incubated at 27°C for 48 h. The medium is harvested at 48 h and stored until required.

7. The cells are refed and observed for signs of infection for a further two days.

8. The supernatant containing the recombinant virus harvested on day 2 is titrated under an agar overlay and a plaque assay performed. If the beta-galactosidase gene has been incorporated, any recombinant virus can be selected by blue/white screening if X-gal is incorporated into the overlay. Several rounds of plaque purification are required and recombinant viruses are selected on the basis of their occlusion body-negative phenotype.

The analysis of protein expression

Protein expression can be analysed in a number of ways. These include PAGE followed by Coomassie blue staining, indirect immunofluorescence, Western blotting and radio-immunoprecipitation. It is imperative that adequate controls are included at all times when performing these assays. For instance, if the levels of recombinant protein expression are monitored at various time points after infection of cells, lysates from cells infected with a wild-type baculovirus or cells alone must be included in any analysis being performed.

Poxvirus expression systems

The expression of antigens in poxvirus was originally described by Mackett et al (1982). Concern over the use of vaccinia virus in humans which has surfaced in recent years has resulted in efforts to overcome this, such as the production of the non-replicating canary-pox virus to express both the fusion and HA proteins of measles virus (Taylor et al 1992) and an attenuated form of vaccinia virus, NYVAC (Tartaglia et al 1992; Cox et al 1993). Further, raccoon poxvirus has been used to express the rabies virus glycoprotein which has been used to vaccinate sheep (DeMartini et al 1993). Cytotoxic T-cells have been induced by inoculation with such viruses expressing the HIV-1 envelope glycoprotein (Cox et al 1993). Pox viruses have the advantage of having a large genome which can accommodate additional genes, high levels of expression, and a cytoplasmic site of transcription. For their construction, the gene of interest is cloned into a non-essential gene locus such as thymidine kinase. Recombinants are selected on the basis of their growth in TK-cells in the presence of the toxic analogue BUdR. Vaccinia virus recombinants have been used extensively for the study of both cellular and humoral immune responses to virus infection. For a review on the use of vaccinia virus on T-cell studies see Bennink and Yewdell (1990). The vaccinia T7 system has been used extensively to transcribe and translate proteins that are encoded under the control of the T7 RNA polymerase promoter. Cells are infected with the vaccinia virus recombinant expressing the T7 enzyme which are then transfected with the plasmid containing the gene under the control of T7. Expression of the protein can be detected using conventional techniques.

Procedure
(Smith 1993)

1. The gene of interest is cloned into a poxvirus expression plasmid under the control of a vaccinia virus promoter (i.e. p11 or p7.5).
2. CV-1 cells are infected with wild-type vaccinia virus at moi of 0.5 and the flask is incubated at 37°C for 2 h.
3. Plasmid DNA is precipitated by the dropwise addition of 6.5 µl 2 M $CaCl_2$ to a 1 ml solution of 1 µg plasmid DNA which has been added to 19 µl carrier DNA while vortexing.
4. The virus is removed and the precipitated DNA is added thus allowing homologous recombination to occur.
5. The flask is incubated at 37°C for 30 min, medium added and further incubated for 3–4 h.
6. The cells are refed and after a further 48 h the cells are harvested.
7. The virus is plaque purified.
8. Cells are freeze–thawed three times and titrated on TK-143 cells by the addition of 0.5 ml inoculum followed by rocking for 2 h.
9. Cells are overlayed with 4 ml medium containing 2.5% FCS, 1% low temperature gelling agarose, and 25 µg BUdR. Plaques are harvested after 48 h and further rounds of plaque purification are carried out. Purified virus is analyzed for the production of the relevant protein.

The transient expression of viral antigens

The transient expression of viral antigens in mammalian expression systems has a number of uses. The location of the protein can be determined, i.e. whether it remains in the Golgi or endoplasmic reticulum or whether it is transported to the surface of the cell. Protein interactions can be studied by co-transfection techniques, and whether the transport of a protein to a different compartment of a cell is dependent on a second transfected protein can be assessed. Eukaryotic expression vectors are available which can be used for these purposes. The gene of interest is usually inserted under the control of a strong eukaryotic promoter such as the major immediate early gene promoter of human cytomegalovirus or the RSV LTR promoter. The SV40 origin of replication is often included to ensure the replication of the plasmid in COS-7 cells. The co-transfection of such a plasmid with a plasmid containing a selectable marker will allow for the production of stably expressing cell lines.

Procedure

DEAE dextran transfection

1. The gene of interest is cloned into the vector of choice (as described previously).
2. 60 mm tissue culture dishes are seeded with COS-7 cells at a concentration of 5×10^5.
3. The next day, the monolayer is washed three times in PBS.
4. 1 μg DNA + 500 μl PBS + 5 μl DEAE dextran are mixed together and added to the cells.
5. The plates are incubated at 37°C for 30 min and rocked gently.
6. 5 ml growth medium containing chloroquin is added and the plate is incubated at 37°C for a further 3–5 hours.
7. The plate is washed and refed with growth medium and incubated for a further 48–72 hours.

Detection of proteins

Antibodies raised against the expressed proteins can be used for detection purposes.

Surface expression

1. Cells are fixed for 5 min with a solution of 2% isotonic paraformaldehyde.
2. The slides are washed three times in PBS.
3. The primary antibody is added and the slides incubated at 37°C for 1 h.
4. The slides are washed three times in PBS and the secondary antibody added and the slide is incubated as before.
5. Slides are washed and mounted in 90% glycerol/10% PBS.
6. Slides are examined using a microscope equipped with a mercury vapour lamp. FITC is excited by blue light at 490 nm and emits a green light at 520 nm. TRITC is excited by green light at 540 nm and emits a red light at 625 nm. The size of the protein can be determined by RIPA or Western blotting.

For the detection of the protein internally, cells are fixed with a 50:50 solution of methanol and acetone for 5 min and stained as described above.

In vitro transcription/ translation systems

It is possible to use a cell-free transcription/ translation system to determine the size of processed and unprocessed forms of viral antigens. The gene encoding the protein of interest is cloned into a plasmid such as pBluescript II KS+ which contains the T3 and

T7 RNA polymerase promoter or psp72 which contains SP6 and T7 promoters. The circular plasmid is transcribed and translated in a rabbit reticulocyte lysate in the presence of the relevant polymerase enzyme. The addition of canine pancreatic microsomal membranes enables the processing of the protein to occur.

Prokaryotic gene expression

The use of bacteria for the expression of either full length or truncated forms of proteins has been described extensively. The carboxyl terminal sequence of the inserted sequence may be modified to contain additional amino acids that can be used for purification purposes such as a histidine tag (His_6) which can be used to bind the protein to a nickel column. One particular system that has been used widely for this purpose is the pGEX system (Smith and Johnson 1988). Here, the sequence of interest is inserted into a plasmid fused with the C-terminus of Sj26, a 26 kDa Glutathione S-transferase (GST) encoded by the parasitic helminth *Schistosoma japonicum*. The protein can then be purified by its affinity with a glutathione-Sepharose column and eluted using reduced glutathione. The pGEX vectors are designed so that GST can be cleaved by site specific proteases such as thrombin or blood coagulation factor Xa, after which excess GST or uncleaved protein can be absorbed on glutathione agarose.

Virus polypeptides may also be expressed as β-galactosidase fusions, and others may be fused with staphylococcal protein A to allow for their purification on IgG-Sepharose. The insolubility of some of these proteins may be overcome by the use of sarkosyl buffer (Grieco et al 1992). pGEX vectors are available for the insertion of the gene or part of the gene in one of three open reading frames.

Other recently described fusion systems include the CHO recognition domain (CRD) of the galactose-specific rat hepatic lectin, which is used to create fusions with eukaryotic pro-

teins using galactose-Sepharose for purification (Taylor and Drickamer 1991). Similarly, the pBR322 derivative pVB2 has the mg1B gene which encodes the galactose binding protein of *E. coli*. An EcoRI restriction endonuclease site allows for in-frame fusions. GBP is taken to the periplasmic space of a bacterial cell and the recombinant protein can be isolated from the periplasm by osmotic shock (Müller et al 1989).

Procedure

1. The gene is cloned into the pGEX plasmid of choice using the techniques outlined above.
2. The plasmid is used to transform JM105 cells.
3. An overnight culture of bacteria is diluted 1/50 with LB broth containing 100 µg ml^{-1} ampicillin.
4. The cells are grown to mid log phase (A600 = 0.6–1.0) and the expression of the fusion protein is induced by the addition of isopropyl-β-D-thiogalactoside (IPTG) to a final concentration of 0.1–10 mM.
5. The cells are grown for 3–5 h at 37°C.
6. 1 ml of culture is centrifuged at 14,000 rpm for 2 min and 100 µl PBS added. 10 µl of this is analyzed by PAGE followed by Coomassie blue staining.
7. Insolubility of the protein may be overcome by the addition of Triton X-100 to a final concentration of 1%, shaking for 30 min and analysis of the protein from the supernatant.

The purified proteins may then be inoculated into animals to raise monospecific antisera. Further techniques include fusion to the heat shock protein.

Purification of proteins to which His6 tag has been attached by affinity chromatography
(Soumounou and Laliberte 1994).

1. Bacteria are resuspended in buffer (500 mM NaCl, 160 mM Tris-HCl, pH 8.0) and lysozyme is added to a final concentration of 2 mg ml^{-1} and incubated at room temperature for 20 min.
2. Cells are freeze–thawed several times and sonicated.
3. The lysate is centrifuged at 15,000 g and the pellet resuspended in 20 ml of the buffer described in 1, containing 6 M guanidine-HCl, 5 mM 2-mercaptoethanol and 0.1% Tween 20 and incubated at room temperature for 30 min with vortexing.
4. Solubilized proteins are recovered by ultracentrifugation (15,000 g for 40 min at 4°C) and incubated with 2.5 ml Ni-NTA Agarose (Qiagen).
5. The resin is washed with buffer described in step 1, containing guanidine, and bound proteins are eluted with this buffer containing 250 nM imidazole.
6. The purified proteins are dialyzed for 24 h at 4°C against 20 mM NaCl, 10 mM Tris HCl, pH 8.0.

References

Alberts B, Bray D, Lewis J, Raff M, Roberts K, Watson JD (1989) Molecular Biology of the Cell, 2nd edn. Garland Publ Co, New York.

Alberts BM, Amodio FJ, Jenkins M, Gutmann ED, Lewis FL (1968) Cold Spring Harbour Symp Quant Biol 33: 289–305.

Ardoin P, Clark DH, Hannoun C (1969) Am J Trop Med Hyg 18: 592–598.

Axen R, Porath J, Ernback S (1967) Nature 214: 1302–1304.

Bennink JR, Yewdell JW (1990) Curr Top Microbiol Immunol 163: 154–184.

Bernardi G (1971) Meth Enzymol 21: 95–139.

Chappell WA, White LA, Gamble WC (1984) Production Manual for Viral, Rickettsial, Chlamydial, Mycoplasmal Reagents, 6th Edn, Centers for Disease Control, Atlanta, GA.

Chicz R, Regnier F (1990) Meth Enzymol 182: 392–421.

Cox WI, Tartaglia J, Paoletti E (1993) Virology 195: 845–850.

Cremer NE, Schmidt NJ, Jensen F, Hoffman M, Oshiro LS, Lennette EH (1975) J Clin Microbiol 1: 262–267.

DeMartini JC, Bickle HM, Brodie SJ, He BX, Esposito JJ (1993) Arch Virol 133: 211–222.

Deutscher M (Ed) (1990) Guide to Protein Purification, Methods in Enzymology 182, Academic Press.

Dowdle WR, Lambriex M, Hierholzer JC (1971) Appl Microbiol 21: 718–722.

Fields BN, Knipe DM, Chanock RM, Hirsch MS, Melnick JL, Monath TP, Roizman B (Eds.) (1990) Virology, Vols. 1 and 2, 2nd Edn. Raven Press, New York.

Gersten DM, Marchalonis JJ (1978) J Immun Meth 24: 305–309.

Grieco F, Hay JM, Hull R (1992) Bio Techniques 13: 856–857.

Harlow E, Lane D (1988) Antibodies – a laboratory manual, Cold Spring Harbor Laboratory.

Hierholzer JC (1976) Virology 75: 155–165.

Hierholzer JC (1993) Immunol Allergy Clin North Amer 13: 27–42.

Hierholzer JC, Anderson LJ, Halonen PE (1990) Med Virol 9: 17–45.

Hierholzer JC, Dowdle WR (1970) J Virol 6: 782–787.

Hierholzer JC, Palmer EL, Whitfield SG, Kaye HS, Dowdle WR (1972) Virology 48: 516–527.

Jarvis DL (1991) Ann N Y Acad Sci 646: 240–247.

Kohn J, Wilchek (1984) Appl Biochem Biotechnol 9: 285–304.

Lennette EH, Halonen P, Murphy FA (Eds.) (1988) Laboratory Diagnosis of Infectious Diseases: Principles and Practice, Vol. II, Viral, Rickettsial, and Chlamydial Diseases, Springer Verlag, New York.

Mackett N, Smith GL, Moss B (1982) Proc Nat Acad Sci USA 79: 7415–7419.

March SC, Parlch I, Cuatrecasas (1974) Anal Biochem 60: 149–152.

Muller N, Vogel M, Gottstein B, Scholle A, Seebeck T (1989) Gene 75: 329–334.

Norrby E (1962) Proc Soc Exp Biol Med 111: 814–818.

Powell KL, Purifoy DJM (1977) J Virol 24: 618–626.

Purifoy DJM, Powell KL (1976) J Virol 19: 717–731.

Randall RE, Killington RA, Watson DH (1980) J Gen Virol 48: 297–310.

Randall RE, Souberbielle BE (1990) In: Controls of Virus Diseases. Dimmock NJ, Griffiths PD, Madeley CR (Eds.) Cambridge University Press, Cambridge, pp. 21–51.

Randall RE, Young DF (1988a) J Gen Virol 69: 2505–2516.

Randall RE, Young DF, Southern JA (1988b) J Gen Virol 69: 2517–2526.

Schmidt NJ, Emmons RW (Eds.) (1989) Diagnostic Procedures for Viral, Rickettsial and Chlamydial Infections, 6th edn. American Public Health Assn, Washington, D.C.

Schneider C, Neman RA, Sutherland DA, Asser U, Graves MF (1982) J Biol Chem 257: 10760–10769.

Sever JL, Castellano GA, Pelon W, Huebner RJ, Wolman F (1964) J Lab Clin Med 64: 983–988.

Simanis V, Lane DP (1985) Virology 144: 88–100.

Simon M (1962) Acta Virol 6: 302–308.

Sisk WP, Bradley JD, Leipold RJ, Stoltzfus AM, Ponce de Leon M, Hilf M, Peng C, Cohen GH, Eisenberg RJ (1994) Virology 68: 766–775.

Smith CEG, Holt D (1961) Bull Wld Hlth Org 24: 749–759.

Smith DB, Johnson KS (1988) Gene 67: 31–40.

Smith GL (1993) In: Molecular Virology. A Practical Approach, Davison AJ, Elliot RM (Eds.) IRL Press, Oxford, pp. 257–283.

Soumounou Y, Laliberte J-F (1994) J Gen Virol 75: 2567–2573.

Tartaglia J, Cox WI, Taylor J, Perkus M, Riviere M, Meignier B, Paoletti E (1992) Aids Res Hum Retro 8: 1445–1447.

Taverne J, Marshall JH, Fulton F (1958) J Gen Microbiol 19: 451–461.

Taylor J, Weinberg R, Tartaglia J, Richardson C, Alkhatib G, Briedis D, Appel M, Norton E, Paoletti E (1992) Virology 187: 321–328.

Taylor ME, Drickamer K (1991) Biochem J 274: 575–580.

Tessier DC, Thomas DY, Khouri HE, Laliberte F, Vernet T (1991) Gene 98: 177–183.

Vialard G, Lalumiere M, Vernet T, Briedis D, Alkhatib G, Henning D, Levin D, Richardson C (1990) J Virol 64: 37–50.

Wilchek M, Miron T, Kohn J (1984) Affinity Chromatography, in Methods in Enzymology 104: 3–55.

Virus purification

R. A. Killington
A. Stokes
J. C. Hierholzer

Virus purification is the physical separation of virus in a concentrated form from the host cell milieu in which it has grown. Viruses need to be purified for many studies in which properties or structure of the virus must be distinguished from those of the host cells or culture medium, such as analyses of structure of viral polypeptides, function of membrane glycoproteins, etc.

In this review, we will describe proven methods of purifying enveloped versus nonenveloped viruses, and labile versus stable viruses, as these properties constitute important differences in the methods. We will also discuss those criteria used by various laboratories for determining the degree of purity achieved in virus preparations.

Virology Methods Manual
ISBN 0–12–465330–8

Principles of ultracentrifugation

Ultracentrifugation is the usual technique of choice for the purification of particles of defined size (i.e. virions) from their contaminating materials. In any suspension of particles their rate of sedimentation depends not only on the size, density and morphology of the particles but also on the nature of the medium in which they are suspended and the force applied to the particles during centrifugation.

One important contributory factor to consider in the separation and ultimate purification of virions from contaminating materials is therefore the viscosity of the medium in which they are centrifuged and this chapter addresses such an issue later.

Types of centrifugal separations

It is of course theoretically possible to separate particles solely on the basis of *differential pelleting*, where asymmetrical particles will sediment slower than spherical particles of the same mass and density. By increasing the time of centrifugation or the centrifugation speed smaller particles will also pellet. Differential centrifugation also separates particles on the basis of their density. Whilst the procedure can be successful in achieving good separation of a variety of particles as long as there are large differences in their mass and/or densities, the yield of such a procedure is likely to be low and the purity of the particles questionable. The technique is however often used as a starting point designed so as to enrich populations of particles before further purification. Virus purification is more likely to be achieved by the technique of density gradient centrifugation, where separation of the components is achieved by sedimentation through a density gradient, (i.e. a solution which increases in density with increasing distance down the centrifuge tube).

Two types of approach are routinely used – rate-zonal centrifugation and isopycnic centrifugation.

In rate-zonal centrifugation the problem of co-sedimentation of particles is overcome by layering the sample in the form of a narrow layer on top of a density gradient. During centrifugation the sample particles separate as a series of bands or zones, each with its own characteristic sedimentation rate. Centrifugation is stopped before the particles pellet and the separated components are collected by fractionation of the gradient. The rate at which the particles sediment depends on their size, shape, density, the centrifugal force, and the density and viscosity profile of the gradient.

Isopycnic centrifugation separates particles solely on the basis of their different densities. The sample is loaded directly on to a preformed density gradient and then centrifuged or is mixed with the gradient medium to give a solution of uniform density and the density gradient forms during centrifugation (e.g. Dea and Tijssen 1988).

In rate-zonal centrifugation the density of the gradient must not exceed that of the particles being separated whereas in isopycnic centrifugation the maximum density must always exceed the density of the particles.

The above procedures are carried out in *preparative* ultracentrifuges which are usually grouped on the basis of their speed. Routinely one would wish for a machine capable of 40–80 $\times$ 10^3 rpm and 600 $\times$ 10^3 g.

Centrifuge rotors come in various sizes but would routinely be swing-out rotors for rate-zonal centrifugation and fixed angle or vertical rotors for isopycnic centrifugation.

PEG precipitation

Concentration of viral suspensions by precipitation techniques is a useful starting point for virus purification.

Advantages over other concentration methods

Precipitation of macromolecular proteins such as viruses by high molecular weight polyethylene glycol–6000 (PEG), pioneered by Yamamoto et al (1970) for bacteriophages, is an effective concentration method because the viruses are slowly precipitated in a cold, high-salt environment which protects them from chemical and physical denaturation.

PEG precipitation is more gentle than physical concentration by ultracentrifugation or molecular sieve filtration. These are also done in the cold, but ulltracentrifugation often packs the virions so tightly, even atop sucrose cushions, that they cannot be resuspended without significant loss of virus, and ultrafiltration requires magnetic mixing to keep the filter cleared and loses a great deal of virus trapped in the filter itself. PEG is also more effective, in our hands, than ammonium sulfate precipitation, although the latter has been used with good results for astroviruses, caliciviruses, coronaviruses, picornaviruses and many others (Ashley and Caul 1982; Tannock 1973; Wadey and Westaway 1981; Minor 1985). The PEG precipitation procedure outlined below has been performed with good results for coronaviruses (Hierholzer 1976; Lanser and Howard 1980), rhabdoviruses (Obijeski et al 1974), parainfluenzaviruses (Hierholzer et al 1993), respiratory syncytial virus (Anderson et al 1984; Cash et al 1977; Hierholzer et al 1994), rubella virus (Fuccillo and Sever 1989), and picornaviruses (Hasegawa and Inouye 1983; Hierholzer et al 1984).

Protocol and follow-up

1. It is best to start with a large-volume virus culture in which calf serum and other protein additives have been withheld from the maintenance medium.
2. At complete CPE, the cells and medium are harvested by scraping with a rubber policeman. (Multiple cycles of freeze–thawing can effectively break up the cells if the virus is stable to such treatment.) The pooled harvest is clarified by large-volume, low-speed centrifugation, such as in a Beckman JA-14 rotor in a J2-21 centrifuge at 10,000 rpm (15,300 g) or a J-21 rotor in an L8-70 centrifuge at 12,000 rpm (15,000 g), for 20 min at 3°C.
3. Transfer the supernatant to a large beaker in an ice bath on a magnetic stirrer.
4. *Slowly* add NaCl to a final concentration of 2.3%, with constant but gentle stirring.
5. *Slowly* add PEG-6000 to a final concentration of 7.0%, also with constant and gentle stirring. Cover the beaker and stir for about 1 h more to ensure complete solubilization of the PEG. (Others have used higher salt [to 2.7%] and lower and higher PEG (6.0–10.0%) with good results (Fuccillo and Sever 1989; Hasegawa and Inouye 1983; Hierholzer et al 1984; Lanser and Howard 1980; Yamamoto et al 1970).)
6. Transfer the beaker and ice bath to a refrigerator, and allow the virus (and other proteins) to precipitate overnight at 4°C.
7. Collect the precipitate by the same

centrifugation method used for clarification (step 2). Aspirate or drain the centrifuge bottles thoroughly to remove as much PEG as possible.

8. Resuspend the precipitate in a small volume of TES buffer (0.01 M Tris-HCl, pH 7.2, 0.002 M EDTA, 0.15 M NaCl). The buffer should be added at about 2 ml per centrifuge bottle and aspirated thoroughly with a syringe and 22-gauge needle. The suspension is then transferred to a clean tube, and each bottle is rinsed with an additional 1 ml of buffer which is added to the pooled suspension.

9. Finally, the PEG is removed (pelleted) by centrifugation of this pooled suspension at 13,000 g for 4 min at 23°C in a Beckman Microfuge or similar device. The supernatant now contains approximately 100–fold concentrated virus in isotonic TES buffer; the virus preparation may be considered enriched, but not purified.

Sucrose gradients

Sucrose is suitable for most rate-zonal centrifugation procedures and is often the ideal method for the formation of sharp, easily isolated bands of pure virus. Sucrose is however very viscous at densities greater than 30% w/v and some laboratories use Ficoll or Dextran (Pharmacia Fine Chemicals) as an alternative. The procedures for gradient formation are, however, the same. The gradient solution is usually made up in an aqueous buffer at neutral pH; borate buffer should never be used. The gradients are usually of the continuous type, i.e. the density of the sucrose solution increases smoothly with increasing distance from the axis of rotation. In designing gradients it is essential that the top of the gradient is of sufficient density to support the virus sample whereas the density at the bottom must exceed that of the virus particles. Step gradients (e.g. 5–30%, 10–40% or 15–45%) should be used whenever possible as they result in better separation of virus particles from contaminating materials. Gradients should also never be overloaded with sample, and whilst this procedure is of course a 'learning curve' for different viruses Hull (1985) suggests that SW27 (large swing out rotors) should never be loaded with more than 5 mg virus whereas the smaller tube (SW50) should contain 1 mg of virus or less.

Gradients are either produced by the diffusion method, where a series of differing sucrose concentrations are layered one on top of the other and allowed to diffuse, or by the use of gradient makers, which range from home-made devices put together by the local glass-blower to sophisticated commercially acquired apparatus.

The diffusion method relies on the aliquoting, by underlaying or overlaying, of identical volumes of a series of sucrose solutions to produce a step gradient. Once prepared the tube is stood either vertically or horizontally and the sucrose allowed to diffuse to form the gradient. If left vertically the tubes should be allowed to stand overnight at 4°C.

Typical volume examples for preparation of a variety of different sized gradients are shown below (reproduced from Hull, 1985).

Gradients made by means of a gradient maker can be used immediately. The gradient maker consists of two vessels of equal cross-sectional area joined by a connecting channel which is opened or closed by means of a stopcock. The outlet or mixing chamber has a fine tube exit which, via a piece of flexible tubing, leads to the centrifuge tube. Vessels are constructed for various volume gradients. Whilst sucrose will flow by gravity many workers prefer to use a peristaltic pump between the glass exit tube and the centrifuge tube (see Fig. 4.1)

The methods for gradient preparation are well documented by Hames (1984) but a brief description of the 'dense end first' method is given here.

1. Always use clean dry vessels and tubing.

Table 4.1

| Tube size (inches) | Rotor | ml of sucrose | | | |
		40%*	30%	20%	10%
3 × 1	SW25	7	7	7	4
3.5 × 1	SW27	8	8	8	6
3.5 × 9/16	SW41	3	3	3	2
2 × 0.5	SW50.1	1	1	1	1

* percentages as given by w/v.

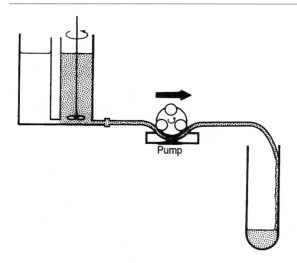

Figure 4.1. Preparation of sucrose gradients (from Hames 1984).

2. Connect the vessel outlet tubing to the top of the centrifuge tube. The tubing may be held in place but as long as care is taken can often be left 'lodged' against the inner side of the top of the centrifuge tube.

3. Ensure stop-cock between chambers is closed and introduce required volume of less dense solution into the reservoir chamber. Add appropriate volume of the more dense solution to the mixing chamber.

4. Stir the solution in the mixing chamber using a helix stainless steel wire (or similar device) driven by an overhead motor.

5. Set a peristaltic pump to give a steady flow rate and open connecting stop-cock (watch out for trapped air). The solution flowing into the centrifuge tube becomes progressively more dilute, thus establishing a gradient.

6. The gradient is stored at the required temperature but should normally be used within an hour.

A gradient preformed in such a way is ready for use in rate-zonal centrifugation, hopefully leading to the formation of a visible band of pure virus. Such a band can often be observed by shining a beam of light up through the bottom of the clear centrifuge tube, this being carried out in a darkened room. For some purposes the band can be harvested by puncturing the tube with a hypodermic syringe and withdrawing the band, the sample being pelleted later by ultracentrifugation.

It is however often necessary to collect appropriately volumed fractions from sucrose gradients. For this purpose, again, commercial apparatus is available, but great success is achieved easily by the construction of a home-made apparatus. The authors have used the three designs discussed by Minor (1985) but prefer the apparatus referred to as 'c' in his article. This is briefly discussed below (see Fig. 4.2.)

The apparatus consists of a rubber bung, a bleed tube of steel tubing attached to a short piece of silicone rubber tubing (i), and a glass inlet tube attached to a repeating syringe adjustable to deliver

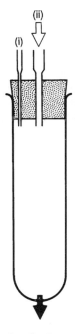

Figure 4.2. Apparatus for harvesting sucrose gradients (from Minor 1985).

0.5–2.0 ml of liquid paraffin (ii).

1. Clamp the centrifuge tube vertically.
2. Insert the rubber bung.
3. Pump liquid paraffin into the tube until it emerges from the bleed tube. Clamp the bleed tube.
4. Pierce the bottom of the centrifuge tube.
5. Collect fractions of appropriate volume by displacement with a known volume of liquid paraffin delivered by the repeating syringe.

Such a method is capable of giving good separation of 'bands', of e.g. empty and full capsids, etc.

Sucrose density gradient rate-zonal centrifugation has been used for the purification of a whole range of viruses, e.g. influenza virus (Barrett and Inglis 1985), adenovirus (Precious and Russell 1985), coronavirus (Collins and Alexander 1980), parainfluenzavirus (Ito et al 1987), rotavirus (McCrae 1985), rhabdovirus (Wunner 1985), togavirus (Gould and Clegg 1985), picornavirus (Minor 1985), and herpes viruses (Killington and Powell 1985).

Specific purification methods for a small capsid virus (e.g. picornavirus) and a large enveloped virus (e.g. a herpes virus) are detailed below.

Picornavirus

(Minor 1985)

Preparations of virus for purification are usually derived following high m.o.i. of appropriate cell cultures (e.g. HeLa suspension cultures) which are freeze–thawed two or three times and then centrifuged to remove the debris. The supernatant is often treated with either ammonium sulphate or polythene glycol prior to purification. Picornaviruses are however often associated with membranes and thus detergent is usually added (e.g. 1% NP40) to free the virus particles. The purification process is as follows:

1. Prepare a solution to give final concentrations of 15 g of sucrose per 100 ml, 10 mM Tris-HCl pH 7.4, 50 mM NaCl. Prepare a similar solution at final concentrations of 45 g of sucrose per 100 ml, 10 mM Tris-HCl pH 7.4, 50 mM NaCl.
2. Prepare 30 ml linear gradients of sucrose from 15% to 45% in an ultracentrifuge tube of 35–40 ml capacity (e.g. Beckman SW28) using 15 ml of each of these solutions per gradient and a suitable gradient maker.
3. Prepare a solution of 10% NP–40 (BDH) in PBS. Add one-tenth of a volume to the sample, whose volume should not exceed 6 ml. The sample should clarify visibly as it is shaken with the detergent.
4. Layer the sample carefully onto the preformed gradient. Balance the tubes with liquid paraffin.
5. Centrifuge the tubes at 4°C at 80,000 g for 4 h (for example at 25,000 rpm in a Beckman L8 ultracentrifuge, SW28 rotor).
6. Harvest the gradients as described above. Assay for virus. The infectious virus peaks should be about $\frac{2}{3}$ down the gradient.

Virus purified in such a way is suitable for most purposes. However some impurities may remain and if extreme purity is required it may be necessary to re-purify on caesium chloride gradients.

Herpes simplex virus

(Killington and Powell 1985)

Herpes simplex virus provides a more difficult challenge than most viruses with regard to the preparation of pure virus particles. Techniques which work well with one virus strain in a particular cell line do not work for other strains of virus in the same cells or for the same strain of virus in different cells. For this reason we give two methods here. Method 1 relies on the virus strain being released into the extracellular medium of e.g. Hep-2 infected cells. Method 2 appears to work for most strains.

Method 1

(Powell and Watson 1975)

1. Infect confluent monolayers of Hep-2 cells in roller cultures at a m.o.i. of 20–25 (pfu cell^{-1}).
2. Wash the infected cells after virus adsorption, add fresh medium and incubate the cells at 32°C for 2–3 days.
3. At the end of the incubation, centrifuge the medium at low speed to remove cell debris.
4. Harvest the virus either by precipitation from the medium with polyethylene glycol (PEG, molecular weight 6000, 8% w/v in the presence of 0.5 M NaCl) or by centrifugation (12,000 rpm, 2 h in a GSA rotor, Sorvall RCS-5B centrifuge).
5. Resuspend the virus in a low molarity Tris buffer pH 7.8 containing 50 mM NaCl. It is preferable to allow re-suspension overnight if this is convenient.
6. Layer the suspension of virus over a 30 ml gradient of 5–45% sucrose in the same buffer and centrifuge for 1 h at 12,500 rpm (Sorvall AH627 rotor). At the end of this period a fluffy white band of purified virus should be clearly visible at the centre of the gradient. This visible band contains the single peak of infectious virus in the gradient.

At this point the virus is of adequate purity (about 50 μg of protein/10^{10} particles virus) for many purposes including the preparation of virus DNA. The virus may be recovered by simple sedimentation. To produce high quality preparations of virus a wide variety of other techniques can be used, including a second sucrose gradient or caesium chloride gradients. Both these techniques yield virus with a protein/particle ratio better than 20 μg/10^{10} particles.

Method 2

(Spear and Roizman 1972; Heine et al 1972; Killington et al 1977)

1. Infect the cells exactly as described for method 1.
2. Incubate the cells at 37°C for 18–24 h and harvest by scraping from the glass and low-speed centrifugation.
3. Resuspend the cell pellet so obtained in Reticulocyte Standard Buffer (RSB) and allow the cells to swell for 10 min. The cytoplasm may then be obtained from the cells by Dounce homogenization.
4. Centrifuge the Dounce-homogenized cells at low speed to remove nuclei and cell debris.
5. Layer the supernatant (containing the majority of the infectious virus) on to a 5–40% Dextran gradient in Tris buffer and centrifuge at 12,500 rpm for 1 h (Sorvall AH 627 rotor); the virus is obtained by removing the visible band in the centre of the gradient.
6. Collect the virus from this band by sedimentation (20,000 rpm for 1 h, Sorvall AH 627 rotor).

At this point the virus is of adequate purity for many purposes but can easily be improved by the methods mentioned above. Purified virus derived by either method may be resuspended in distilled water or a suitable buffer and aliquots taken for infectivity assay, total particle count and protein estimation. Virus can be frozen at −70°C, but on thawing this leads to partial disintegraton of the viral envelope.

Chapter 4

Caesium chloride gradients

Caesium chloride (CsCl) is one of the materials of choice used for the purification of viruses by a technique referred to as buoyant density-gradient sedimentation, isopycnic centrifugation or equilibrium density gradient centrifugation. This method is based on the premise that the layering of a virus suspension on to a pre-formed gradient followed by ultracentrifugation will result in the migration of virus particles until they reach an equilibrium according to their buoyant density. Alternatively, the gradient may be field formed by mixing the virus suspension with a known amount of CsCl in a suitable buffer prior to centrifugation when the gradient is produced. This technique contrasts with the procedure of rate-zonal centrifugation which separates particles on the basis of size. Other materials used in isopycnic centrifugation include organic molecules such as sugars (sucrose) or polysaccharides (Ficoll), iodinated aromatic compounds (Nycodenz) or colloidal silica (Percoll). Hence no one particular compound is of universal application. More far reaching applications of CsCl gradients include the purification of plasmid DNA and the separation of subviral components.

The widespread use of CsCl is attributed to the fact that solutions of up to 1.91 g cm^{-3} can be prepared from it which is highly desirable for the purification of viruses whose buoyant densities range from 1.28–1.45 g cm^{-3} (non-enveloped) to 1.18–1.25 g cm^{-3} (enveloped). Suggestions for the concentrations of CsCl to be used for gradient formation range from 1.32 g cm^{-3} (32% w/v) for a virus containing 5% RNA to 1.7 g cm^{-3} (55.5%) w/v for a DNA virus.

In addition to its high level of solubility and density, CsCl is able to form solutions of low ionic strength and viscosity. Also, at a suitable pH its presence does not affect the biological activities of the virus. Optical grade CsCl does not absorb UV light allowing direct photometric analysis of gradient fractions. Further it does not interfere with the activity of scintillation fluids, thereby allowing analysis of radioactively labeled virus preparations taken from the gradient. CsCl can easily be removed from the virus fraction by dialysis, filtration or ultracentrifugation.

CsCl gradients may either be self formed or preformed and the latter type of gradient may either be discontinuous or continuous. For the discontinuous gradient, often referred to as a step gradient, different densities of CsCl are layered into a centrifuge tube, beginning either by underlaying the least dense with a more dense preparation or by layering the less dense preparation on the top of the more dense. The virus sample is loaded on to the top of the gradient and centrifugation begun immediately. The continuous gradient is prepared in the same manner but additionally it is held at 4°C overnight, allowing diffusion to occur. More often however, a gradient maker is used to form the continuous gradient thus saving time. For the self-forming gradient, the virus sample, the gradient solute and the buffer are mixed together in proportions that will generate a suitable density range on centrifugation.

Swing out, fixed angle and vertical rotors can all be used for the purpose of CsCl centrifugation. If limited time is available, the various fractions of the gradient are collected and their densities can be measured in an Abbé refractometer. Alternatively, known volumes of liquid may be weighed using a pycnometer. Some methods for virus purification using CsCl gradient centrifugation are given below.

The purification of picornaviruses on a preformed CsCl gradient

(Minor 1985)

1. Prepare a 40% w/w solution of CsCl by dissolving 4 g of solid CsCl in 6 ml of 0.01 M Tris-HCl pH 7.4.

2. Prepare a 5% w/w solution of CsCl by dissolving 0.5 g of solid CsCl in 9.5 ml of 0.01 M Tris-HCl pH 7.4.
3. Pour a 10 ml 5–40% linear CsCl gradient in an ultracentrifuge tube of 12 ml capacity (e.g. Beckman SW41 tube) using 5 ml of each solution and a suitable gradient maker.
4. Layer the sample containing 1% NP-40 on to the gradient in a volume of 1 ml. Balance centrifuge tubes using liquid paraffin.
5. Centrifuge at 120,000 g for at least 4 h and preferably overnight at 4°C in, for example, a Beckman L8 ultracentrifuge, SW41 head at 30,000 rpm.
6. Harvest the gradients.

The purification of Brome mosaic virus on a self forming CsCl gradient

(Hull, 1985)

1. Precipitate a suspension of virus extracted from infected leaves with polyethylene glycol 6000 (10% in 0.1 M NaCl and centrifuge at 10,000 g for 10 min, resuspend in 1/10 the volume of 0.1 M sodium acetate pH 5.0 and centrifuge at 10,000 g for 10 min to recover the supernatant.
2. Add CsCl to give a density of 1.36 g cm^{-3} and centrifuge at 36,000 rpm for 18 h in a Beckman R40 rotor.
3. Recover the virus band from the gradient and dialyse against at least 100 volumes of 0.1 M sodium acetate pH 5.0 for 3–4 h to remove the CsCl.
4. Repeat steps 1 and 2 and resuspend the final product in 1 ml of sodium acetate pH 5.0 per 100 g of starting leaf material.

The use of CsCl gradient centrifugation in the isolation and purification of viruses from tissue samples

Following the treatment of tissue samples to extract a virus of interest, CsCl gradient centrifugation can then be used for its purification. One such example of this was an examination of the structure of fish lymphocystis disease virus from skin tumours of pleuronectes following their purification on CsCl gradients (Samalecos 1986).

1. Tissue is homogenized (1–5 g) in TNE buffer and the suspension clarified by centrifugation at 3000 rpm for 20 min twice.
2. The cell free supernatant is centrifuged through a 30% (w/w) sucrose cushion in a Spinco SW 27 rotor at 25,000 rpm for 120 min at 4°C.
3. The virus pellets are resuspended in TNE buffer and layered on to 35 ml gradients of 25–60% (w/w) sucrose and recentrifuged for 20 h in a Spinco SW27 rotor at 25,000 rpm at 4°C.
4. The virus band is collected and centrifuged in a CsCl gradient (10–35% w/w) for 24 h in a Spinco SW41 rotor at 30,000 rpm at 10°C. The virus band in the middle of the gradient is harvested, dialyzed against TNE buffer and used for electron microscopy.

A second example of the use of this technique for the purification of a virus from biological material was in the isolation of rabbit picobirnaviruses from faecal material. These particles co-sediment with 32 nm virus particles which have a buoyant density of 1.39 g cm^{-3} (Gallimore et al 1993).

1. A 10% faecal suspension is clarified by centrifugation at 1500 rpm for 15 min.
2. The supernatant is extracted with an equal volume of trichlorotrifluoroethane.
3. The virus present in the aqueous phase is concentrated by centrifugation through a 45% sucrose cushion at 45,000 rpm for 2 h at 5°C in a Beckman SW55Ti rotor.
4. The pellet is resuspended in Tris/Ca buffer and loaded on to a 30% (v/v) CsCl gradient and centrifuged at 35,000 rpm for 17.5 h.
5. The gradient is harvested into 0.3 ml fractions and the buoyant density of each fraction is calculated from its refractive index.
   The sample is then ready for further examination by such techniques as polyacrylamide gel electrophoresis (PAGE).

Finally, CsCl centrifugation has been used for the separation on the basis of buoyant density of viruses isolated from faecal material whose description had previously been limited to that of 'small round viruses'. These were then further examined by electron microscopy and could be classified in more detail (Oliver and Phillips 1988).

1. 0.3 ml of virus supernatant was layered on to 4.5 ml of 45% aqueous CsCl and centrifuged at 100,000 g for 18 h in an MSE 65 Superspeed ultracentrifuge using a swing out rotor.
2. 2.5 μl of 0.3 ml fractions with densities between 1.2 and 1.5 g cm^{-3} were placed on agar coated slides and allowed to dry. Samples were stained and examined by electron microscopy. By carrying out this retrospective study, small round viruses found in faecal samples were classified into groups such as astrovirus, 'Norwalk-like' virus, parvovirus, enterovirus and hepatitis A.

The purification of viruses by CsCl density centrifugation for use in immunological assays

CsCl density gradient centrifugation was used for the production of purified preparations of rotavirus antigens for use in T-cell proliferation assays (Bruce et al 1994). Virus was pelleted from 400 ml of clarified (5000 g for 30 min) cell culture lysates and resuspended in 3 ml of 20 mM-Tris-HCl pH 7.5 buffer containing 5 mM calcium chloride. The virus was purified further by differential centrifugation on a five-step caesium chloride gradient. Double and single-shelled rotavirus particles were harvested from the gradient, pooled and washed by ultracentrifugation. The virus purified thus was then used in T-cell proliferation assays.

The purification of subviral components using CsCl gradient centrifugation

CsCl gradient centrifugation is effective in the production of purified subviral components from either biological fluids or from systems which over-express the protein. Three examples of this are given below.

1. HBsAg was purified from the plasma of high-titre chronic carriers of HBsAg

(Gavilanes et al 1990). Following treatment with octyl glucoside the suspension was layered onto a 12.8 ml CsCl linear gradient (density 1.15–1.32 g cm^{-3}). The CsCl had been previously filtered through GSWPO4750 Millipore filters before use.

2. Gradients were centrifuged for 4 h at 154,400 g in a Beckman SW40 rotor.
3. Fractions of 0.4 ml were collected beginning from the bottom of the gradient and their absorbance at 280 nm measured. Antigen-positive fractions were pooled and dialyzed against 10 mм-Tris (pH 7.0)/50 mм NaCl.

Hepatitis B core antigen is composed of an envelope carrying the surface antigen and an internal capsid containing the circular, partially dsDNA genome and the viral polymerase. Empty cores have been produced in baculo-virus and one cycle of CsCl gradient centrifugation was used for their purification. Three species were found in sedimentation velocity studies of a 3 mg ml^{-1} solution. These had migrations of 71.3S, 62.5S and 11.0S respectively (Hilditch et al 1990).

Hepatitis delta virus antigen was expressed in a eukaryotic cell line (Macnaughton et al 1990) and the density of the antigen was found to be 1.19 g cm^{-3} by equilibrium centrifugation in caesium chloride. The procedure was as follows:

1. A 200 µl sample of ammonium sulphate precipitated recHDAg was overlaid on a 10 ml gradient of preformed caesium chloride (1.1–1.5 g cm^{-3} and centrifuged (120,000 g) for 25 h at 20°C and 0.5 ml fractions collected).
2. Fractions were tested for HDAg activity by RIA and its density was estimated from the refractive index.

Positive density/negative viscosity gradients

Rationale

Positive density/negative viscosity gradients were first proposed by Barzilai et al (1972) as a means of effectively separating viruses from cytoplasmic components with similar densities. His studies used CsCl to provide density and glycerol for viscosity, and the gradients were employed to purify foot-and-mouth disease virus, a picornavirus, from the host cell milieu in which it was grown. The method described here is patterned after Obijeski et al (1974), who found that potassium tartrate provided a gentler chemical environment than caesium or rubidium salts for enveloped viruses.

The gradients are constructed such that the potassium tartrate yields increasing density from the top of the gradient to the bottom, while the glycerol yields decreasing viscosity from the top to the bottom; thus the designation 'positive density/negative viscosity'. The method is gentle and does not destroy labile viruses either by pelleting them or by a harsh chemical milieu. It has been found particularly useful for purifying enveloped viruses such as rhabdoviruses (Obijeski et al 1974), coronaviruses (Hierholzer 1976), parainfluenza and mumps viruses (Hierholzer et al 1993), and respiratory syncytial virus (Hierholzer et al 1994), and non-enveloped but nonstable viruses such as caliciviruses and astroviruses (Ashley and Caul 1982). In the 30% (v/v) glycerol-to-40% (v/v) potassium tartrate gradients used for enveloped viruses, the top of the gradient after centrifugation contains a band of flocculent material with a refractive index of ~1.356; followed by a faint, hazy band (~1.377); a sharp, compact virus band (~1.379); another faint, hazy band just below the virus (~1.380); and two very flocculent bands near the bottom of the tube (RI 1.381 and 1.385, respectively). The RI values correspond to a range of 15–32% sucrose. For non-enveloped viruses, the gradient is constructed with 30% glycerol and 60% tartrate to provide the greater density needed for these viruses (Ashley and Caul 1982).

Protocol and interpretation

1. Construct gradients in cellulose nitrate centrifuge tubes holding at least 10 ml. The directions here will be for the Beckman SW41 tubes, which hold 12.5 ml to the top, and allow for 10 ml of gradient and 2.5 ml of previously-concentrated virus. The tubes should be situated vertically, as with all gradients.
2. To make three identical gradients, place 16 ml of 40% di-potassium tartrate in TES buffer, pH 7.2 (see page 176), in the right-hand cylinder to prevent an air trap, and then lead it into the three lines of tubing leading to the pump and centrifuge tubes. This provides a small cushion of 40% tartrate (highest density) which will prevent viruses with densities around 1.18 g cm^{-3} from passing through.
3. Commence stirring in the right-hand cylinder, either with a stainless steel agitator rod or a magnetic mixing bar. Adjust the stirrer so that excessive air bubbles are not formed and forced into the tubing going to the pump and centrifuge tubes. Excessive bubbles can create air traps and also disrupt the linearity of the gradients.

4. Add 15 ml of 30% glycerol in the same TES buffer to the left-hand cylinder, open the stopcock at the bottom of the chamber joining the two cylinders, and allow the glycerol to begin feeding into the mixing chamber as the pump is slowly filling the tubes.

5. The linear gradients are best formed over a 40–50 minute period at ambient temperature.

6. Gently load the gradients with 2.5 ml of concentrated virus per tube.

7. Load the tubes onto the SW41 rotor and spin at 41,000 rpm (208,000 avg. g) for 18 h at 3°C. (Alternatively, for larger volumes, Beckman SW27.1 cellulose nitrate tubes can be filled with 15 ml of gradient and 3 ml of virus concentrate, and spun in an SW28 rotor at 27,000 rpm (130,000 avg. g) for 18 h at 3°C).

8. After centrifugation, study the tubes with a strong, narrow-beam light aimed upward from below the bottom of the tube in a darkened room. The virus band should stand out as a narrow, condensed band sandwiched between two hazy bands of cellular material of the same density.

9. Harvest the virus band, either by careful pipetting from the top of the gradient downwards, or by puncturing the bottom of the tube and collecting the bands dropwise.

10. Verify the virus band by refractive index, electron microscopy, some appropriate antigen or nucleic acid test, or preferably by all three.

Filtration methods

Gel filtration, also referred to as size exclusion liquid chromatography (SEC), gel chromatography or gel permeation chromatography has proven to be one of a number of methods of choice for the purification of viruses and is extensively used in the purification of subviral components including antigens and virally encoded enzymes often expressed in either prokaryotic or eukaryotic systems. SEC is used in the separation of simple mixtures conveniently and rapidly when the components of the mixture have a sufficient difference in size. The technique uses a solid phase composed of a column packing of beads with pores of a defined average size. The beads have a specific size exclusion so that the separation of solute entering the column is dependent on its ability to enter the pores. The smaller components are able to enter the pores and are retained in the column and are eluted first. Solutes of intermediate size are less able to approach the walls of the pores and spend less time in the pores. These move through the column at speeds dependent on their relative size. Thus separation in SEC is strictly on the basis of molecular size. The retention of solutes by adsorption is undesirable and usually does not occur with the correct combination of substrate and mobile phase. A differential elution, proportional to the particle size (and consequently to the particle molecular weight) can be obtained.

The beads are composed of various materials. The ideal surface must be neutral and hydrophilic to minimize the possibility of adsorption. Highly cross-linked, mechanically stable, macroporous matrices from neutral, hydrophilic polymers such as dextrans or agarose have been used for such purposes. The commercially available Sepharose CL (Pharmacia) is a beaded agarose matrix which has been cross-linked. However, cross-linking agents introduce hydrophobic character into the matrix. Pore diameter and pore volume can also be reduced during cross-linking.

Sepharose gel filtration media give a broad range of fractionation (10,000–40,000,000 M_r) and have a high exclusion limit for the separation of biomolecules. The particle size is from 45–200 μm. The beaded agarose matrix shows low non-specific binding and the cross-linked forms have good chemical and physical stability. Sepharose is available with three different agarose contents: 2%, 4% and 6%. Increasing the agarose concentration decreases matrix porosity thus altering the fractionation range while increasing the rigidity.

Operating instructions and gel selection depend on the application and the desired resolution. The technique can be broadly separated into two categories, desalting or group separation and fractionation. For desalting, the molecule of interest is eluted in the void volume whilst smaller molecules are retained. Thus the exclusion size should be smaller than the molecule of interest. For fractionation, molecules of varying molecular weight are separated within the gel matrix and thus the molecules of interest should fall within the separation range of the gel. Gel filtration is a non-interactive technique which means that the conditions can be chosen to maintain the stability of the molecules being separated. This is a valuable means of separating unknown samples but, more pertinent here, can also be used for the purification of viruses such as poliovirus or rabies virus (van Wezel et al 1979). Filtration on Sephacryl S300 has also been used for the purification of influenza neuraminidase fragments.

The more efficient method of high performance SEC (HPSEC) is now frequently used where the system is closed and operated at high pressures. Thus separations take 10–20 min compared to hours. High pressure, rapid flow rates and sophisticated equipment are characteristic of this procedure. However, small more rigid porous particles will be used for column packing as opposed to the ones used for SEC which would collapse at high pressure. For details on these systems see Snyder and Kirkland (1979) and Yau et al (1979).

The steps involved in gel filtration are:

a) bed preparation;
b) sample application;
c) sample flow-achieved by gravity feeding of the column;
d) detection and quantitation of the purified virus particle or protein.

Some applications of SEC are given below. McGrath et al (1978) used a Sepharose 4B chromatographic method for the purification of a retrovirus. This method gave increased purified virus yields, conserved the virus glycoprotein and the preparation had an increased recovery of biological infectivity in comparison with the previously used method of sucrose density gradient centrifugation.

1. Viruses are harvested from infected cells and cell debris pelleted by centrifugation at 10,000 g.
2. Clarified supernatant is concentrated 10–50 fold in an Amicon ultrafiltration apparatus using a PM10 membrane at an ultrafiltration rate of 1 ml/min. The concentrate is spun through a discontinuous sucrose gradient (25% to 40% w/w) in TEN buffer (20 mM Tris, 1 mM EDTA, 0.1 M NaCl, pH 7.5) for 2.5 h at 90,000 g and the virus band collected.
3. The supernatant concentrated by ultrafiltration corresponding to 5% of a pre-sterilized Sepharose C1 4B (Pharmacia) column bed volume is chromatographed at 4°C in TEN buffer. Virus appears in the void volume at a flow rate of 0.5 to 1.0 ml min^{-1}. The fractions containing the virus peak are monitored by optical density at 280 nm and by radioactivity.

Pinto et al (1991) used gel filtration techniques for the recovery and purification of a virus from the erythrocytes of sea bass.

1. Red blood cells from 40 ml of blood are collected by centrifugation at 2000 g for 20 min and resuspended in 40 ml of TNE (50 mM Tris-HCl, 150 mM NaCl and 1 mM EDTA, pH 7.4) buffer with 0.1% SDS.
2. Samples are freeze–thawed and sonicated three times and clarified by two centrifugation steps at 3000 g and 6000 g for 10 min.
3. The supernatant is concentrated to a final volume of 8–10 ml by ultrafiltration through CX30 immersible units. The complete removal of haemoglobin is accomplished by Sephadex G-100 gel filtration in a 20 × 6.5 cm column, with TNE/0.1% SDS as the eluent.
4. The volume of the first peak of UV light absorbing material to emerge corresponds to the first 10 ml of the void volume. The eluted volume is reconcentrated to 1 ml by ultrafiltration through immersible filters. The presence of virus particles is determined by staining with 2% phosphotungstic acid and electron microscopy. Protein concentration determined by the Lowry's method ranges from 25–250 µg ml^{-1}.

Whilst being useful for the purification of whole virus particles, gel filtration can be manipulated so that subviral components can be obtained in a pure form. One such example is work carried out on the oligomeric form of the gp160 glycoprotein of simian immunodeficiency virus. It is possible to purify oligomeric forms of SIV gp160 to greater than 90% purity using a simple gel filtration method (Rhodes et al 1994). Concentrated samples of CHO supernatants from cells expressing gp160 are filtered through Sepharose 6B (Sigma). 0.5 ml volumes from the column are collected and analysed for the presence of gp120/160 by ELISA. These results demonstrated that the major form of sgp160 existed as a 660 K species (tetramer). Gel filtration was then used to purify this further. To do this, protein from one-litre batches of supernatant was precipitated with 85% ammonium sulphate, resuspended in 30 ml of water and dialyzed for 24 h against 3 changes of PBS. Six-millilitre aliquots (0.5 mg gp160) were separated by gel-filtration chromatography using a Sephacryl S-400HR column (90 × 2.5 cm). Three-millilitre fractions were collected and each screened for gp 160 by ELISA. Fractions containing gp160 were pooled and concentrated by ultrafiltration centrifugation through a Centricon filter with a 10 K size exclusion. Protein was stored at −20°C in 50 mM Tris-HCl pH 7.6.

For further applications of gel filtration techniques for the purification of viral proteins see HSV-1 UL8 protein (Parry et al 1993), Epstein-Barr virus Nuclear Protein 2A (Tsui and Schubach 1994), HTLV1 recombinant protease (Daenke et al 1994), HIV-1 reverse transcriptase (Sharma et al 1994), HIV-2 Nef Protein (Du Bois et al 1993).

Criteria of purity

When designing a purification protocol it is essential to apply stringent tests to ensure that the virus particles produced are pure. Once the protocol has been tried and tested the purity of each batch of virus should be assessed by at least one criterion.

Protein/particle ratios are good indications of purity. Estimations of particle weight and percent protein allows the calculation of a target protein/particle ratio, e.g. for herpes simplex approximately 13.5 μg/10^{10} particles. Whilst such figures are not totally accurate they do give a valid target for which to aim. The observation of particles in the electron microscope, whilst not a good criterion of purity, does allow the detection of 'unwanted structures'.

It would be expected that constituents of the medium would form a major part of the contaminants of purified virus preparations. This can be monitored by gel diffusion tests, where antisera raised against e.g. calf serum, or uninfected cells can be reacted with virus preparation.

Another method designed to detect free antigen contaminants in the purified virus is non-SDS electrophoresis, where pure virus should yield no detectable stained bands moving into the gel.

Comparison of radioactively labeled polypeptide profiles with stained profiles on SDS polyacrylamide gels can also be a useful monitor of purity.

Finally, another method of assaying virus purity is to use prelabeled cells. Cells are labeled with e.g. ^{14}C-amino acids for a considerable period prior to infection and then chased with unlabeled amino acids. Following infection, infected cells are labeled with ^{3}H-amino acids. The degree of incorporated label is monitored throughout the purification procedure. This method, again, is a rough guide to the degree of purity.

References

Anderson LJ, Coombs RA, Tsou C, Hierholzer JC (1984) J Clin Microbiol 19: 934–936.

Ashley CR, Caul EO (1982) J Clin Microbiol 16: 377–381.

Barzilai R, Lazarus LH, Goldblum N (1972) Arch Virusforsch 36: 141–146.

Barrett T, Inglis SC (1985) In: Virology: a practical approach. BWJ Mahy (Ed.) IRL Press, Oxford.

Bruce MG, Campbell I, Xiong Y, Redmond M, Snodgrass DR (1994) J Gen Virol 75: 1859–1866.

Cash P, Wunner WH, Pringle CR (1977) Virology 82: 369–379.

Collins MS, Alexander DJ (1980) Arch Virol 63: 239–251.

Daenke S, Schramm HJ, Bangham CRM (1994) J Gen Virol 75: 2233–2239.

Dea S, Tijseen P (1988) Arch. Virol. 99, 173–186.

Du Bois GC, Hodge DR, Hanson CA, Samuel KP, Zweig M, Showalter SD, Papas TS (1993) Aids research and human retroviruses 9: 1225–1231.

Fuccillo DA, Sever JL In: Schmidt NJ, Emmons RW (Eds.) (1989) Diagnostic Procedures for Viral, Rickettsial and Chlamydial Infections, 6th edn., American Public Health Assn., Washington, D.C., pp. 713–730.

Gallimore C, Lewis D, Brown D (1993) Arch Virol 133: 63–73.

Gavilanes F, Gomez-Gutierrez J, Aracil M, Gonzalez-Ros JM, Ferragut JA et al (1990) Biochem J 265: 857–864.

Gould E, Clegg J (1985) In: Virology: a practical approach. BWJ Mahy (Ed.) IRL Press.

Hames D (1984) In: Centrifugation: a practical approach. D Rickwood (Ed.) IRL Press.

Hasegawa A, Inouye S (1983) J Clin Microbiol 17: 458–462.

Heine J-W, Spear PG, Roizman B (1972) J Virol 9: 431–439.

Hierholzer JC (1976) Virology 75: 155–165.

Hierholzer JC, Bingham PG, Castells E, Coombs RA (1993) Arch Virol 130: 335–352.

Hierholzer JC, Bingham PG, Coombs RA, Stone YO, Hatch MH (1984) J Clin Microbiol 19: 826–830.

Hierholzer JC, Tannock GA, Hierholzer CM, Coombs RA, Kennett ML, Phillips PA, Gust ID (1994) Arch Virol 136: 133–147.

Hilditch CM, Rogers LJ, Bishop DL (1990) J Gen Virol 71: 2755–2759.

Hull R (1985) In: Virology: a practical approach. BWJ Mahy (Ed.) IRL Press, Oxford.

Ito Y, Tsurudome M, Hishiyama M (1987) Arch Virol 95: 211–224.

Killington RA, Powell K (1985) In: Virology: a practical approach. B Mahy (Ed.) IRL Press, Oxford.

Killington RA, Yeo J, Honess RW, Watson DH, Duncan BD, Halliburton IW, Mumford J (1977) J Gen Virol 37: 297–310.

Lanser JA, Howard CR (1980) J Gen Virol 46: 349–361.

Mcgrath M, Witte O, Pincus T, Weissman IL (1978) J Virol 25: 923–927.

McCrae M (1985) In: Virology: a practical approach. B Mahy (Ed.) IRL Press, Oxford.

Minor PD (1985) In: Virology: a practical approach. B Mahy (Ed.) IRL Press, Oxford.

Obijeski JF, Marchenko AT, Bishop DH, Cann BW, Murphy FA (1974) J Gen Virol 22: 21–33.

Oliver AR, Phillips AD (1988) J Medical Virol 24: 211–218.

Parry ME, Stow ND, Marsden HS (1993) J Gen Virol 74: 607–612.

Pinto RM, Jofre J, Bosch A (1991) Arch Virol 120: 83–96.

Powell K, Watson D (1975) J Gen Virol 29: 167.

Precious B, Russell WC (1985) In: Virology: a practical approach. BWJ Mahy (Ed.) IRL Press, Oxford.

Rhodes AD, Spitali M, Hutchinson G, Rud E, Stephens PE (1994) J Gen Virol 75: 207–213.

Samalecos CP (1986) Arch Virol 91: 1–10.

Sharma SK, Basu A, Fan N, Evans DN (1994) Biotech Appli Biochem 19: 155–167.

Snyder LR, Kirkland JJ (1979) Introduction to modern liquid chromatography. 2nd Edition. John Wiley & Sons Inc., New York.

Spear PG, Roizman B (1972) J Virol 9: 143–159.

Tannock GA (1973) Arch ges Virusforsch 43: 259–271.

Tsui S, Schubach WH (1994) J Virol 68: 4287–4294.

Van Wezel CW, van Herwaarden JAM, van de Heuvel-de-Rijk EW (1979) Develop Biol Standard 42: 65–69.

Wadey CN, Westaway EG (1981) Intervirology 15: 19–27.

Wunner WH (1985) In: Virology: a practical approach. B Mahy (Ed.) IRL Press, Oxford.

Yamamoto KR, Alberts BM, Benzinger R, Lawhorne L, Treiber G (1970) Virology 40: 734–744.

Yau WW, Kirkland JJ, Bly DD (1979) In: Practice of Gel Permeation Gel Filtration Chomatography. John Wiley & Sons Inc., New York.

Electron microscopy

5

I. L. Chrystie

The aim of this chapter is to provide a detailed methodology of some of the basic electron microscopic (EM) techniques currently used in virology. It does not, however, cover operation of the electron microscope or of other equipment for which the manufacturers' instructions would be more appropriate. The chapter is subdivided into four sections: a general introduction (detailing necessary equipment, safety precautions, etc); negative staining procedures; thin sectioning procedures; and briefly scanning EM. Following a brief discussion of the principles, each technique is given in sufficient detail to be followed as a recipe. Modifications are included within the methodology or in a following paragraph. However, it is not intended to be a comprehensive text and readers are directed to the bibliography for more complex techniques. Finally, it must be stated that the total novice should ensure that they receive their initial instruction from a competent electron microscopist, ideally on a recognized academic or manufacturer-run course.

Safety

Most of the chemicals used in EM are hazardous and should be handled with appropriate precautions.

All fixatives are poisonous by ingestion, inhalation or contact, and some are volatile, especially osmium tetroxide (OsO_4) and acrolein. Many are flammable. The majority of resins are thought to cause dermatological problems and some are known carcinogens.

When mixed with solvents (e.g. during infiltration procedures) they are absorbed into the skin much faster. Solvents are flammable and propylene oxide is carcinogenic. Some buffers are poisonous (veronal contains barbiturate and cacodylate contains arsenic). Stains contain heavy metals which are cumulative poisons and uranyl salts are radioactive as well as toxic.

Sensible precautions involve: adequate storage (small amounts, safety containers, labeling); appropriate personal protection (laboratory coat, gloves, safety goggles); appropriate containment (fume cupboards, working over absorbent paper); spark and flame free environment; spillage protocols; correct (and legal!) disposal procedures.

In addition to the above it must be remembered that viruses are potentially pathogenic and must be handled accordingly.

Basic equipment

The size, equipment and organization of an EM unit will naturally vary according to the service requirements. However, there are some basic requirements which need to be considered. At least three separate rooms will be required, a microscope room, a preparation room, and a photographic dark room. An additional room for ultrathin sectioning has considerable advantages. Necessary equipment includes a fume hood (for resins, solvents. etc.), a safety cabinet (for handling of infectious material), a vacuum evaporation

Virology Methods Manual
ISBN 0–12–465330–8

unit (for preparation of carbon-coated grids), a bench and ultracentrifuge, 30–90°C oven (for curing blocks), glass knifemaker, an ultramicrotome, a sonicator (for cleaning EM parts), an enlarger, and a photographic processor. Some companies provide 'starter kits' of chemicals and/or basic equipment such as grids and tweezers.

Negative staining

Principles

Simplicity and rapidity, coupled with high resolution, have ensured that the negative staining technique is of major importance in virus morphology and diagnosis.

Virus particles do not scatter electrons to any appreciable extent and thus are not visible in the electron microscope. Negative stains provide an electron opaque background against which particles can be visualized. The penetration of the stain into the virus reveals its morphology. Negative stains must contain an electron dense element (a heavy metal), be water soluble, and, on drying, must form a non-crystalline sheet. Ideally they should not react with virus particles. Table 5.1 lists a number of commonly used negative stains.

Support films

Plastic films tend to decompose under the electron beam and move somewhat when irra-diated. Carbon films are more rigid but very fragile. Carbon coating of plastic films provides an ideal compromise for all but very high resolution work, for which carbon films are to be preferred. Specialist literature should be consulted for methods of production of carbon films, carbon/carbon-platinum films for cryo EM, and holey carbon films.

Preparation of carbon-coated, plastic films

1. Clean a microscope slide with detergent, rinse with distilled water (dH_2O), and dry.
2. Place the slide in a solution of plastic. Suitable plastics include Formvar (0.1–0.5% in chloroform); Butvar (0.2–0.4% in chloroform), pioloform (0.3–1% in chloroform) and collodion (0.5–1.5% in amyl acetate).
3. Remove the slide and allow it to drain vertically until all the solvent has evaporated.

Table 5.1. Negative stains commonly used in routine electron microscopy of viruses.

Stain*	Conc.	pH	Comments
Phosphotungstic acid	1–3%	5.0–8.0	Stain most commonly used by animal virologists. Can tolerate relatively high concentrations of salts in the virus suspension. Has detrimental effect on some viruses (Fig. 5.1).
Uranyl acetate	1.0–2.0%	4.4	pH can only be altered over very narrow range. Sensitive to salts in virus suspension. Often preferable to use two-step staining technique.
Uranyl formate	1.0–2.0%	4.4	
Uranyl nitrate	0.5–1.0%	4.4	
Uranyl oxalate	0.5–1.0%	5.0–7.0	
Ammonium molybdate	1–4%	6.0–8.0	Useful for negative staining of whole cell preparations and osmotically sensitive structures (Figure 5.2). Adjust pH with ammonium hydroxide.
Sodium silicotungstate	2–4%	5.0–8.0	
Methylamine tungstate	1.0–2.0%	6.0–8.0	Low buffering capacity

* All stains will benefit from the addition of bacitracin (0.1%) as a wetting agent to aid spreading.

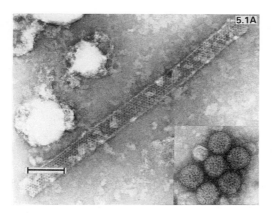
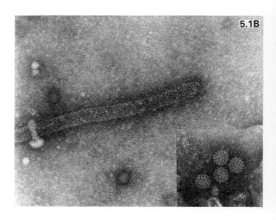

Figure 5.1. Tubules formed from viral capsid material are often present in preparations of rotavirus and papovavirus. Such tubules are rarely seen with phosphotungstate (PTA) stains but are readily visible with other stains. **A.** Faecal preparation containing rotavirus stained with 1% methylamine tungstate pH 6.5 (inset stained with 3% PTA pH 6.5). **B.** Sample of urine containing polyomavirus stained with 1% methylamine tungstate pH 6.5 (inset stained with PTA pH 6.5). Bar = 50nm

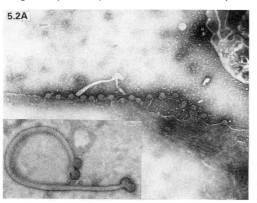
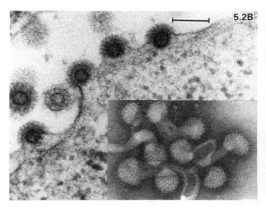

Figure 5.2. Spumavirus (SFV 11) from an orang-utan growing in Sup-T1 cells. **A.** Stained with 4% ammonium molybdate pH 6.0 showing virus budding from cell membrane. **B.** Thin section electronmicrograph of the same preparation. (Inset negatively stained as A. showing distinct virus fringe which is not easily visible when stained with PTA). Bars = 50nm

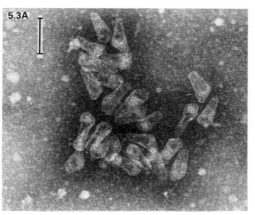
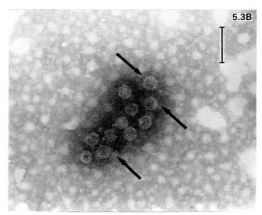

Figure 5.3. **A.** Negatively stained immune complex of HIV-2 cores and a serum from an HIV-2 positive patient (3% PTA pH 6.0). **B.** Negatively stained immune complex of BK virus from urine and patient's serum (3% PTA pH 6.0). IgM molecules can easily be visualised (arrows). Bar = 50nm

4. Score a rectangle in the film along one surface about 5 mm in from the edge and insert the slide, scored side uppermost, into a dish of dH_2O at a shallow angle. The film should float on the surface of the water. Breathing on the film may facilitate release.

5. Place grids on the film. Opinion varies as to whether grids should be matt or shiny side down. The author's personal opinion is that it does not matter.

6. Cover the film and grids with a square of filter paper. When the paper is fully wetted remove it gently. The film, plus grids, should remain attached to the filter paper, which should be allowed to dry, grids uppermost, at room temperature.

7. When dry, the coated grids, on the filter paper, are placed into a suitable vacuum coating apparatus, and a thin film of carbon is evaporated onto the grids. No further details are given as different machines vary and all that is necessary is to follow the manufacturer's instructions. The thickness of the carbon film may be estimated by observing its deposition on a thickness indicator (a piece of white porcelain with a drop of vacuum oil on it). The carbon is only visible on the porcelain – not the oil.

8. The grids are then ready for use.

Carbon films are notoriously hydrophobic. This can be reduced by subjecting the films to ion bombardment in a glow-discharge apparatus (see manufacturer's instructions), by exposing to UV light for 30 min, or by treating with 1% Alcian blue for 5 min. The use of wetting agents (e.g. bacitracin) in stains/buffers is also recommended.

The plastic film often sticks to the glass surface. Its release can be facilitated by abrading the glass with scouring powder while cleaning or by polishing the glass with a small amount of detergent rather than washing and rinsing. Alternatively, freshly cleaved mica can be used instead of glass.

As an alternative to casting films on a solid surface, collodion films may be cast directly on the surface of the water by allowing one drop of the plastic in amyl acetate (which floats on water) to drop onto the surface. Once the solvent has evaporated the grids may be placed on the resultant film.

Negative staining methods

The more frequently used techniques are described below. Specialist literature should be consulted for such methods as the negative staining carbon film technique developed by Horne and Pasquali-Ronchetti (in which suitable virus preparations are simultaneously crystallized and negatively stained), shadowing, and low temperature techniques such as freeze drying, freeze etching, and examination of viruses frozen in thin layers of ice.

One step method

This is the simplest and most widely used method.

1. Using fine, clean forceps and fine-bore pipettes, mix equal amounts (approximately 25 µl) of virus suspension and negative stain on a glass slide or a waxed surface.

2. Place a drop on a coated EM grid or float grid on surface of stain/virus drop.

3. After a few seconds remove the bulk of the fluid with the edge of a strip of filter paper. The longer the grid is in contact with the suspension the more virus will be absorbed. However, the

need for any greater sensitivity must be balanced against any deleterious effects of the stain on the virus.

4. Air dry the grid.
5. Examine in the EM: an initial examination will indicate if more/less stain is required.

Two step method

Some specimens contain high salt concentrations which are likely to mask virus particles. In addition longer adsorption times might be necessary (e.g. with low virus concentrations).

1. Apply virus suspension alone to the coated grid or float grid on a drop of virus suspension for from a few seconds to several hours (use a humidified chamber for adsorption times greater than 1 min).
2. Wash the grid gently with one or more drops of distilled water.
3. Add a drop of the negative stain. Penetration of stain into virus can be controlled by varying the staining time.
4. Remove the bulk of the fluid with the edge of a piece of filter paper.
5. Air dry the grid and examine in the EM.

Agar technique

This is another technique for either removing unwanted salts or increasing the adsorption of virus particles to the grid.

1. Prepare 1% agar in dH$_2$O on a glass slide. Agarose is equally useful. Gels can also be prepared in a disposable

microtitre plate which can be sealed, stored, and wells cut off as required.

2. Slightly dry the agar/agarose block (15 min in air) and place a drop of virus suspension onto the solidified agar or agarose.
3. Invert a coated grid on top of the drop. (Some workers recommend placing the grid under the sample, coated side uppermost.)
4. When the drop has been absorbed by the agar (up to 60 min), remove the grid.
5. Wash, stain, and examine as above.

Pseudo-replica technique

Yet another technique for reducing the effects of salt or improving virus adsorption.

1. Prepare 1% agar or agarose on a glass side.
2. Cut out a 1 cm^2 block, and dry slightly (15 min).
3. Place a drop of virus suspension on the block and allow to dry.
4. Flood the block with 0.5% formvar in ethylene dichloride or chloroform and allow to dry. Any other suitable plastic may be used (see Support films, page 93).
5. Trim the block slightly to facilitate release of the film and float the film (which now contains the virus particles) onto a suitable negative stain.
6. Pick up the film with a bare copper grid or place the grid onto the film and pick up both with filter paper.
7. Air dry the grid and examine in the EM.

Airfuge

Beckman Instruments Inc. produce a rotor (the EM-90) for use in their Airfuge centrifuge. This rotor is specifically designed for sedimenting virus particles onto coated grids for subsequent examination by EM. Sensitivity may be increased by up to 1000-fold over the usual 1-step technique, although cellular debris can be a problem with some clinical samples. In addition the rotor must be scrupulously washed after use to avoid contamination. This is of particular importance if the rotor is used for diagnostic purposes. The manufacturer provides excellent instructions.

Particle counting

A reasonably accurate determination of numbers of virus particles per unit volume requires a preparation of polystyrene latex particles of known size and concentration (commercially available).

1. Dilute a commercial preparation of latex particles to a concentration of approx 10^8 particles per millilitre.
2. Mix the virus preparation with an equal volume of latex particles.
3. Carry out a standard negative staining procedure. Some workers recommend the use of spraying procedures, however the hazards associated with spraying pathogenic organisms must not be underestimated.
4. Count the virus particles and latex particles per unit area. Counts may be performed either directly in the microscope or on electron micrographs. Measurements should be taken from different parts of the grid and from more than one grid.
5. Determine virus concentration by the following equation

$$\text{concentration of virus} = \frac{\text{concentration of latex} \times \text{virus count}}{\text{latex count}}$$

Calibration

The importance of an accurately calibrated EM cannot be overstated. One cannot accept the figures quoted by the manufacturer, and individuals are encouraged to treat calibration as a routine procedure.

Some commercially available calibration specimens are listed in Table 5.2.

Preparative techniques

To be detected by negative staining electron microscopy, the concentration of virus particles must be over 10^6 per ml. Also, non-viral debris must not obscure the virus particles.

Table 5.2.

Method	Comments
Diffraction grating replicas	Most useful have 2160 lines mm^{-1} and are cross-hatched. Useful up to 50–100,000× magnification.
Polystyrene latex particles	Particles of certified diameter within the range of 20–1000 nm are available. A statistically significant number of particles should be measured.
Holey single crystal gold film	Can be usefully employed up to 900,000×.
Negatively stained catalase crystals	Lattice plane spacings of 8.75 nm and 6.85 nm are clearly visible.

However the major advantage of negative staining EM in the clinical environment is its rapidity, thus any preparative techniques used need to be considered in this light. Specimens may be examined:

Directly, if virus is present in relatively high concentration and is unlikely to be significantly obscured by debris. Such specimens include preparations from vesicular lesions and faecal specimens.

After concentration, if virus is present in low amounts. Such specimens include urine, blood, and CSF. Concentrative methods include ultracentrifugation (100,000 g for 30 min) and Lyphogel.

After semi-purification, if virus is likely to be obscured by non-viral material in the specimen. Such specimens include faecal samples (especially when looking for the smaller viruses), and biopsy specimens. Techniques involve clarification by low speed centrifugation (5000 g for 10 min) followed by ultracentrifugation of the resultant supernatant.

Preparation of clinical specimens

Vesicular lesions

Dry vesicular fluid or scrapings from vesicles onto the centre of a microscope slide. Transport to the EM laboratory in a sealed container.

Resuspend the material in a drop of sterile distilled water.

Negatively stain and examine.

Viruses detected include herpes simplex and varicella zoster, molluscum contagiosum, and, rarely, Coxsackie virus (hand, foot, and mouth lesions).

Faeces

Resuspend faecal sample in dH_2O to 10% (the specimen may be examined at this stage with only a slight reduction in sensitivity).

Centrifuge at 5000 g for 15 min.

Centrifuge the supernatant at 100,000+ g for 60 min. Alternative concentration techniques include the use of Lyphogel and precipitation with ammonium sulphate.

Resuspend the pellet in a drop of single distilled water (sufficient to form an opalescent suspension).

Negatively stain and examine.

Viruses detected include: rotavirus, adenovirus, calicivirus, astrovirus, an assortment of small smooth round viruses (SSRV) and small round structured viruses (SRSV, including Norwalk virus), coronavirus-like particles, and reovirus.

Respiratory secretions

Some authors have described techniques for examining respiratory secretions for such viruses as influenza, parainfluenza, adenovirus, and respiratory syncytial virus. However such specimens are not examined by EM in the majority of laboratories.

Serum, urine, CSF

Centrifuge at $\geq$ 100,000 g for 60 min.

Resuspend the pellet, negatively stain, and examine.

Hepatitis B virus and human parvovirus may be detected in serum. Cytomegalovirus and BK virus (papovavirus) may be detected in urine.

Biopsy specimens

Grind the sample in single distilled water, or disrupt by freezing and thawing. Either use the sample directly or following a brief clarification at 5000 g.

Negatively stain and examine.

Papillomavirus or molluscum contagiosum may be detected in skin lesions. Herpes virus has been detected in brain biopsy samples from patients with suspected herpes encephalitis.

Cell culture

Centrifuge cells plus culture fluid at $\geq 100,000$ g for 60 min.

Resuspend the pellet in dH$_2$O (the osmotic shock releases the virus from the cells).

Negatively stain and examine.

Used to confirm cytopathic effect in cell culture. Routine screening of uninoculated cell cultures will often identify adventitious virions (paramyxovirus, foamy virus, polyomavirus), especially in simian cultures. Mycoplasma may also be detected.

Immune electron microscopy

Immune electron microscopy (IEM) is the visualization of the reaction between an antigen, usually a virus, and an antibody, and may be used to detect either component of this reaction. Thus the technique has been used to detect serological responses to such viruses as Norwalk virus; has assisted in the identification of rubella virus; and has been used diagnostically to identify hepatitis B virus infection and viruses associated with diarrhoea. The technique is also used routinely by some workers to serotype such viruses as rotaviruses, enteroviruses and adenoviruses. (See Fig. 5.3. for examples of use)

Classical technique

Mix equal volumes of virus and antiserum.

Incubate at 37°C for 60 min, then at 4°C overnight (although clumping can often be visualized after 15–30 min at 37°C).

Centrifuge at 20,000 g for 60 min, resuspend the pellet in single distilled water, stain and examine.

Clumping of virus particles indicates a positive result. However, some virus particles may clump naturally and care must be taken in interpretation. Concentrations of virus and antiserum may need to be modified as too little antibody and clumping will not occur; too much and virus particles will be obscured by the antibody.

Direct examination of clumping is often possible using the one or two step techniques. In addition, the agar technique (above) can be employed.

Clumps may also be picked up with protein A-coated grids (see below).

Serum in agar

This technique is a modification of the agar technique described above.

> Add antibody to molten agar or agarose (at approx. 40°C). Antibody concentration will need to be determined for each batch.
>
> Add to disposable microtitre plates and seal (can be stored for several months at 4°C).
>
> Cut off the required number of wells and place a drop of virus preparation on agar surface.
>
> Continue as for agar technique, page 96. Clumping of virus denotes a positive result.

Solid phase IEM (SPIEM)

The attachment of antibody molecules to EM support films, and the use of such antibody-coated films to trap virus particles, was a logical development of solid phase enzyme immunoassays.

> Float a coated grid on a drop of *Staphylococcus aureus* protein A in PBS for 30 min at RT (0.25–2 mg ml^{-1} is normally adequate).
>
> Wash in 5 drops of PBS.
>
> Float grid on a drop of antiserum in PBS for 30 min. The technique can be started at this point but with less sensitivity. Time may be increased (although some have suggested that 5 min is adequate).
>
> Wash as before (some workers recommend adding 0.1–1% bovine serum albumin and/or gelatine to the wash at this stage).

> Grids may be dried and stored at this stage for later use.
>
> Place grid on a drop of the specimen for a further 30 min. Time may be increased to overnight for more sensitivity.
>
> Wash as before (final wash in dH$_2$O).
>
> Stain and examine. A positive result is indicated by a higher number of virus particles attached to the grid compared with suitable controls.
>
> The grid can be floated on a second antibody before staining (SPIEM with decoration). A positive result to the second antibody is indicated by a halo around each virus particle.

Colloidal gold enhancement of IEM techniques

Identification of the immune reaction can be enhanced by labeling antibody molecules with electron dense markers. Such markers include ferritin or colloidal gold (which is available in a variety of well defined sizes). Although the primary antibody may be labeled, it is more usual, and more efficient, for a secondary anti-immunoglobulin to be labeled. Alternatively a cell wall component of *S. aureus*, protein A, which reacts with the Fc part of IgG, may be labeled. Colloidal-gold-labeled antisera (GLA) or protein A (PAG) may be used in the various protocols described above to enhance the visualization of the virus/antibody reaction.

> With the classical technique add GLA or PAG to reaction mixture for 10 min to 1 h after initial incubation, then proceed with the centrifugation or agar technique.
>
> With SPIEM use GLA as secondary antibody.

Thin section techniques

While negative staining techniques provide the resolution necessary to study viral morphology, the many interactions between viruses and cells (adsorption, uptake, morphogenesis, release) are best studied by thin section methods. In addition, viruses which do not demonstrate a well defined structure by negative staining are often more readily studied in thin section (for example rubella virus or the Retroviridae). The following basic methodology should prove adequate for most situations. Not included are techniques involving ultrathin cryosections.

Sample preparation

Tissue samples should be immersed in fixative and chopped with a scalpel or razor blade into cubes approximately 1 mm thick. Cell suspensions should be centrifuged gently (500 g for 10 min). The resultant pellet, if handled carefully, may be teased into 1 mm^3 'blocks' and treated as tissue. (Fixation will stabilize the cell pellet, especially if there was protein in the tissue culture medium.) Small pellets can be retained in centrifuge tubes and embedded *in situ*. A suitable cell pellet can also be formed with a haematocrit centrifuge.

Fixation, dehydration and embedding

Carry out primary fixation in 2.5% glutaraldehyde in phosphate buffer (pH 7.2) for 60 min.

Wash in PBS (three washes of 10 min each) and then post fix in 1% osmium tetroxide in PBS for 60 min.

Wash with three changes of dH_2O (10 min each).

Dehydrate in an ethanol series of 50%, 75%, 95%, 100%, 100%, each stage for 15 min.

Following 10 min in propylene oxide, infiltrate with resin/propylene oxide mixtures of 1:1 for 1 h followed by three changes in neat resin for 1 h each. Note that a variable speed rotator assists greatly in infiltration of specimens with resin. Blocks of tissue will sink when fully impregnated.

Place in capsules/trays with fresh resin, label.

Polymerize at 60° for 24 h.

Trim block and cut sections.

Modifications to the above procedure

A variety of fixative formulations have been employed. For example some workers recommend the use of 0.2 M cacodylate buffer for glutaraldehyde fixation and 0.2 M cacodylate, s-collidine, or veronal acetate buffers may be used with OsO_4. Other commonly used primary fixatives include glutaraldehyde/formaldehyde, glutaraldehyde/formaldehyde/acrolein, and glutaraldehyde/osmium tetroxide mixtures.

Treatment of tissue with 1% tannic acid in cacodylate buffer for 15–45 min prior to postfixation can both improve fixation quality and enhance electron contrast, especially of viral surface projections. The use of phosphate buffers is not recommended for this procedure and tissues should be washed (2 × 30 min) in cacodylate buffer prior to tannic acid treatment. A post treatment wash in 1%

sodium sulphate (5 min) is often employed. Tannic acid treatment may also be employed post-OsO_4 fixation.

Tissue may be stained with 0.5% uranyl acetate prior to dehydration (from 15 min to several hours) or with 2% uranyl acetate in the first (50% ethanol) dehydration step from 15 min to 1 h.

Dehydration may also be carried out by using acetone or by immersing the samples in 2,2-dimethoxypropane (DMP) for 2 × 15 min. (But note that block staining with uranyl acetate cannot be used with DMP.)

Infiltration times may be shortened with the use of low viscosity resins. For example, infiltration with Spurr's resin may be accomplished within 30 min and the resin will cure in 2–8 h at 70°C.

Sectioning

A full description of sectioning techniques is outside the remit of this chapter. Indeed, the methodology can only really be learnt from an experienced microscopist. Briefly, the cured resin block is trimmed to reveal the embedded sample. Semi-thin sections are cut to establish specimen orientation and morphology, and the block re-trimmed as necessary (to a surface area of approximately 1 mm^2). Ultrathin sections are cut with diamond, sapphire, or glass knives, and the sections are stained and examined.

Staining

Contrast is enhanced by staining sections. The commonest staining protocols utilize double staining with a uranyl salt followed by a lead salt. Staining is best performed on drops of stain placed on dental wax or parafilm in a small petri dish. Placing several NaOH pellets in the dish will ensure a CO_2-free environment which will avoid contamination of lead stains. A suitable schedule follows:

Filter or centrifuge all stains before use.

Place grid (with sections) face down on a drop of 1% uranyl acetate in single distilled water for 2 min.

Wash with 20 drops of single distilled water (boiled to remove CO_2).

Place grid face down on a drop of lead citrate (e.g. Reynold's) for 4–6 min. Dilution of the stain may be necessary to avoid overstaining.

Wash with 20 drops of boiled single distilled water. A first wash in 0.02 N NaOH assists in preventing contamination.

A double lead staining protocol of lead citrate (up to 10 min), uranyl acetate (up to 60 min), lead citrate (up to 30 min) has been recommended for poorly staining sections.

Immune EM

As with negative staining techniques, the visualization of the immune reaction is widely used for the detection of virus particles and antigens, and is of particular use in determining stages of viral morphogenesis. Both gold and ferritin labeled markers may be employed. In addition, enzyme labeled markers may be detected by visualizing the reaction product. There are two basic techniques, labeling either before or after embedding procedures.

Labeling prior to embedding

Surface antigens may be labeled prior to fixation and embedding (although a brief, mild fixation may assist in stabilizing antigens). The following protocol is for cells in suspension tissue culture.

Prefix in 0.5% glutaraldehyde for 5–10 min (not essential).

Wash cells in PBS.

Add a suitable dilution of primary antibody in PBS for 30 min.

Wash three times in PBS.

Add a suitable dilution of gold-labeled conjugate for 30 min. Gold labeled protein A can be used.

Wash in PBS.

Fix and embed as described above.

Post embedding labeling

Internal antigens are best detected by staining sections. However fixation and embedding techniques must be adjusted to retain antigenicity. The following technique is recommended.

Prepare formaldehyde freshly from paraformaldehyde.

Fix in 3% formaldehyde/0.1% glutaraldehyde in PBS for 30 min.

Wash in PBS.

Embed in LR White resin. Infiltration

schedule is: 75% ethanol/resin 3:1, 60 min; 100% resin, 60 min; 100% resin, 12 h.

Polymerize at 55°C for 24 h.

Cut sections. Collect on carbon coated plastic films (nickel grids are recommended).

Float on a drop of 1% BSA in PBS (PBSA) for 2 h to overnight (1% non-fat dried milk or 1% bacitracin in PBS may be used).

Float on a drop of antibody in PBSA for 2 h.

Float on PBSA for 10 min (×3).

Float on PAG for 1 h (GLA may also be used).

Wash with PBSA (×3) then dH$_2$O.

Stain with uranyl acetate and lead citrate and examine. Note that post-fixation with 2.5% glutaraldehyde, washing with dH$_2$O, and staining with 1.8% uranyl acetate containing 0.2% methylcellulose has also been recommended. Note also that, for visualization of gold particles, overstaining at this stage must be avoided.

Lowicryl resins may also be used. Their advantage is that tissues may be embedded at low temperatures (−30°C).

Photography

Photographic techniques are an essential aspect of EM. Although specific details are impossible to give, the following general recommendations should be considered.

Micrograph quality is a function of: negative size (the larger the negative, the less the enlargement required), emulsion type (must be fine grain and provide sufficient contrast), development (timing and temperature are vital for consistency), fixation and washing (if not performed correctly negatives will deteriorate), and enlargement procedures (the use of a point light source, condenser enlarger and glossy paper will increase print contrast). The use of poly-contrast paper, coupled with a print processor is most useful, however many electron microscopists prefer hand-produced prints, especially for publication purposes. The production of prints by non-electron microscopists should be discouraged.

Scanning EM (SEM)

Although available for some time, SEM has only recently been recognized as an effective technique for visualizing viruses budding from cell membranes. Of the many methods published, the following has produced some excellent results.

The technique requires the use of poly-L-lysine coated coverslips. These are prepared by floating coverslips on poly-L-lysine (1 mg ml^{-1} in dH$_2$O) for 10 min and air drying.

Pellet cells gently (500 g for 5–10 min), resuspend in a small volume of medium.

Flood a poly-L-lysine coated coverslip with cells, leave for 5 min (note that cells may be grown on coverslips and fixed *in situ*).

Fix in 2.5% glutaraldehyde in isotonic cacodylate buffer (pH 7.4) for 1 h at 37°C and overnight at 4°C.

Processing is best performed in a continuous flow apparatus to avoid drying artifacts.

Wash in PBS.

Post-fix in 1% OsO$_4$ in isotonic cacodylate buffer (pH 7.4) for 1 h. Treatment with 1–5% tannic acid in dH$_2$O for 30 min followed by a further post-fixation in 1% OsO$_4$ for 30 min has also been recommended.

Dehydrate rapidly in ethanol (25%, 50%, 75%, 100%, 100%; 1–2 min each stage).

Critical point dry in CO$_2$ following the manufacturer's instructions. Air drying has been used but with considerable shrinkage.

Mount coverslip on a specimen stub.

Sputter coat with gold/palladium (5 nm) (again following the manufacturer's instructions).

Examine.

Bibliography

Madeley CR, Field AM (1988) Virus Morphology (2nd Ed.) Churchill Livingstone.

Nermut MV, Steven AC (Eds.) (1987) Animal Virus Structure, Elsevier Science, New York.

Doane FW, Anderson N (1987) Electron Microscopy in Diagnostic Virology. A Practical Guide and Atlas. Cambridge University Press.

Hayat MA (Ed.) Principles and Techniques of Electron Microscopy. Van Nostrand Reinhold.

Glauert AM (Ed.) Practical Methods in Electron Microscopy, Volume 3 part 1: Fixation, Dehydration and Embedding of Biological Specimens (Glauert AM); Part 2: Ultramicrotomy (Reid N); Volume 5: Staining Methods for Sectioned Material (Lewis PR and Knight DP); Volume 6 part 1: Autoradiography and Immunochemistry (Williams MA); Volume 10: Low Temperature Methods in Biological Electronmicroscopy (Robards AW and Sletyr UB); Volume 13: Sectioning and Cryosectioning for Electron Microscopy (Reid N and Beesley JE). American Elsevier Publishing Company, New York, USA.

Bozzola JJ, Russell LD (1992) Electron Microscopy: principles and techniques for biologists. Jones and Barttell, Boston, USA.

Traditional serological tests

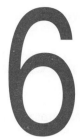

M. A. Chernesky

Serological tests have the dual capacity to be used for diagnosing recent infection or determining a patient's immunity status. Both structural and nonstructural components of viruses usually induce antibodies during infection. Over the past 30 years many traditional techniques have been developed and applied for several viruses. The following tests could be considered traditional: neutralization, complement fixation (CF), hemagglutination inhibition (HI), single radial hemolysis (SRH), particle agglutination with latex (LA) or labeled erythrocytes (called passive hemagglutination – PHA), immunodiffusion, counter immunoelectrophoresis (CIEOP). Some of these have been replaced as routine tests by immunoassays but they are still often used as reference tests.

Virology Methods Manual
ISBN 0–12–465330–8

Neutralization

Neutralization tests can be performed with any virus and especially with those which neither hemagglutinate nor react in CF tests (Schmidt 1979). In principle, virus and antiserum are mixed and allowed to react for an appropriate time. The mixture is then inoculated into a susceptible host system which is observed for signs of infection. By the use of specific antisera, unknown viruses may be serologically identified. Conversely, specific viruses may be used to test for serum antibodies. Cross-neutralization tests between two viruses and their antisera may be used for antigenic comparison of the viruses, for which they are particularly suitable because neutralization tests are usually more narrowly specific than other serological tests. Variations of the test are possible, utilizing different hosts and indicator effects. Examples of systems for demonstrating neutralization are as follows: counting 'pocks' on the chorioallantoic membrane of embryonated eggs inoculated with vaccinia serum-virus mixtures; counting deaths in groups of newborn mice inoculated intraperitoneally with Coxsackie group A serum–virus mixtures; observing inoculated tubes of cell cultures for the development of specific cytopathic effects (CPE), hemagglutinins (HA) or hemadsorption (HD) effects, or counting focal 'plaques' of cell degeneration in monolayers of cell cultures overlaid with agar gel medium after inoculation (see page 33).

Methods

Most viruses grow in one or other type of cell culture, usually producing CPE, and can be conveniently tested by inoculation of culture tubes either as a 'constant virus-varying serum method' or 'constant serum-varying virus method'. The first method, in which a constant predetermined dose of virus is allowed to react with various dilutions of one or more sera, allows the antibody level to be expressed as a 'titer' (calculated as the final dilution of serum in initial serum–virus mixture at endpoint). The second method makes serial dilutions of virus which are mixed with a single dilution of serum. The virus is titrated in the presence of control non-immune serum, and unknown or specific antiserum. The difference between these titers is the 'neutralization index' (NI), usually expressed as the $\log_{10}$ NI. It is calculated by subtracting the $\log_{10}$ titer with the test serum from the $\log_{10}$ titer with non-immune control serum.

Materials and reagents

Viruses

The most commonly used neutralization test measures protective antibodies or recent infection with enteroviruses (by showing a four-fold or greater rise in titer between acute and convalescent sera in a paired test). A pool of infectious virus suspension is prepared in cell cultures, clarified and freed of aggregates by centrifugation, divided into aliquots, and preserved by freezing. For each neutralization test, a fresh aliquot of virus is thawed and diluted as indicated by preliminary titration. As a routine, one hundred 50%-infectious-units (ID_{50}) per inoculum is used for constant virus-varying serum tests.

Sera

Suitable initial dilutions of sera are heat-inactivated (56°C, 30 min) before use in order to destroy complement and other labile non-specific neutralizing or potentiating factors. When testing some weakly reactive viruses or nonavid sera, higher titers may be achieved by adding fresh, unheated, antibody-free guinea-pig serum before mixing with virus. Specificity of reference antisera should have been established by previous tests against homotypic and heterotypic viruses.

The neutralization reaction

Equal volumes of serum and virus are mixed and held for an appropriate time and temperature to allow virtually complete reaction to take place without significant thermal destruction of virus. As a rule, 1 h at room temperature (or in a refrigerator for labile viruses) is sufficient.

Controls

(a) Virus controls are always required to check the infectivity of virus suspensions used in the test.
(b) Specificity controls: the possibility of nonspecific neutralization of viruses is controlled by testing them with several different antisera or with 'normal' nonimmune serum of the same species. These conditions are easily satisfied in the preliminary 'screening' test of an unidentified virus isolate since it is then tested against several antisera. Errors of identification or deterioration of reference reagents can be controlled by testing the prototype virus and corresponding antisera against one another. This can be done in the confirmatory test of identification of an 'unknown' virus isolate.
(c) Serum toxicity controls may be necessary, especially in cell cultures, and sometimes with other host systems.

Assay for neutralization

After completion of the reaction, mixtures should be inoculated immediately, or held in the refrigerator for a short time if delay is unavoidable. Significant differences in time from preparation of mixtures to their inoculation should be avoided. Control virus titrations should be inoculated last as a check on deterioration during the test (intelligible results may often be obtained with too high a virus dosage, but rarely with too low). The standard volume of the various mixtures inoculated into appropriate test-hosts are as follows: 0.2 ml per cell culture tube, 0.03 ml intraperitoneal or intracerebral per day-old mouse, 0.1 ml on to the chlorioallantoic membrane of a 12-day egg.

Quality control

Inoculated eggs, animals or cultures are held under appropriate conditions until the indicator effect has fully developed (this is judged by previous virus titrations, and is indicated by the behaviour of virus controls in the test run).

Interpretation

Inoculated animals are scored for paralysis, death, etc., eggs for numbers of chorioallantoic pocks, etc. cell cultures for specific CPE or for HA or HD reactions or other appropriate indicator effect. Provided the controls are satisfactory, interpretation of the test is usually straightforward. Titers are conveniently calculated by simple methods such as the Karber or the Reed and Muench, both of which can be found in most text books on statistics (also see page 37). The presence of neutralizing antibodies is the best measure of viral immunity. A change in neutralizing antibody titers between paired sera from a patient tested in the same test on the same day is indicative of recent infection.

Complement fixation

The complement fixation (CF) test measures CF antibodies to a particular virus in a patients' serum by mixing the serum with an optimal amount of antigen. If antibodies are present they will attach to the CF antigens. When this occurs in the presence of added complement the immune complex 'fixes' it and eliminates it from solution, so that it is not available to react with an added indicator system consisting of sheep erythrocytes sensitized with antiserum to self (hemolysin). Elimination of the free complement by the virus-antibody complexing prevents lysis of the sheep erythrocytes. The test is made quantitative by diluting serum specimens in serial two-fold steps and then testing each dilution for CF activity.

Materials and reagents

Hemolysin

Hemolysin is anti-sheep erythrocyte antiserum produced in rabbits or horses and is normally supplied as a 50% solution. It is used as a 1/100 working stock solution which can then be further diluted on the day of the test.

Complement

Complement is supplied lyophilized in ampoules and must be reconstituted immediately before use to 1/8 which corresponds to a dilution of 1/10 of the original guinea-pig serum.

Erythrocytes

Sheep erythrocytes are supplied washed and stabilized as a 10% suspension of packed cells which can be stored for up to 2 weeks at 4°C if formalinized or up to 4 weeks if preserved in Alsever's solution (dextrose-citrate buffer). On the day of the test the cells are washed and resuspended in veronal buffer to a concentration of 4%.

Buffer

Veronal (sodium barbital) buffer is pH neutral, in the range 6.8–7.4, and contains Mg^{2+} and Ca^{2+} ions. The cations are important for complement binding and allow the reaction to occur even at high dilutions of serum when the naturally occurring divalent salt concentration would be suboptimal. Correct formulations for veronal buffer are available commercially in the form of tablets which are dissolved in sterile distilled water.

Antigens

Antigens for diagnostic serology are available commercially in lyophilized form. CF antigens can be prepared from laboratory animals, embryonated eggs or cell cultures of high potency. They must have a minimum amount of host cell material which might give anti-complementary activity and other non-specific reactions. Viruses such as rubella, the herpes viruses and arboviruses require extraction in alkaline buffer (glycine or borate) to improve potency. Some viruses such as respiratory syncytial virus and adenoviruses release antigen into the medium of infected cultures to a sufficiently high titer to allow the use of the culture medium as CF antigen. Control antigens should be prepared in the same manner from the same lot of uninfected cells that are used for viral antigens. Well prepared antigens should have a titer in the region of 32–128. Anti-complementary activity can usually be removed by heat treatment or absorption with guinea-pig complement.

Sera

Test sera must be collected in sterile containers containing no preservatives or anti-coagulants. Ideally 5–10 ml blood is collected which should yield at least 2–3 ml serum for testing. Plasma cannot be used in the CF test since it will be anti-complementary. When collecting and separating the blood, hemolysis should be avoided. In order to make a diagnosis using the CF test, it is usually necessary to obtain two specimens. The first (acute phase) blood should be taken as soon as possible after onset of illness, the second (convalescent) blood should be taken 10–14 days later. Standard sera with known antibody titers to specified antigens are included in the test as positive control sera. They are supplied in lyophilized form and should be reconstituted to 2–4 times the stated titer for the test.

Microplates

Plastic plates as 96-well ('U'-shape) microplates, using multiwell diluters and disposable plastics for convenience and safety are used for the test.

Methods

Reagent standardization, (complement, hemolysin, antigen and control sera) is performed before carrying out the test. Both the sensitivity and the specificity of the test are affected by the relative concentrations of the reagents used. The optimum concentrations for all the reagents are determined in 'checkerboard' titrations and each new batch of the reagents has to be standardized.

1. Determination of the optimum concentrations of hemolytic serum (hemolysin) and complement is performed as follows:
   (a) 2 volumes of diluent are added to the wells of a 96-well microplate. (This represents 1 volume of serum and 1 volume of antigen in the test proper.) A third volume of diluent is added to the wells of one of the columns in place of complement control wells.
   (b) Dilutions of complement are prepared in tubes containing veronal buffer and 1 volume of each dilution is added to the appropriate wells. The plates are incubated overnight at 4°C or at 15°C.
   (c) The next day, a series of dilutions of hemolysin are prepared in tubes from the 1/100 stock solution and mixed with a series of dilutions of a 4% suspension of sheep RBCs in a checkerboard titration. The cells and the hemolysin dilutions are mixed 1:1 and placed at 37°C for 10–30 min. After the plates are warmed to 37°C the hemolytic system is added to the appropriate wells, covered and incubated at 37°C for 30 min with intermittent shaking, then read. Complete hemolysis is scored as 0 and no hemolysis as 4. The optimal sensitizing concentration (OSC) of the hemolysin is defined as the dilution which gives complete lysis with the highest dilution of complement. Similarly, the minimum hemolytic dose (MHD) of complement is defined as the dilution of complement giving complete lysis with 1 OSC of hemolysin. Some laboratories

read the CF test at 50% hemolysis and 1 unit of complement is then defined as the dilution giving 50% lysis (HD_{50}) with 1 OSC of hemolysin.

2. Titrations of antigen and standard serum are carried out, using a similar procedure as that used for complement and hemolysin as follows:

(a) Before serum specimens are diluted for testing they are heat-treated at 56°C for 30 min to inactivate native complement.

(b) The test procedure is started by adding 3 unit volumes of barbitone buffer to the first column of wells of a 96-well microplate and 1 volume of buffer to each of wells 2–12 in each row. One volume of heat-inactivated patient's serum is added to the first well and dilutions are then made across the plate to column 10 to give a series of doubling dilutions from 1/4 to 1/2048. One volume of serum dilution is drawn from well 1 and transferred to well 11 and a further volume is likewise transferred to well 12. These wells provide the serum control and the control antigen.

(c) The freeze-dried antigens are reconstituted with sterile distilled water and diluted to double their optimal concentration (2 units). One volume is added to each of the wells up to column 10 as appropriate. One volume of diluent is added to well 11 in place of antigen as the 'serum control'. Control antigens are diluted and added to well 12 as appropriate.

(d) In addition to serum and antigen controls, a control titration of standard positive serum, with the matching antigen, is set up as for the test sera, including a control for anti-complementary activity.

(e) The complement is diluted to working strength and 1 volume is added to all the wells, including the control wells. The complement controls are set up in three wells to contain dilutions of the complement from working strength, e.g. 3, 1, 0.5 HD_{50}.

(f) A fourth well containing just 4 volumes of buffer without complement) is prepared as the sensitized erythrocyte control for autolysis. The plate is covered with a lid or adhesive film and incubated overnight.

(g) The next morning a 4% washed erythrocyte suspension is prepared in barbitone buffer, mixed with hemolysin (1 OSC) and placed at 37°C. The test plate is removed from the incubator and allowed to warm. The sensitized cells are added to each well, including all the controls, and the plate is sealed and placed at 37°C for 30 min. During incubation the plate should be agitated at 10-min intervals on a shaker.

(h) The plate is removed from the incubator and read immediately if the 100% end-point is used or, after allowing the erythrocytes to settle, if the 50% end-point is used.

Quality control

The cell control must show no lysis. The serum controls and control antigen wells should show lysis. The standard antiserum control should give the right titer and the complement control should show the right potency. Inaccuracies in the titrations of antigen (or antibody), complement or hemolysin or in the standardization of sheep erythrocytes may be compounded by errors during test performance. It may be necessary to titrate complement in the presence of test antigen at the concentration to be used in the test. Commercially prepared complement should be tested for the presence of specific antibodies to certain viruses. Complement obtained in lyophilized form after reconstitution, should be divided into samples large enough for one run and kept frozen, preferably at −70°C. Each sample must be thawed only once just before use. Sheep erythrocytes must be washed and standardized carefully to prevent cell lysis or enhanced sensitivity of the cell membrane to complement. A hemolysin titration should be performed each time a new lot of hemolysin is used. If heat inactivation is ineffective, to eliminate inherent anticomplementary activity in sera, absorb them by mixing 150 μl of serum with 50 μl undiluted complement. The mixture is left for 30 min at 37°C and then 1 ml of veronal buffer is added to make a 1/8 dilution of the serum. If the serum continues to be anticomplementary, an additional serum specimen should be requested and tested.

Interpretation

Results of the CF test are meant to confirm the physician's provisional clinical diagnosis and should be considered within the larger context that includes the epidemiologic background, past medical history, previous immunizations, pertinent laboratory data, and current physical examination findings.

The antibody titer of a serum is expressed as the reciprocal of the highest dilution of serum showing 100% or 50% lysis, whichever is used in the test. An infection is diagnosed using the CF test by demonstrating a seroconversion in antibody status or a greater than 4-fold rise in the antibody titer, between paired sera collected during the course of the illness. The use of high CF titers as a method of diagnosis generally must be regarded as unreliable in individual patients. Complement-fixing antibodies in many cases appear later than those detected by other tests (e.g. hemagglutination inhibition and neutralization) and are generally short-lived, becoming undetectable after a few years in most cases. This characteristic regarding the kinetics of CF antibodies can be useful in timing the activity of certain infections (e.g. rubella). Timing of infectious activity can also be ascertained by the use of different preparations of CF antigens. In mumps, for example, antibodies to the soluble antigens (i.e. mixture of virion components and virus-directed proteins released upon the disintegration of viral particles or infected cells) appear and disappear earlier than those produced against the viral antigens (i.e. intact virions), which rise later and persist for years. Another approach to determining the recent onset of a primary infection is the detection of IgM CF antibodies after the removal of IgG by a number of procedures (e.g. staphylococcal protein A or G). This approach does not always lead to conclusive results, since IgM antibodies may recur upon reactivation of a latent infection (e.g. cytomegalovirus), remain for more than a year (e.g. rubella virus), or persist at very low levels for many years in chronic carriers (e.g. hepatitis B virus). In any case, IgM antibodies against viral antigens can rarely be detected in the CF test.

Hemagglutination–inhibition

The principle of the hemagglutination–inhibition (HI) test is to measure, by dilution, the level of inhibiting antibodies in a patients' serum that will prevent agglutination of susceptible erythrocytes by viruses that are able to attach to erythrocyte receptors. It is really a neutralization test with erythrocyte agglutination as the indicator system. The classical HI test is best described for measuring rubella antibodies (Chernesky and Mahony 1995).

Materials and reagents

Microtiter plates

The test is conveniently performed in disposable plastic or vinyl V or U-bottom microtiter plates.

Antigen

Rubella hemagglutinating (HA) antigen is titrated each time the test is performed. HA antigen is available commercially but to prepare it infect monolayers of BHK-21 cells grown in 32-oz (960 ml) bottles with 5–10 ml of rubella stock containing 10^4 or more 50% tissue culture infective doses per ml. After the virus has adsorbed for 2 h at 37°C, the monolayers are covered with Eagle medium containing 2% fetal calf serum that has previously been adsorbed with kaolin. The medium is changed after 24 h and then harvested for HA antigen after days 5 and 7 of incubation. High-titered antigen can be extracted from the monolayers by extracting the cell-associated antigen with alkaline buffers (e.g. 0.1M glycine buffer, pH 9.6).

Erythrocytes

Whole blood is collected by drawing a sample from a pigeon wing vein into modified Alsever solution. The erythrocytes are washed three times in HEPES (N-2-hydroxyethylpiperazine-N-2-ethanesulfonic acid)-saline-albumin-gelatin buffer (HSAG) (pH 6.2), and the packed cells are suspended in an equal volume of HSAG to make a 50% suspension.

Buffer

HSAG is made from three different stock solutions: (i) 5X HEPES-saline, (ii) 2X BSA, and (iii) 100X gelatin. HEPES-saline is made by adding 29.8 g of HEPES powder, 40.95 g of NaCl, and 0.74 g of $CaCl_2$ to 1 liter of water and adjusting the pH to 6.2. BSA is made by adding 20 g of BSA powder to 1 liter of water. Gelatin is made by adding 25.0 mg of gelatin to 2 liters of water. All solutions are filtered. A working solution of HSAG is made by adding 200 ml of HEPES-saline to 500 ml of BSA solution and 100 ml of gelatin stock solution. The volume is made up to 1 liter by adding 200 ml of sterile distilled water. The pH of the working solution should be 6.25. The solution can be stored for 2 months if it remains sterile. HSAG may be purchased from commercial sources.

Test sera

Test sera are pretreated with kaolin. Acid-washed kaolin powder can be purchased from most scientific supply companies. Kaolin (25 g) is washed with Tris buffer until a pH of 7.0 or greater is achieved. The Tris buffer is made by mixing 12.1 g of Trizma base, 80 ml of 1 N HCl, and 0.85 g of NaCl and bringing the volume to 1 liter. This solution is then further diluted 1:10 in distilled water for washing the kaolin. After the final wash in Tris buffer, the kaolin pellet is suspended in 100 ml of Tris-bovine albumin buffer. Tris buffer is made by adding to 96.67 ml of Tris buffer the following ingredients: 0.33 ml of a 35% sterile solution of bovine serum albumin, 1 ml of a 0.5% $MgCl_2$ $6H_2O$ solution, 1 ml of an 8% NaN_3 solution, and 1 ml of a 0.5% $CaCl_2$ solution.

Methods

Dilution of antigen and calculation of HA

Serial twofold dilutions of the antigen are made in 0.025 ml of HSAG (pH 6.2) to which 0.05 ml of a 0.25% washed suspension of pigeon erythrocytes is added. Control cups containing no antigen are included. The plates are sealed and placed at 4°C for 1 h, after which time they are placed at room temperature for 15 min before being read. The highest dilution that produces a pattern of complete hemagglutination is considered 1 HA unit; 4 HAU are used in the HI test.

Washing and absorption of erythrocytes

Part of a 50% suspension of a pigeon erythrocytes suspension is used to absorb nonspecific agglutinins from the test sera. A 10% working suspension is made in HSAG, from which the 0.25% suspension to be used in the test is prepared.

Removal of nonspecific inhibitors

Before the HI test is performed, nonspecific inhibitors of hemagglutination and nonspecific agglutinins must be removed from sera. Test serum (0.1 ml) is added to 0.1 ml of HSAG and 0.6 ml of a 25% suspension of kaolin. The suspension is mixed and allowed to sit at room temperature for 20 min with frequent agitation. The kaolin is pelleted in a clinical centrifuge, and the supernatant fluid is transferred to a clean tube containing 0.05 ml of a 50% suspension of pigeon erythrocytes. After 60 min of incubation at 4°C, the erythrocytes are centrifuged; the supernatant fluid is removed and heated at 56°C for 30 min. This final sample, which represents a dilution of 1:8, is ready to be incorporated into the test. Alternatively, nonspecific inhibitors may be removed by precipitation with heparin and manganous chloride. The serum sample is diluted 1:4 with 0.15 M NaCl. To each 0.8 ml of diluted serum are added 0.03 ml of sodium heparin (200 U) and 0.04 ml of 1 M manganous chloride. The sample is held at 4°C for 20 min, and the precipitate which forms is pelleted by centrifugation. The supernatant fluid is then absorbed with pigeon erythrocytes as described above. Known positive and negative control sera are treated similarly.

Performing the HI test

Serial twofold dilutions of each serum are made in 0.025 ml amounts of HSAG. An area of the plate is reserved for duplication of the first three dilutions of each serum. These dilutions receive HSAG in place of antigen and serve as serum controls. To each other dilution of serum is added 4 HAU of antigen in a volume of 0.025 ml. The antigen is back-titrated in a separate section of the plate by doubling dilutions in 0.025 ml of HSAG to represent 4, 2, 1 and 0.5 HAU. The plates are incubated for 1 h at room temperature, after which 0.05 ml of a 0.25% suspension of pigeon erythrocytes is added to each well and the plates are mixed on a plate vibrator. The hemagglutination pattern is read after 1 h at 4°C. The highest dilution of serum that completely inhibits hemagglutination is taken as the endpoint or rubella titer.

Quality control

Quality control of the HI test is not as crucial as in the CF test but care needs to be taken in the use of fresh reagents. All reagents used in the HI test must be carefully controlled from one test to the next. The World Health Organization provides HI antibody standards which can be used for the rubella HI system. All pretest procedures and appropriate controls described above must be observed to enable valid testing and interpretation.

Interpretation

Interpretations are made for the declaration of immunity, or in the case of paired sera testing, recent infection. The presence of HI antibodies to a dilution of at least 10 international units is generally accepted as immune to rubella. Correct interpretation of HI results at lower dilutions requires inhibition in at least the first two wells of the tray and an accurate back titration of antigen in the test. A four-fold difference in titer between acute and convalescent sera performed in the same test on the same day is required to be declared representative of a recent infection. All other controls in the test must be as expected.

Particle agglutination

Materials and methods

Particle agglutination tests come in several forms. Most commonly used in the clinical laboratory is the slide agglutination procedure, in which the particle reagents are added to the surface of a slide. Generally, the particles are white and the background slide is black. After the particle reagent which is coated with antigen, is added to the slide, the serum or cerebrospinal fluid sample is placed next to it and the mixture is shaken. Clumping represents the combination of antigen and antibody.

Slide agglutination reactions have several major advantages; they are very fast and easy to perform, their use in the laboratory can be decentralized so that they may be performed as needed without interference with the work flow, and they are usually cost efficient. Disadvantages of the slide test include the need for reading skills, the particular care needed to ensure that clumping is not due to nonspecific interactions or that antibody is missed because of a prozone effect. Many antigens will directly adsorb onto the surface of latex particles or erythrocytes. Erythrocytes are subject to degradation and must be treated to provide stability and to enable optimal adsorption of antigen onto the surface. Formalin can be used to increase the adsorption of polysaccharides, proteins, and haptens. Tannic acid and pyruvic aldehyde can be used to stabilize the cell membrane through the tanning process.

Quality control

Commercial manufacturers follow quality control production procedures to ensure consistency of their products, and it is important that users follow the protocols in the package insert for obtaining quality results. Reagents should be stored appropriately and not used beyond the expiration date unless steps have been taken to ensure accuracy of results. In the daily performance of these tests, the laboratory protocol must allow for appropriate controls to be performed. Alongside each specific reagent (i.e. carrier with detecting antisera or antigen), the patient specimen must be run with a nonspecific control reagent (i.e. carrier with irrelevant antisera or antigen). Care must be taken to ensure that the control reagent used is similar in immunoglobulin components to the specific or test reagent (e.g. equine polyclonal antisera for both or mouse monoclonal IgG1 for both).

It is also important that both test and control reagents be tested with positive and negative controls.

An additional potential problem is lot-to-lot variation in sensitivity and specificity. It is good laboratory practice to make limited in-house evaluations of each new lot of materials. This can easily be done either by making serial dilutions of the positive control from each lot and running a comparison with both lots or by maintaining a laboratory-standardized pool of specimen and determining the titer of this pool with each new lot of reagents.

Interpretation

Interpretation of the pattern of agglutination is subjective and hence an additional source of error. Most manufacturers provide instructions that use a 1+ to 4+ grading system as compared with either the positive or negative controls. Strict adherence to the labeling, package inserts, and recommendations of the manufacturer for interpretation is important for both accurate and consistent results. In laboratories in which more than one technologist performs these tests, each positive finding in body fluids should be confirmed by an additional reader.

When used to detect the presence of antibody, agglutination tests are screening tests; that provide a yes or no answer to the presence of antibody. In some circumstances, this result can be interpreted as immune or susceptible (e.g. in determining immune status to rubella virus). Although IgM is a very good agglutinating agent, the methodology for determining this specific class of antibody is generally not performed for agglutination tests.

Serial dilutions of patient serum can be used to obtain a semi-quantitative concentration of antibody. This has some clinical value if one has performed epidemiological studies to determine normal limits. As with many other serological tests, demonstration of a change in titer can provide evidence for a recent infection. The decision to use most agglutination tests generally rests on the need for rapid results or the nature of a particular clinical setting. The issue of cost may at times also be decisive.

Single radial hemolysis (SRH)

Radial hemolysis can be used to screen large numbers of sera by preparing plates in advance and storing them at 4°C. The most widespread use of this test is for rubella serology.

Material and methods

Freshly drawn sheep erythrocytes are washed with dextrose-gelatin-Veronal buffer, treated with 2.5 mg of trypsin per milliliter in dextrose-gelatin-Veronal for 1 h at room temperature, and sensitized with rubella HA antigen (240 HAU in HSAG buffer, pH 6.2, for 1 h at 4°C). Sensitized erythrocytes (0.15 ml of a 50% suspension) are mixed with 0.4 ml of guinea pig complement and then added to 10 ml of 0.8% agarose preheated to 43°C and poured into a petri dish (100 mm by 15 mm). Plates can be stored at 4°C and used for up to 14 days. Prepoured radial hemolysis plates are available from commercial sources. Sera are inactivated at 56°C for 30 min, pipetted into 3-mm-diameter wells punched in the agarose, and allowed to diffuse overnight at 4°C in a humidified atmosphere. Plates are then incubated for 2 h at 37°C. Plates with incomplete hemolysis are flooded with 4 ml of guinea pig complement (diluted 1:3) and reincubated.

Quality control

All sera are tested in control plates containing unsensitized erythrocytes to monitor non-specific hemolysis. Zones of hemolysis in control plates may range from 3.5 to 5 mm in diameter.

Interpretation

Zone diameters of > 5 mm are taken to indicate immunity for rubella. Significant differences in zone diameters between acute and convalescent sera may suggest titer change. Sera may also be titrated in the system.

Immunodiffusion

This method permits the comparison of antigen–antibody reactions between an antigenic solution and various antisera or antiserum and various antigenic solutions on the sample plate. Through the agar-gel medium contained in a petri dish, antigen and antibody diffuse towards each other from separate wells. One well is centrally located and the others are peripheral to it at equal distance. The antigen solution may be placed in the central reservoir and the various antisera in the others, or vice versa. Patterns of lines of precipitate form between the central and one (or more) of the peripheral wells containing serologically related materials. The number of precipitate lines indicates the minimum number of antigen–antibody reactions present.

Materials and methods

Agar-gel diffusion medium is prepared to contain 1.0–1.5% agar in PBS solution, pH 7.4. After autoclaving and cooling to 45°C, merthiolate and methyl-orange are added in a final concentration of 0.01% and 1:300,000 respectively. Portions of agar-gel diffusion medium (15 ml) are poured into petri dishes and allowed to harden at room temperature. Cups of 7 mm in diameter, 7 mm apart are cut from the agar with the aid of a cutting template. Each cup is filled with 0.05 ml of antigenic solution[s] and antisera. The plates are incubated at room temperature or at 35°C in a humidified chamber and observed daily for signs of precipitation bands for a period up to two weeks.

Quality control

Sera with any particulate matter should be clarified by centrifugation before testing. Optimal antigen and antibody concentration should be determined previously for the system.

Interpretation

A precipitation line between the serum test well and the antigen well joining in identity (position in the agar) with a known serum reacting with the diffused antigen indicates the presence of antibody to the antigen.

Immunoelectrosmophoresis (IEOP)

In this technique, antigen and antibody are electrophoresed toward each other in agar or agarose so that they interact and form a precipitate. At pH 8.6, negatively charged antigens will have anodic mobility, whereas the electroendosmotic effect will give antibody molecules cathodic mobility. Thus, under the influence of the electric field, the antigen and antibody molecules will migrate toward each other. However, because the reactants are being forced to move, once they meet there will be little time available for the lattice to develop. Consequently, the antibodies used must be of high affinity.

Material and methods

IEOP kits have been provided from commercial sources which contain clear instructions for performing the test and interpreting the results. Internal controls are provided and the instructions of the package insert should be followed carefully.

Quality control

The ionic strength of the buffer should be low to promote precipitation (barbital buffer, pH 8.6, with ionic strength of 0.05 is appropriate). Since the reactants will be close to their original concentrations when they meet, they need to be at near equivalence ratio to begin with; the reactants cannot diffuse to achieve equivalence ratio as in double diffusion. Antigen excess can therefore be a serious problem. When the antigen concentration is unknown, several different antigen/antibody ratios should be used to try to bracket the equivalence ratio. The plate should be watched closely during electrophoresis. A precipitate may become visible within 10 min of the start; the power should then be switched off and the lattice allowed to build up. If no precipitate is seen, the electrophoresis should be continued for a limited time only, usually 30 min, and the plate should then be left for 10–20 min to permit any lattice to form. It is a mistake to continue electrophoresis beyond about 30 min, since the reactants will have moved through each other. The advantage of this procedure is that the time taken for precipitation is decreased greatly. In addition, there is considerably less dilution of each reactant per unit distance travelled than in passive immunodiffusion, and this procedure is thus more sensitive than simple diffusion procedures.

Interpretation

According to the instructions in the kit package insert, a precipitation line after appropriate electrophoresis indicates the presence of antibodies at a unit dose in the serum tested, or antigen present if a clinical specimen is assayed.

Comments

Although these traditional serological tests have been replaced by enzyme immunoassays and therefore have been eliminated from many working laboratory manuals, they will continue to serve as reference standard tests for comparative purposes. This is especially true for the neutralization test which remains the closest measurement of humoral immunity for any viral infection.

References

Chernesky MA, Mahony JB (1995) In: Manual of Clinical Microbiology, 6th edn., Murray PR, et al (Eds.), ASM Press, Washington, D.C., pp. 968–973.

Hsiung GD (1994) Complement Fixation Test: Hsiung's Diagnostic Virology, 4th edn., Hsiung GD (Ed.) Yale Univ Press, New Haven, Conn and London, pp. 76–82.

Schmidt NJ (1979) In: Cell Culture Techniques for Diagnostic Virology: Neutralization Tests in Diagnostic Procedures for Viral, Rickettsial and Chlamydial Infections, 5th edn. Lennette EH and Schmidt NJ (Eds.) Am Pub H Assoc, Washington D.C., pp. 104–111.

Immunoassays: principles and assay design

7

M. A. Chernesky
J. B. Mahony

Immunoassays may be constructed as liquid phase (LPIA) or solid-phase (SPIA) types. LPIA were popularized in the field of chemistry but have not been extensively explored for microbiology. Most LPIA are competitive between assayed sample and labeled sample. After determination of the fraction of labeled sample bound by antigen or antibody the concentration of sample can be calculated by comparison with results for appropriate standards. In the absence of a solid phase to separate labeled and unlabeled samples the procedure depends upon a change in the specific enzyme activity when antibody-antigen complexes form. SPIA for the detection of antigens or antibodies use as reaction indicators: a radioactive label for the radioimmunoassay (RIA), an enzyme which will react with a substrate in an enzyme immunoassay (EIA), or a fluorescent dye used in a fluorescent immunoassay (FIA). The substrate to be acted on by an enzyme may be fluorescent, radioactive, chemiluminescent or chromogenic.

Virology Methods Manual
ISBN 0–12–465330–8

Antigen detection

Most SPIAs for the detection of antigen employ one of three methods: (1) competitive; (2) direct (double-antibody sandwich method); or (3) indirect (double-antibody sandwich-antiglobulin method). In competitive assays, labeled antigen is mixed with the test sample that may contain antigen and they compete for a limited amount of antibody attached to the solid phase. A negative control sample containing only labeled antigen is included. Unbound antigen is washed away and the difference in indicator activity between the specimen and control is measured. A direct SPIA for detection of antigen involves adding the clinical specimen to a capture antibody (CA) attached to the solid phase. Unbound antigen is washed away before the addition of a labeled detector antibody (DA). The DA is measured and the more labeled substrate detected, the more antigen is present in the sample. The indirect test is similar to the direct assay employing a CA and DA, but the DA is not labeled. Instead, a third indicator antibody (IA) that is anti-species to DA is labeled; the remainder of the assay is similar to the direct procedure. This approach has become the most popular because of the availability of IA conjugates from commercial sources. The indirect test provides some amplification of the binding reactions. They may create some problems, however, as they are very sensitive and anti-species antisera may cross-react nonspecifically.

Competitive assay

Specific antigen present in a test specimen inhibits the binding of a predetermined amount of labeled antibody to antigen immobilized on a solid phase. The detector antibody can be labeled with enzyme, ^{125}I or biotin and the solid phase can be beads, plates or tubes.

The following protocol describes the detection of rat rotavirus using biotinylated antibody and peroxidase labeled avidin–biotin complex (Vonderfecht et al 1985):

1. Coat wells of a polystyrene microtiter plate (Immulon 2; Dynatech Laboratories Inc., Alexandria, VA) with 100 µl of either rat rotavirus antigen or control antigen diluted optimally in carbonate buffer, pH 9.6 overnight at 4°C. The optimal concentrations of viral antigen and biotin-labeled antibody are determined by checkerboard titration.
2. Mix an equal volume (50 µl) of the test specimen, diluted 1:5 in fetal bovine serum (FBS), with biotin-conjugated antirotavirus antibody diluted in phosphate buffered saline (PBS) containing 0.05% Tween 20 and 0.5% gelatin and incubate for 1 h at 37°C then place into precoated microtiter plate wells. Incubate for 1 h at 37°C then wash wells three times with PBS.
3. Add 0.1 ml of preformed peroxidase-avidin-biotin complex (Vector Laboratories, Burlingame, CA) and incubate for 1 h at 37°C.
4. Wash the wells, add the substrate (0.4 mg OPD and 0.4 µl of 30% H_2O_2 per ml of 0.01 M citrate buffer, pH 5) and read at 450 nm. Subtract the OD of wells with control antigen from the OD of wells with rotavirus antigen to determine specific activity and determine percent inhibition as 100 × (1 − net specific activity divided by negative control). The specificity of the inhibition reaction can be verified by blocking with specific immune serum.

Comment

Despite the relative ease of performing the competitive assay and its excellent sensitivity this assay has not been widely adopted in clinical laboratories.

Sandwich assay

The assay can be either a direct (using an enzyme-labeled detector antibody as the indicator) or an indirect (using a second enzyme-labeled anti species antibody following the detector) assay and employ either polyclonal or monoclonal antibody reagents. Assays with the combination of polyclonal capture and monoclonal detector antibodies usually provide the best performance. Sandwich assays have been developed for a number of viruses (rotavirus, influenza, RSV) and several are available as commercial kits. The following protocol describes the detection of rotavirus antigen in stool specimens using 96-well microtiter plates (Yolken et al 1980).

1. Coat alternate rows of microtiter plates with goat antirotavirus antiserum and non-immune goat serum (0.1 ml) diluted 1:10,000 in PBS (0.5 $\mu g\ ml^{-1}$) and incubate overnight at 4°C. Wash plate five times with PBST.
2. Add 50 μl diluted stool filtrate and 50 μl N-acetylcysteine (to decrease binding of stool material to non-immune globulin) in duplicate to the antirotavirus antibody and control antibody coated wells, and incubate for 2 h at 37°C. Wash the plate five times with PBS.
3. Add 100 μl enzyme-labeled antirotavirus antibody optimally diluted (approximately 1:2000) in PBS containing 2% fetal bovine serum and incubate for 1 h at 37°C. Wash five times.
4. Add freshly prepared substrate (p-nitrophenyl phosphate for alkaline phosphatase or OPD for peroxidase)

and incubate for 30 min at room temperature.
5. Calculate specific reactivity by subtracting the mean activity of the specimen in wells coated with non-immune serum from the mean activity of wells coated with antirotavirus antiserum. A specimen is considered positive if its mean reactivity is greater than 2 standard deviations above the mean of the negative controls.

Comment

The direct assay has the advantage of requiring only a single detection antibody. The indirect assay may be more convenient if the laboratory is doing a number of different EIAs and wants to use a single enzyme-labeled indicator antibody. The indirect assay is generally more sensitive than the direct EIA.

Immunodot assay

The immunodot assay (IDA) for antigen is similar to Western blotting for antibody as both use nitrocellulose membranes. In IDA viral antigen in a clinical specimen is detected by dotting the specimen onto nitrocellulose and reacting the strip with antiviral antibody in either a direct or indirect format. IDA has been used to detect HIV following amplification of virus in H9 cell culture (Blumberg et al 1987) and to detect rotavirus antigen in stool specimens. A modification of IDA called immune complex dot assay (ICDA), where antigen is allowed to react with specific antibody and the antigen-antibody complex is spotted onto nitrocellulose and detected with colloidal gold-labeled anti species antibody, has been described (Wu et al 1990). ICDA was more sensitive than IDA for detecting rotavirus antigen in stool specimens.

The following protocol describes the detection of rotavirus antigen by IDA:

1. Spot 1 µl of stool specimen (10% stool filtrate in dH$_2$O) together with positive and negative controls onto nitrocellulose strips with a Drummond microdispenser and allow to dry for 15 min at room temperature.
2. Block the strips with 2 ml of 1% BSA–0.5% gelatin in PBS for 20 min at 37°C.
3. React the strips with rabbit anti-rotavirus antiserum diluted 1:1000 in blocking solution for 90 min at 37°C then wash strips with PBS twice for 5 min each.
4. React the strips with gold labeled-anti rabbit IgG antiserum (GAR G15, Janssen Chimica) diluted 1:10 for 2 h at room temperature on an orbital shaker (50 rpm). Wash twice with PBS and once with dH$_2$O.
5. Place the strips into silver enhancement solution (Janssen Chimica) for 20 min then wash with tap water and air dry.

Antibody detection

Competitive measurement

In a competitive assay format human antibody against a viral antigen(s) can be measured by combining the sample with a predetermined amount of conjugated antibody directed against the same viral antigen(s) and incubating the mixture with the antigen-coated solid phase. Specific antibody, if present in the sample, will compete with the conjugated antibody for binding sites on the solid phase and lead to a reduction in signal. The signal generated will be inversely proportional to the amount of sample antibody.

Antibodies against the antigens of interest can be prepared in animals or purified from human serum. Alternatively, specific monoclonal antibodies can be developed. The antibodies must be purified, conjugated with the appropriate label (fluorochrome, enzyme, lanthanide, or radioisotope), and rigorously evaluated before use. An important aspect of conjugate evaluation involves the serial titration of the conjugate against serial dilutions of antigen to measure activity and define the titration curve of the conjugate across several antigen concentrations. Each conjugate titration curve will exhibit a point at which the next dilution of conjugate will exhibit a substantial drop in signal (Fig. 7.1). Several conjugate-antigen dilution pairs that meet the basic criteria should be selected then further characterized with respect to sensitivity, using preparations containing known amounts of antigen-specific antibody. The goal is to select the conjugate antigen pair that contains the highest dilution of conjugate and antigen which will:

(i) permit the generation of high signal
(ii) exhibit a substantial reduction in signal in the presence of sample antibody
(iii) allow the measurement of small amounts

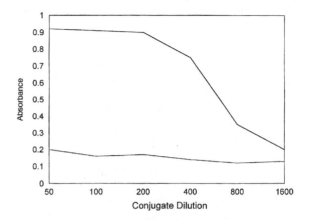

Figure 7.1. Titration of anti IgG conjugate. BK virus antigen (top line) or control antigen (bottom line) were coated onto wells of a 96-well microtiter plate. Mouse anti BK virus antiserum diluted 1:1000 was the detection antibody. Goat anti-mouse IgG antibody conjugate was serially diluted and detected with OPD substrate.

of sample antibody against all important antigenic determinants.

Competitive assays are based on a limiting-reagent concept where solid-phase antigen and conjugate concentrations are minimized so that even small quantities of sample antibody can effectively block the binding of conjugate. An advantage to using the competitive format for antibody measurement is the relative ease with which highly specific antibodies, especially monoclonal antibodies, can be purified and conjugated. In general, antibodies are easier to purify than antigens, and since the specificity of the test is conveyed by the conjugate relatively impure antigen can be used on the solid phase. Another advantage is a reduction in the number of procedural steps since sample and conjugate can be incubated with the antigen on the solid phase. Competitive assays are generally more sensitive than indirect assays. Competitive RIAs and EIAs have been used to measure antibody to HB core Ag (anti-HBc). The anti-HBc assay has been commercialized by Abbott Diagnostics and has been used extensively in clinical laboratories for over twenty years (Mushahwar et al 1978; Purcell et al 1984).

The following procedure describes the detection of anti-HBc by competitive RIA using plastic beads.

1. Viral antigen is used to coat 6 mm polystyrene beads by passive adsorption using carbonate buffer pH 9.6 (with or without the use of initial capture antibody coated to the solid phase).
2. An aliquot of serum undiluted (0.1 ml) is mixed with 0.1 ml of ^{125}I-anti-HBc solution, the mixture is added to an antigen coated bead and incubated overnight at room temperature.
3. The bead is washed with water and counted in a gamma counter. A reduction of 50% in the count compared to a negative control sample is considered positive for anti-HBc.

Comment

The format of this assay has been changed over the years from RIA to EIA and more recently to microparticle EIA but the principle of the assay has remained unchanged. The competitive assay format can be used to measure antibody to any virus and provides a simple (one-step) sensitive assay.

Non-competitive IgG or total antibody measurement

Either direct or indirect approaches may be used to construct a SPIA to measure antibodies in a patient's specimen. The solid phase is usually coated with either antigen(s), or anti-immunoglobulins (anti-total or anti-

class, i.e. anti-IgG, -IgM, -IgA etc.). If the solid phase is coated with antigen all classes of antibodies in the specimen will be trapped. A conjugated DA which is anti-species can then be used to detect all antibody classes trapped or the DA can be specific for a class such as anti-human IgM or IgG. This approach usually requires the pre-adsorption of the sample with anti-rheumatoid factor (RF) or aggregated IgG to eliminate RF interference (described in more detail below). When anti-species antibodies are used on the solid phase they are usually anti-IgM. This approach will capture only IgM, which will be available for the DA which can be labeled antigen available to act on an added substrate. Alternatively at this stage an unlabeled antigen is added then detected by a virus-specific DA (which may be labeled for a direct assay) or followed by a labeled anti-species antibody.

A further modification of the antibody class capture assay, and one that will permit the measurement of antigen-specific IgG, involves the use of labeled antigen and a solid phase coated with RF-IgM. A sample containing antigen-specific IgG is mixed with labeled conjugate and incubated with the solid phase coated with RF-IgM. Only antigen-specific IgG complexed with labeled antigen is bound by the RF-IgM; therefore, only a single incubation step is required. Antigen quality, as well as the quality of RF-IgM coating the solid phase, must be carefully assessed.

The noncompetitive technique has been widely used to measure specific anti-viral antibody because it requires only a few reagents, is easy to perform and provides an objective quantifiable result. The assay is most often performed in microtiter plates or on plastic beads although it can be adapted to plastic tubes, microparticles, paramagnetic beads or other solid surfaces. This format has allowed commercial companies to develop automated instrumentation with increased throughput for processing several hundred specimens per day.

The following procedure describes the detection of BK papovavirus antibody (Mahony et al 1989) but it can be used to detect either IgG or

IgM antibody to any virus for which antigen can be obtained:

Procedure

1. BK virus purified by CsCl ultracentrifugation from infected cell culture is diluted in carbonate buffer, pH 9.6 and passively adsorbed to wells of 96 well polystyrene microtiter plates for 2 h at 37°C.
2. The plates are washed with phosphate buffered solution (PBS) and blocked with PBS containing 10% FBS for 2 h at 37°C. The blocking reagent is removed and the plate dried by tapping on paper towels. Control antigen-coated wells are prepared in the same way using mock-infected cultures.
3. Serial two fold dilutions of sera to be tested (50 µl) diluted in Buffer G (0.01 M phosphate buffer pH 7.2, 0.3 M NaCl, 0.001 M $MgCl_2$, 0.5% gelatin, 0.1% FBS) are incubated in duplicate in BKV antigen and control antigen coated wells for 3 h at 37°C.
4. BKV IgG or IgM antibody is detected by adding 50 µl of HRP-conjugated goat anti human IgG or IgM immunoglobulin diluted optimally in buffer G (usually 1:400–1:1200 depending on the supplier) for 1 h at 37°C.
5. OPD substrate (50 µl) is added and the plates are incubated for 30 min followed by 3 N HCl stop solution (50 µl). The plates are read in a microtiter plate ELISA reader at 492 nm. The cutoff for positivity is established as twice the mean (or X + 3 SE) of 5–10 representative negative specimens (obtained from a similar patient population).

Comment

There are many variations of this EIA protocol. Some use blocking solutions and diluents containing Tween-20 or NP40 detergents, some incubate at room temperature, 37°C or 4°C, some use HRP-conjugate, while others use alkaline phosphatase conjugates (see below). We have successfully used the above protocol with minor modification to measure specific antibody to BKV, *Chlamydia trachomatis*, Parvovirus B19 and CMV.

Immunoblotting

Immunoblotting or Western blotting has been used to detect specific antibodies to a number of viruses. Viral proteins are first separated by polyacrylamide gel electrophoresis and trans-blotted to nitrocellulose or nylon membranes then reacted with clinical specimens usually sera, but saliva or urine can be tested. Recombinant immunoblot assays (RIBA) use recombinant proteins expressed in prokaryotic or eukaryotic expression systems instead of viral polypeptides in the form of purified viral antigen prepared from infected cell culture. Western blot and RIBA have been successfully commercialized and supplementary or confirmatory kits are available for detecting antibody to a number of viruses including HIV-1, HTLV-I and HCV. These assays can also be used for typing herpes simplex virus and HIV. The following protocol describes a Western blot assay for detecting HSV-1 and HSV-2 specific antibody as described by Ashley and Militoni (1987).

1. HSV-1 (strain KOS) and HSV-2 (strain 333) viruses are used to infect separate cultures of human diploid fibroblast cells (MOI of 1). Cells are harvested at 3+ CPE by gently scraping with a rubber policeman.
2. Cells are washed in PBS, collected by low speed centrifugation (5 min at 500 *g*) and suspended in a small volume (0.25 ml for each 75 cm^2 flask) of lysis buffer (0.125 M tris, pH 6.8, 20% glycerol, 8% SDS, 10%

2-mercaptoethanol, 0.025%
Bromphenol Blue) and frozen in
aliquots at −70°C.

3. Aliquots of HSV-1 and HSV-2 are
thawed, boiled for 10 min, and
electrophoresed on a 9%
polyacrylamide gel with a 4°C stacking
gel at 100 volts for 2 h. Proteins are
electrophoretically transferred to
nitrocellulose at 100 V for 1 h (Bio Rad
mini Protein gel transblotter).

4. Reactive sites are blocked by
incubating the NC paper in 5% (w/v)
Blotto in PBS for 1 h at room
temperature on an orbital shaker.
Rinse with 0.1% Tween-20 in PBS
(PBST) twice for 10 min each and cut
NC into strips 3 mm wide.

5. Dilute serum to be tested 1:50 in PBS
and incubate for 1 h at room
temperature with one HSV-1 and one
HSV-2 strip. Rinse the strips twice in
PBS then incubate in HRP-conjugated
goat anti human IgG antibody diluted
1:500 in PBS for 1 h with gentle
shaking. Rinse the strips again and
incubate in freshly prepared 4-chloro-
1-naphthol (0.5 mg ml^{-1}) substrate
containing 0.025% hydrogen peroxide
in PBS and allow color to develop for
5–10 min then stop with distilled
water. Dry and store strips in the
dark.

Comment

For the detection of HSV-1 and HSV-2
specific antibody each serum must be
tested on an HSV-1 and HSV-2 strip (Fig.
7.2). Interpretation is based on the
following criteria (Ashley et al 1993). A
predominance of antibody to either
HSV-1 or HSV-2 blots is interpreted as
infection with HSV-1 or HSV-2
respectively. HSV-1 positive sera will
contain antibodies to 11–18 HSV-1
proteins (gB, gG, gC-GE, VP16, gD, p45)
and lack antibody to the 92 kDa HSV-2
glycoprotein G (gG-92) on the HSV-2
blot. HSV-2 positive sera generally show

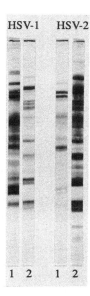

Figure 7.2. Immunoblot detection of HSV-1 and
HSV-2 type-specific antibody. Serum from two individuals with culture-documented HSV-1 and HSV-2
infections were reacted with immunoblot strips of
HSV-1 (1) or HSV-2 (2) infected cell lysates. Antibodies were visualized with HRP-anti human IgG
antibody conjugate and 4-chloro-1-naphthol.

fainter bands than HSV-1 positive sera
therefore, some sera showing strong
reactivity on the HSV-2 blot will require
preadsorption to clarify the HSV-1 type.
HSV-2 positive sera react primarily with
proteins in the HSV-2 strip, have a gG-92
band and will show 16–24 HSV-2 bands
(major bands of 150 kDa, gG-92, gG-70,
52 kDa, 49 kDa, 47 kDa, 45 kDa) and
fewer than 6 HSV-1 bands. Sera with
both HSV-1 and HSV-2 antibodies have
full antibody profiles on both strips and a
clear gG-92 band. Some sera will require
adsorption with type 1 or 2 virus for
typing.

Radioimmuno-precipitation (RIPA)

In RIPA specific anti-viral antibodies are detected by immunoprecipitation of radio-labeled viral proteins followed by either scintillation counting of washed precipitates or immune complex dissociation, polyacrylamide gel electrophoresis and autoradiography to identify specific proteins. This method has not had widespread application in virology but is still used by some laboratories in place of Western blotting as a confirmatory test for HIV. The following protocol for HIV antibody has been adapted from Tersmette et al (1988).

1. HIV-1 is propagated in H9 cells in the presence of ^{35}S-methonine or ^{35}S-cysteine (10 µCi ml^{-1}) for 8 h and a cell lysate is prepared by scraping and homogenizing cells in 0.125 M Tris-HCl, pH 6.8, 8% SDS, 0.1 M 2-mercaptoethanol.
   An alternative approach is to purify HIV on a sucrose gradient, treat with 0.2% Triton X-100 and label with ^{125}I using chloramine-T (the preparation can be enriched for HIV glycoproteins by adsorption to lentil-lectin sepharose beads and elution with 0.3 M α-methyl-D-mannoside).
2. An aliquot of viral lysate containing 5×10^4 cpm of labeled protein is incubated with 5 µl of serum for 16 h at 4°C.
3. An aliquot of protein A-Sepharose beads (5 mg) is added and the mixture incubated 90 min, pelleted and washed four times with PBS followed by a final wash in 10 mM Tris-HCl, pH 6.8.
4. Bound immunoprecipitates are eluted with 8% SDS and 0.1 M 2-mercaptoethanol and analyzed by polyacrylamide gel electrophoresis and autoradiography.

Comment

RIPA is a labour intensive test employing metabolic or surface radiolabeling and immunoprecipitation techniques that are usually restricted to research laboratories. It has the advantage of being more sensitive and specific than Western blot especially for the detection of high molecular weight glycoproteins of HIV.

IgM measurement

The most common assays for IgM use a standard indirect solid-phase ELISA with the antigen immobilized and an IgM-specific secondary DA. As mentioned above false positivity is common due to the presence of IgM rheumatoid factor (RF) in the patient sample. False negativity can also occur from competitive inhibition of IgM binding in the presence of high levels of specific IgG. One way to approach these problems is to use an isolated IgM preparation from the patient sample, removing IgG which acts as a substrate for IgM RF and competes with the specific IgM for binding to the antigen or remove all of the IgG with the addition of a precipitating anti-IgG. An alternative approach is to remove the RF itself by using an aggregated IgG preparation. RF false positives can be eliminated by treatment of serum with commercial adsorbents such as RF sorbent (Behringwerke) (Zapata et al 1984).

A second approach is to modify the type of immunoassay by using an IgM capture assay. In this procedure, a polyclonal anti-IgM antibody is bound to the solid phase. Upon incubation of the patient sample, all IgM will be captured on the plate. The test antigen is then added, binding any specific IgM present on the plate. An enzyme-labeled secondary antibody is then added, and the reaction is completed. This assay obviates the problems with false-negative results due to competitive inhibition with IgM, as all of the IgG in the patient sample is washed away in the first step. False positive results, however, may still occur as a result of bound IgM RF either reacting with the IgG conjugate or binding any antigen-specific IgG in the sample. One way to avoid the problem with conjugate binding is to use F(ab')$_2$-conjugated antibodies. Alternatively, the assay can be modified to a direct technique by employing enzyme-labeled antigen in the second step, thus eliminating any immunoglobulin that could bind RF. Even with these modifications, problems can still occur with borderline and low positive IgM results.

Antibody capture assays can be used to measure antiviral IgG, IgM or IgA antibody. The following RIA procedure has been used to detect IgM antibody to parvovirus B19 (Cohen et al 1983), but the method can be modified to detect either IgG or IgM antibody to other viruses.

Procedure

1. Wells of microtiter plates are coated with sheep anti-human IgM antibody diluted 1:200 in carbonate buffer, pH 9.6 for 2 h at 37°C. All reagent volumes are 50 μl per well and washes are with PBS containing 0.5% Tween-20 (PBST).
2. Serial serum dilutions beginning at 1:200 are prepared in buffer G (as above but containing 2% normal sheep serum) and inoculated in plates overnight at 4°C.
3. Parvovirus B19 antigen is prepared by ultracentrifugation of viremic serum is diluted optimally in buffer G (usually 1:200–1:800) and added to the wells. The plates are incubated for 3 h at 3°C.
4. A mouse monoclonal antibody to parvovirus B19 viral capsid protein diluted in buffer G is added at optimal dilution and the plate is incubated for 1 h at 37°C.
5. HRP-conjugated affinity purified goat anti mouse IgG antibody optimally diluted in buffer G is added and the plate is incubated for 1 h at 37°C followed by OPD substrate.
6. The plates are read in an ELISA plate reader and the cut-off determined as twice the mean absorpance of 5–10 IgM negative sera. IgM antibody titers are determined as the highest serum dilution with an absorpance greater than the cut-off.

Comment

Capture assays can be formatted as an EIA or RIA. For RIA, a ^{125}I-labeled anti species antibody (2–10 μCi ug^{-1}; usually 10,000 cpm per assay) is substituted for enzyme-labeled conjugate and the assay is run on other polyvinyl chloride plates and individual wells are cut apart with scissors or on plastic beads and the beads counted in a gamma counter. Specific reactivity is expressed as a Binding Ratio (cpm for viral antigen divided by cpm for control antigen).

Solid phases

A number of surfaces can be used for SPIAs: plastic, polyvinyl chloride, nitrocellulose, agarose, glass, cellulose, polyacrylamide, and dextran. Plastic is by far the most popular, especially with the frequent use of 96-well microtiter plates. These plates can be purchased in intact form or as 8- or 12-well individual strips for running a small number of samples. Plastic beads are also popular, especially with some commercial companies. Most antigens and antibodies are bound through hydrophobic interactions. Proteins generally are used at a concentration of 1–50 μg ml^{-1}. A high-pH (9.6) carbonate coating buffer is often used as the diluent (1.59 g of Na_2CO_3; 2.93 g of $NaHCO_3$; 0.2 g NaN_3 made up to 1 l distilled water and stored at 4°C for 2 weeks); however, the optimal buffer should be determined experimentally for each system. In addition to passive absorption, immunoreactants can be coupled covalently by a variety of methods.

Absorption depends on the concentration and type of antigen, surface characteristics of the plastic, time, and temperature. Several studies have shown that use of too much antigen may actually result in the stacking of several layers of antigen, which results in a protein-plastic layer that is subsequently covered by a second layer formed by protein-protein interactions. To avoid this problem, at least three washes, and preferably more, should always be performed between assay steps. Both the isoelectric point and chemical composition of the antigen may affect its ability to adhere to the solid phase. Lipid antigens may pose difficulties in obtaining reproducible coating to the wells of the solid phase. It is critical with these types of antigens that several plates be screened for optimal coating. In addition, the physical characteristics of 96-well microtiter plates have important variables such as an 'edge effect' in which the perimeter wells of plates may absorb more protein than the inner wells, thereby causing an assay bias. Different plates from several manufacturers should be screened for this effect when an assay is set up. When the lot of a plate is changed, they should be reevaluated to ensure that none of the assay parameters need to be modified. Coated plates generally are stable for a few weeks to several months, depending on conditions. Most antigens have the greatest stability when dessicated in a foil pack. Commercial kits usually have plates packaged in this way, providing a longer shelf life. For in-house assays in which stable packaging may be more difficult to achieve, the integrity of the solid phase should be closely monitored. A procedure which should always be conducted is to wash stored plates prior to use so as to remove any free antigen that may have desorbed during storage.

Conjugate

Depending on the assay, if it is an EIA it must contain either an antibody or an antigen conjugated with an enzyme. The desirable properties of such an enzyme include a high turnover rate, stability, low cost, ease of conjugation, lack of endogenous enzyme in the patient sample, easy detection, and compatibility with the standard conditions used. The most popular enzymes are alkaline phosphatase (AP) and horseradish peroxidase (HRP). A variety of other enzymes are also available, but they are not as frequently used. These include B-galactosidase, glucose oxidase, urease, and carbonic anhydrase, which are primarily used in immunohistochemistry and for assays with a fluorometric or other end point.

There are a number of choices available for an antibody conjugate: whole polyclonal antibodies, immunoglobulin G (IgG) fractions or F(ab')$_2$ fragments of polyclonal antibodies, affinity-purified polyclonal antibodies. It is best to screen several antibody preparations and choose the conjugate that provides optimal results for the least cost. The least purified antibodies, such as whole polyclonal conjugates, are inexpensive, but they frequently give a high background. This problem can often be alleviated with the use of an IgG fraction of the same antisera. If one is performing an IgM assay or using an antigen source containing Fc receptors, use of F(ab')$_2$ antibodies may significantly improve results. Overall, affinity-purified antibodies often give the best results, with high detectability and low background levels. In addition, they are available from several commercial companies and are relatively inexpensive. AP conjugated affinity-purified antibodies are generally more expensive than HRP conjugates. Monoclonal antibodies are the most expensive but some assays require the specificity that they offer.

In choosing the proper dilution of an antibody conjugate, one can run a checkerboard titration using a high and low positive standard along with buffer alone. The optimal conjugate dilution is one in which the absorpance of the high positive control is 1.0 or greater, coupled with background levels of less than 0.1 absorpance unit. A checkerboard titration is performed as follows:

1. The plate is coated horizontally. Four different antigen or antibody coating concentrations can be tested, with each concentration added to duplicate horizontal rows.
2. Following this coating step, unreactive sites are blocked by using a nonspecific protein, i.e. BSA, gelatin, or nonfat dry milk. For test samples, we use a high positive patient control, negative control, and PBS alone. For control specimens, a 1:100 dilution is often used since most analytes can be measured at this level and nonspecific binding is decreased.
3. Following an incubation of 1–2 h at RT, the plate is washed 3–6 times with PBS.
4. The conjugate is added in a vertical fashion to the plate. Four dilutions in triplicate wells can be used per 96-well plate, in rows 1 to 12. The conjugate dilution will vary greatly with the type of antibody used (dilutions may range from 1:50 to 1:100,000).
5. After incubation for 1–2 h, the enzyme reaction is developed with the appropriate substrate. The optimal choice for the assay is a combination of antigen concentration and conjugate dilution that gives a PBS value of < 0.05, a negative control of <0.2, and a high positive control value of >1.0 absorpance unit.
6. This checkerboard titration may have to be modified if a positive control serum is not available. In this case, the antibody conjugate titration can be performed by coating the solid phase with the immunoglobulin protein to which the antibody conjugate is directed. Following determination of an appropriate conjugate dilution, the solid phase can be coated in a range from 1 to 50 μg ml^{-1}, as this is the most commonly used range of concentrations in all EIAs.
7. Once these optimal concentrations are determined, a large number of patient samples can be screened and a pool of positive controls can be obtained.

Enzyme-antibody conjugation

Excellent enzyme-labeled antibodies of various specificities are available from several commercial sources. However, in some circumstances it may be necessary to label antibodies in the laboratory. The procedure begins with enrichment of the antibodies from serum or ascites fluid. This initial step is required so that proteins other than antibodies will not be labeled and give false-positive results. Antibody enrichment is conveniently performed by using ammonium sulfate fractionation, ion-exchange chromatography, or protein A columns. The second stage represents coupling of the enzyme to antibody. Several methods, including periodate oxidation and gluteraldehyde procedures are widely used. The conditions used ordinarily result in optimum labeling of the antibody. Blocking solutions and wash buffers containing detergent are required to decrease nonspecific color intensity in EIA procedures. When the concentration of protein in the coating solution is suboptimal for saturation of microwell binding sites, an immunologically irrelevant protein is used to occupy (block) the remaining plate surface. Buffers containing bovine serum-albumin or gelatin are commonly used for this purpose. To prevent nonimmunological interactions in the microwell plate wells, all subsequent reagents are added in buffers containing detergent (usually 0.1% Tween-20). In addition, all washing steps between reagent additions are also done in buffers with Tween-20.

An example of an enzyme antibody conjugation is the periodate method.

To 4 mg of peroxidase in 1 ml of distilled water, add 0.2 ml of freshly prepared 0.1 M NaIO$_4$ and stir gently for 20 min.

(On addition of the periodate, the solution should change color from gold to green; if it does not do so, additional $NaIO_4$ is required.) Dialyze the mixture against 1 mM sodium acetate buffer, pH 4.4, overnight at 4°C. Raise the pH by addition of 20 μl of 0.2 M sodium carbonate–bicarbonate buffer (pH 9.5). Immediately add 8 mg of antibody in 1 ml of 0.01 M sodium carbonate buffer, pH 9.5. Stir for 2 h at room temperature. Add 0.1 ml of freshly prepared sodium borohydride (4 mg ml^{-1} in distilled water). Leave for 2 h at 4°C. Precipitate with saturated ammonium sulfate.

Substrates

When deciding on a substrate for an enzyme conjugate, there are several factors to consider. First, the substrate must produce a measurable soluble reaction product. For most EIAs this is a colored reaction product, although fluorescent substrates can be used. Other variables to consider include sensitivity, background absorpance, stability of the compound, toxicity, and cost. Toxicity is a particular concern, since a number of substrates have been suggested to be potentially carcinogenic. If the color will be monitored spectrophotometrically, the maximum wavelength of the absorpance is also a factor, since readers generally come with a limited number of filters.

A variety of substrates are available for HRP (Table 7.1). The enzyme reduces hydrogen peroxide (H_2O_2) and oxidizes a second substrate, which produces a colored reaction product; thus, H_2O_2 is always required along with another substrate. The most popular substrates include o-phenylenediamine (OPD), 5-aminosalicylic acid, 2,2-asinodi-(3)-ethyl-benz-o-thiazoline-6-sulfonate, and 3,3′,5,5′-tetramethylbenzidine (TMB). Although various studies have shown some substrates to be preferable to others, generally they all perform adequately in most assays. In setting up a new procedure, several substrates may be evaluated to determine the optimal compound. Regardless of the secondary substrate used, the most critical variable in catalyzing HRP is the concentration of H_2O_2. This is usually kept as a 30% solution; however, it has limited stability and may account for significant inter-assay variability.

For AP, the most popular substrate is p-nitrophenyl phosphate (pNPP), which absorbs strongly at 405 nm. pNPP is generally dissolved in a high-pH diethanolamine buffer with magnesium added. Use of phosphate-buffered saline (PBS) as a wash buffer in AP-based EIAs may result in low optical density (OD) values. Phosphate is a potent inhibitor of AP, so any phosphate left in the plate wells after washing may cause an inhibition of the enzyme reaction. Although many laboratories report few problems with use of PBS as the

Table 7.1. Commonly used enzymes and substrates for enzyme immunoassays.

Enzyme (Source)	Substrate	Colour Change/Reading
Peroxidase (Horseradish)	o-phenylenediamine (OPD) 5-5′-tetramethylbenzidine (TMB) 5-aminosalicylic acid	Clear to yellow (490 nm)
Alkaline phosphatase (Calf intestine)	p-nitrophenylphosphate	Clear to yellow (405 nm)
Beta lactamase (B. cereus or E. coli)	starch-potassium iodide	Purple to clear (590 nm)
Urease (Jack bean)	urea and a pH indicator bromocresol purple	Yellow to purple (590 nm)

wash buffer in AP-catalyzed EIA, it is a variable to consider if the color reaction does not develop sufficiently. One can substitute a Tris buffer for PBS, as Tris may actually increase AP activity.

Enhancement of SPIA signals

Bacterial proteins

Cell wall proteins in Cowan strains of *Staphylococcus aureus* bind to immunoglobulins from several species in a nonimmunological fashion. Each protein A molecule has four regions that bind to the Fc portion of immunoglobulins. The immunoglobulin-binding properties of protein A make this molecule useful as a developing reagent in enzyme immunoassays. Protein A covalently bound to enzymes is available from several commercial sources and can substitute for enzyme-labeled second antibodies in EIA. Protein A binds poorly to human IgG3 and some immunoglobulins from other mammals. Protein G, a cell wall constituent of some Streptococcus strains, exhibits high-affinity interactions with these immunoglobulins. Protein G is used in EIAs much like protein A and is available in a genetically engineered form designed to reduce nonspecific interactions. It is also used to detect IgA and IgM responses to microbial antigens. In this method, IgG is removed from sera by using protein G coupled to agarose. The residual antibodies are then incubated with the target antigen. The use of enzyme-labeled second antibodies that recognize the heavy chain of IgM or IgA allows a resolution of immune responses of these isotypes.

Avidin–biotin

The strong interaction between avidin from egg white protein; and biotin, a low-molecular-weight vitamin, has been used to amplify the sensitivity of EIA. Each of the four subunits of avidin contains a site that interacts with the ureido ring of biotin. The remaining valeric acid side chain of the biotin molecule can be chemically modified to generate reactive groups without altering avidin interactions. The length of the spacer between the ureido group and the chemically reactive group is sufficient in several commercially available forms of biotin to allow attachment of the biotin to antibodies or enzyme and still permit interactions with avidin. Avidin itself may be covalently linked to enzyme reporter molecules by using several available methods. Streptavidin from *Streptomyces avidinii* as a result of its lower isoelectric point, is used more widely than egg white avidin because of lower background intensity. EIA using avidin–biotin interactions is performed in two major variations. The first method makes use of a biotinylated second antibody. Avidin–enzyme conjugates are then used to detect bound biotinylated antibodies. The increase in sensitivity over standard EIA methods results from a pyramid-like enhancement of reporter group molecules. The other major format of avidin–biotin EIA takes advantage of the multivalency of avidin. In the procedure, unconjugated avidin serves as a bridge between biotinylated antibody and biotin–enzyme conjugates. Alternatively, complexes of avidin and biotinylated enzyme can be used to detect the biotinylated antibody.

Use of chemiluminescent substrates

The cyclic hydrazide luminol (5-amino-2,3-dihydro-1, 4-phthalazinedione) can be employed directly as a label (for example to avidin) in SPIA or as a substrate to interact with peroxidase enzyme. Oxidation of luminol to a chemiluminescent product is catalyzed by free iron ions or chelated iron in peroxidase. The electronically exited aminophthalate anion decay provides the more sensitive signal. Peroxidase conjugated to antibody may act more effectively on luminol than on chromogenic substrates because conjugation of the peroxidase may destroy substantial amounts of enzymatic activity but still allow the large heme(iron) donation for allowing luminol oxidation to take place in a chemiluminescent test.

Use of radioactive isotopes

Although the use of isotopes for diagnostic tests has fallen from popularity the principles are worth discussing. The use of a radioactive conjugate in a SPIA may facilitate the provision of a more sensitive assay based on the kinetics of reaction of the components in the test. The most commonly used isotope is ^{125}I, a weak gamma-emitter with a half-life of 60 days. ^{125}I can be incorporated effectively into protein molecules of high specific activity by several methods without markedly affecting the immunological activity and specificity of the proteins.

The most commonly used conjugation procedure is the chloramine-T method of Hunter and Greenwood (1962).

In this method, the protein to be labeled is added to a mixture of ^{125}I and chloramine-T (a mild oxidizing reagent). After an incubation of 2 min the reaction is stopped by the addition of $NaHSO_3$ or by the direct application of the reaction mixture to a Sephadex G 25 column, which is used to separate the labeled protein. Other methods are also used. To a lesser extent, beta-emitters ^3H and ^{14}C also have been used in solid-phase RIAs.

Highly specific activities of labeled immunoglobulins have been obtained by using the method of reductive methylation with titrated sodium borohydride. Due to the long half-life of these isotopes, the labeled reagents can be stored and used for years. However, because the liquid scintillation counting is considerably more complicated than the gamma-counting, these istopes have not found wide use in diagnostic virus antibody assays.

The labeled immunoglobulins are usually diluted in a buffer containing protein and deter-gent to decrease their nonspecific binding. Eagle minimum essential medium (E-MEM) supplemented with 10% heat-inactivated calf serum 0.5% lactalbumin hydrolysate, antibiotics, and 1% Tween-20) is usually used. Because the activity of the labeled immunoglobulin preparations decrease continuously due to radioactive decay, frequent standardization is necessary. This is done by diluting the preparations to give a standard cpm value (e.g. 5000 cpm) bound when 200 µl of the label is incubated with the solid phase coated with the homologous antigen.

RIA can be used to determine antibodies from all body fluids. Nonspecific inhibitors of hemagglutination, anticomplementary factors, etc. which seriously disturb some serologic antibody tests, do not interfere in the RIA. Like the labeled immunoglobulins, the specimens should be diluted in a buffer containing protein and detergent; PBS containing 0.5% bovine serum albumin and 0.5% Tween-20 (PBS-BSA-Tween) is often used. The expression of serum antibody concentration with an endpoint titer value is the most commonly used method of expressing RIA results. The specimens are tested in several serial dilutions, and the titer value is interpolated from the cpm versus serum dilution curve as the highest dilution where the cpm value of the test specimen is 2.1 times higher than the cpm value of the negative control at the same dilution. As the negative control, either the test specimen incubated with an uninfected control antigen or a standard negative specimen incubated with the virus antigen is used. Similar creation of standard curves mentioned above for EIA apply to providing a measurement of antibodies in a single tested serum.

Measuring responses in SPIA

Each SPIA will have characteristic methods for measuring and interpreting the reaction. We have selected a typical EIA to illustrate the complexity involved. The color reaction of an

EIA can be monitored visually for a qualitative result. For quantitative readings or a more sensitive qualitative assessment, a spectro-photometer is used. Photometers can be inter-faced with a microcomputer equipped with a data reduction package for direct calculation of results.

It is adequate for most assays to blank the OD measurement with air. However, some investigators prefer to blank the plate by using a well containing either substrate or substrate-antibody conjugate alone. If this procedure is used, it is important to document the absolute absorpance of these wells used for blanking. An OD value much greater than 0.1 may indicate a deterioration in some of the assay components. For reporting the analyte in an absolute amount per ml, a reference preparation is used as the source of calibra-tion. A number of these preparations are avail-able from commercial companies, professional organizations, and government agencies. Instead of utilizing a valuable reference pre-paration, the test can be calibrated against a standard and used for regular assays. A dose–response curve is made, consisting of the concentration of the reference preparation ver-sus its absorpance. When making this curve, one must carefully evaluate the characteristics of the data. Although a standard curve can often be constructed by simply plotting the absorpance against a log of concentration and performing linear regression, this may not be the best treatment for all systems. A variety of computer software packages offer a range of curve-fitting techniques for evaluat-ing EIA data.

One common method of expressing data is to determine the mean absorpance of samples for normal individuals and report patient samples as positive when they are two or three standard deviations above this value. Although this method requires running only one dilution of the patient sample, a number of problems can arise. From a statistical point of view, it may not be correct to apply a mean and standard deviation to this type of data, as they are often not normally distributed and there may be an insufficient sample size to apply nonparametric statistics. The greatest

problem with use of absolute absorpance values is the poor reproducibility of results. To deal with this problem, one can use an adjusted absorpance in which the patient value is presented as a ratio or a percentage of a positive control. These methods are simple and incorporate an internal control, but must be carefully standardized. It is important to monitor the level of absolute absorbancies to ensure that they are relatively constant from day to day and within the linear range of the assay. One can use a reference pool of sera with assigned arbitrary units to establish a dose–response curve and then determine patient values from the curve. In addition to extrapolating the values directly from the curve, some investigators have suggested determining the ratio of the area under the dose–response curve of the test serum and the reference serum. These techniques offer much improved reproducibility and a quan-titative answer but the required calculations are more time-consuming and may neces-sitate several dilutions of patient sera to obtain a value falling on the linear portion of the curve. Use of a microcomputer interfaced with the reader greatly simplifies the calcula-tions.

Controls and assay standardization

The basic controls in all assays should include PBS, a negative control, and low and high positive controls. However, additional con-trols should be incorporated when the assay is set up. Initially, one should assess the back-ground absorpance of all reagents alone. One important control is to assess the binding of patient sera to the uncoated solid-phase ma-terial. In a minority of samples, one can find significant binding to the solid phase even when it is coated with a nonspecific protein. This may be a problem, especially in IgM assays, and may require running all samples in both coated and uncoated wells, with sub-traction of the OD reading in the uncoated wells. Whenever any new reagents are used, comparative studies should be performed. There can be significant variability within different lots of the plates and the conjugate, and one can never assume that the assay parameters will remain unchanged. Factors such as alterations in RT and the quality of the water can also significantly affect day-to-day variability in assays. For this reason, reliance on standard curves will yield more reproducible results.

The absorpance in PBS control wells should be less than 0.1 (optimally less than 0.05) OD unit. If the absorpance is higher, the most likely reasons are either inadequate washes or a problem with the enzyme conjugate. It may be important to increase the number and efficiency of the wash steps. If this is not effective, the dilution and purity of the enzyme conjugate should be evaluated. If the conjugate cannot be diluted further without affecting the sensitivity of the assay, one should look for either a higher-avidity or an affinity-purified conjugate. Another way to deal with the problem is to add normal serum (1–5%) of the same species as the conjugate to the conjugate dilution buffer. In addition, use of 1–5% bovine serum albumin (BSA) or another nonspecific protein to bind unreacted sites on the solid phase may correct the problem. Another problem may occur with a high absorpance (>0.2 OD unit) of a negative patient sample and can be dealt with in the same manner as with the PBS control.

An unexpected fall in the amount of an analyte at the high end of the dose–response curve, (hook effect) resulting in a gross underestimation of the analyte may be a problem in sandwich immunoassays with patient samples that contain an extremely high level of an analyte. The patient samples will give a low to moderately high result when the standard assay dilution is used. Upon further dilution of the sample, the result will either be out-of-range high or, if it is diluted far enough, will give an extremely elevated value. Therefore, if the laboratory ran the sample only at the routine dilution, significant underestimation of the value would be reported. This problem may arise from low-affinity antibody, inadequate washing, and suboptimal concentrations of labeled antibody. Always ensure that adequate washing is performed between all steps, especially between the steps following the addition of each antibody. When one is performing new kit evaluations, testing specimens with high levels of the analyte is important, as the frequency of the hook effect with different kits may be variable.

Heterophile antibodies may interfere with sandwich EIAs. These antibodies can be found directed to several different species (i.e. sheep, goat, mouse, and rabbit). Their presence can have a variable effect on SPIAs. If the analyte is not present, a false-positive result may arise from the heterophile cross-linking the two antibodies of the sandwich. As monoclonal antibody-based assays are often used for diagnostically important analytes, erroneous results can cause significant problems in patient care. Addition of nonimmune immunoglobulin from the appropriate species will eliminate this interference; however, the amount and source of the normal serum may be crucial. By employing a systematic approach using some or all of these tactics, the majority of background problems can be solved.

Quality control

Quality control is important because of the complexity and sensitivity of the procedures. These factors tend to magnify errors in performance or materials, and exacting control standards are needed to ensure accurate and precise test results. Critical elements of a control program are standardization of the serochemistry, continuous monitoring of the test processes, and pre-test inspection of test specimens.

Optimum antigen-antibody concentrations are established by conventional block titrations with reference specimens. From these experiments, the test reagent concentrations for maximum specific reactivity and minimum nonspecific signal are established. Test protocols are further validated by testing of known positive and presumed normal specimens from the target-diagnostic population. From these developmental studies, the test findings that correctly differentiate reactive-positive specimens from nonreactive-negative specimens is identified. This cutoff value is expressed as: (i) a fixed absorbance value determined on the basis of the experience of the test developer; (ii) an absorbance value that is a multiplier of a number of standard deviations above the negative population absorbance; (iii) a fraction or percentage of a known positive reference value; or (iv) a combination of these. In every instance, specimens with absorbance values greater than the cutoff are reactive or positive, and those with values less than the cutoff are nonreactive or negative. Some manufacturers establish a 'grey or equivocal' zone which is neither positive or negative. This approach complicates test interpretation and patient management.

The equipment manuals provided by manufacturers must be consulted for performance characteristics, calibration specifications, and operating procedures of all instruments used with EIA tests. These techniques are very sensitive and therefore require accurate fluid measurements. Pipetting devices, plate washers, and well readers must be calibrated, and schedules for calibration checks and routine main-tenance must be established and recorded. Special attention must be paid to pipetting devices. Accuracy for these devices is maximized by, ensuring correct fit of the tips to the device barrel, prewetting tips, and keeping volume delivery below a reagent level so as not to contaminate the pipette. Washers, like reagent delivery devices, must perform exactly as specified. Vacuum and fluid delivery must be set for and matched to the plate test wells. A simple measure of wash efficiency is a plate-to-plate inspection for residual wash fluid. Either excess residual fluid or excessive aspiration in wash cycles, and thus excessive drying, may adversely affect test reactivity. Since all EIA reactions are temperature and time sensitive, technical protocols must include clocks and thermometers as standard monitoring devices to ensure compliance with the parameters established for each test.

Each EIA run should include controls from the reagent manufacturer, a set prepared in-house or obtained from other sources (external or supplemental controls), as well as, whenever possible, a set of primary standards from a recognized reference laboratory. This set is used initially, and at appropriate intervals, to ensure the optimum level of reactivity in consensus with other laboratories. The control set provided by the manufacturer describes the optimum performance characteristics of the test. The results of this control set, however, apply only to the potency of the reagents in the set in use. Variations in reagents, kit to kit or lot to lot, are monitored by the external control set, which should consist of multiple (duplicate or triplicate) high- and mid-range reactive specimens or specimen pools and a nonreactive specimen or specimen pool. This external control thus serves not only to detect immediate failure but also to monitor both excessive run-to-run variation and long-term trends. Values obtained at each test run are efficiently monitored by charts that show, for example, nonreactive or background as well as levels of specific reactivity over time.

References

Ashley RL, Militoni J (1987) J Virol Meth 18: 159–168.

Ashley RL, Dalessio J, Dragaum J, Koulsky LA, Lee FK, Nahmias AJ, Stevens MA, Holmes KK and Corey L (1993) Sex Trans Diseases 20: 230–235.

Blumberg RS, Hartshorn KL, Ardman, B, Kaplan JC, Paradis T, Vogt H, Hirsch MS, Schooley RT (1987) J Clin Microbiol 25: 1989–1992.

Chernesky MA, Mahony JB (1984) Yale J Biol Med 57: 757–776.

Cohen BJ, Mortimer PP, Pereira MS (1983) J Hyg (Camb) 91: 113–130.

Hunter WM, Greenwood FC (1962) Nature 194: 495–496.

Mahony J, Zapata M, Chernesky MA (1989) J Clin Microbiol 27: 1626–1630.

Mushahwar IK, Overby LR, Frosner G, Deinhardt F, Ling CM (1978) J Med Virol 2: 77–87.

Purcell RH, Gerin JC, Almeida, JB, Holland PV (1984) Intervirology 2: 231–243.

Tersmette M, Lelie PN, van der Peol CL, Wester MR, de Goede REY, Lange JMA, Miedema F, Huisman JG (1988) J Med Virol 24: 109–116.

Vonderfecht SL, Miskuff RL, Eiden JJ, Yolken RH (1985) J Clin Microbiol 22: 726–730.

Wu B, Mahony JB, Chernesky MA (1990) J Virol Meth 29: 157–166.

Yolken RH, Stopa PJ, Harris CC (1980) In: Manual of Clinical Immunology, 2nd edn. NR Rose and H Friedman (Eds.) American Society for Microbiology, Washington, D.C., pp. 692–699.

Zapata M, Mahony JB, Chernesky MA (1984) J Med Virol 14: 101–114.

Cell mediated immunity

8

A. C. Mawle

The measurement of the cell-mediated response to viruses has become of major importance over the last few years. The ability to measure T cell responses is critical to the understanding of pathogenesis and in the design of potential vaccines. It is now possible to determine the major T cell epitopes for a given viral protein and study the characteristics of both a helper T cell and cytotoxic T cell response to that epitope. Recently two subsets of T helper cells have been described, based on the cytokine profiles and function of T cell clones responding to a particular antigen. TH1 cells produce interferon-γ and TNF-β, and are responsible for delayed-type hypersensitivity responses. TH2 cells produce interleukin (IL)-4, IL-5 and IL-10, and are responsible for delivering B cell help and antibody class switching (Mossman and Coffman 1989). These two subpopulations both down-regulate each other and enhance their own activity. Their discovery has allowed a better understanding of pathogenesis in diseases such as leishmaniasis (Sher and Coffman 1992) where there is a wide spectrum of disease, and the potential for modulating the immune response to favor either cell-mediated or an antibody response may become important for future therapies or vaccines.

This chapter will describe methods useful for measuring the cell-mediated response to viruses in humans. All of the techniques are applicable to mouse (or other animal) systems, though obviously the specific reagents and conditions will be different. For further information the reader should refer to *Current Protocols in Immunology* (Coligan et al 1991), which is the definitive practical reference in this field.

All of the following procedures should be carried out under sterile conditions at room temperature, unless otherwise indicated.

8

Virology Methods Manual
ISBN 0–12–465330–8

Preparation of lymphocyte populations

Source of lymphocytes

The usual source of human lymphocytes is peripheral blood. However, lymphocytes can be isolated from other tissues such as lymph nodes, tonsils or spleen, if they are available. These have the advantage that a large number of cells can be obtained and frozen for future use. Lymphocytes can also be obtained from infected lesions, though the number of cells obtained this way is usually small.

All human material must be handled as though it were infectious. The possibility of Human Immunodeficiency Virus (HIV) infection is always present, as well as other blood-borne pathogens. Biosafety level 2 practices are recommended for all work, and anyone routinely working with human blood should receive hepatitis B vaccine.

Isolation of peripheral blood lymphocytes (PBL) from whole blood

PBL are isolated using density gradient centrifugation on Ficoll-Hypaque (F/H). During centrifugation, the red cells and granulocytes pass through the F/H and the lymphocytes remain on the surface of the gradient. Most of the platelets remain in the supernatant. The cell population isolated will typically contain 10–20% monocytes, 0–5% granulocytes and some platelets. The granulocyte contamination will increase with the age of the blood. Platelet contamination does not pose a problem unless the subject has an abnormally high platelet count.

Experimental

1. Place heparinized blood into a 50 ml conical tube and add an equal volume of Hanks balanced salt solution (HBSS). Carefully underlay 10 ml F/H, using a pipette.
2. Centrifuge at 400 g for 30 min with no brake.
3. Remove most of the plasma above the interface and discard. This contains most of the platelets. Carefully aspirate the interface layer and transfer to a 50 ml conical tube. Fill the tube with HBSS to dilute out contaminating F/H.
4. Centrifuge for 10 min at 300 g. Wash cells twice more by centrifugation in 20 ml HBSS.
5. Resuspend cells in appropriate culture medium and count using trypan blue exclusion. Cell viability should be >95%.

Preparation of lymphocyte subsets

There are many reasons to study PBL subsets. These include dissecting a cytotoxic T lymphocyte (CTL) response into CD8- and CD4- T cell-mediated components, removing the non-specific natural killer (NK) cell response from a MHC-restricted virus-specific assay, or using a purified CD4$^+$ T cell population to study TH1 and TH2 responses. There are two basic techniques used for purifying PBL subsets; the traditional method using antibody and complement, and the immunomagnetic cell depletion method, which is the method of choice due to its speed and convenience. Both target the cell to be removed using a monoclonal antibody, and in the latter technique, the monoclonal antibody is attached to a magnetic bead. The cells bound to beads are trapped by a magnet, and the remainder washed free and used for study. Both techniques employ negative selection to separate subpopulations, though it is possible to use a positively selected cell population without removing the beads if the beads do not interfere with the assay. It is also possible to remove cells from the beads if necessary. Negative selection is greatly to be preferred over positive selection when isolating lymphocyte subpopulations, since the cell may be affected in some way by the binding of antibody to its surface, which could interfere with subsequent assays. There will be appreciable cell loss with both techniques due to the multiple steps involved, and this should be taken into account when determining the initial number of cells needed for a given assay.

Cell depletion using immunomagnetic beads

1. All procedures must be carried out on ice using cold reagents to prevent phagocytosis of the beads.
2. The beads are stored in preservative containing azide and must be washed before use. The wash buffer used throughout should be phosphate-buffered saline pH 7.2 (PBS) containing 2% fetal calf serum (FCS). Place the desired volume of beads in a conical tube. Add wash buffer and place on the magnetic particle concentrator (MPC) for 1 min. Remove supernatant and repeat twice. Reconstitute the beads to their original volume in wash buffer.
3. Add the washed beads to separated PBL ($2-4 \times 10^6$ ml^{-1}) at a ratio of 10:1. Incubate for 15–60 min on a

mixer at 4°C. The time necessary will depend on the particular monoclonal antibody being used.
4. Place the tube in the MPC for 2–3 minutes and carefully remove the supernatant containing the unbound cells.
5. Add wash buffer and repeat step 4.
6. Centrifuge unbound cells at 300 g for 5 min and resuspend in the desired medium. The purity of the cell population can be determined by immunophenotyping (page 154). For a highly purified cell population, a second round of cell depletion may be required.
7. For positive selection, a lower bead to cell ratio can be used in step 3. The supernatant would be discarded and the bead-bound population retained.

Cell depletion using antibody and complement

1. Isolate PBL and make up to 5×10^6 ml^{-1} in cold, serum-free RPMI 1640 (RPMI).
2. Add monoclonal antibody at a previously titrated concentration and incubate for 30 min on ice.
3. Wash twice by centrifugation in serum-free RPMI.
4. Make a 1:4 dilution of rabbit Lo-Tox complement (Cedarlane) in serum-free RPMI and resuspend cells at 2×10^6 ml^{-1}. Incubate for 1 h in a 37°C waterbath.
5. Wash twice by centrifugation, and determine efficiency of cell depletion by immunophenotyping.

Cell preservation

Most assays of immune function can be performed on frozen cells. These include proliferation assays, immunophenotyping and cytokine production. The results will differ from those obtained with fresh cells, but if they are made the standard for a given set of experiments, they will give acceptable results. PBL can be stored for several years in a liquid nitrogen (LN_2) freezer. Assays of cytotoxic function do not work well with frozen cells, and fresh cells should be used.

Experimental

1. Isolate cells on F/H and make up to $2-10 \times 10^7$ ml^{-1} in ice-cold FCS.
2. Add an equal volume of ice-cold RPMI 1640 + 20% dimethyl sulfoxide (DMSO) dropwise, while gently vortexing the cell suspension. This will give a final mixture of $1-5 \times 10^7$ cells ml^{-1} in RPMI 1640 + 50% FCS + 10% DMSO.
3. Aliquot cells into previously chilled freezing vials at a minimum of 0.5 ml per vial.
4. To freeze, place the vials in an insulated container (double bookbag or styrofoam). Place the container in a $-70°C$ freezer overnight and transfer vials to a LN_2 freezer the next day. If a controlled rate freezer is available, cool at 1°C min^{-1} to $-30°C$, then at 5°C min^{-1} to $-80°C$. Transfer the vials to a LN_2 freezer.
5. To thaw cells, place the vials in a 37°C water bath immediately on removal from the freezer. As soon as the cells are thawed, transfer them to 10 ml RPMI 1640 + 10% FCS to dilute out the DMSO. Wash the cells three times by centrifugation (7 min at 300 g) and count using trypan blue exclusion to determine the cell viability. This will usually be 85% or greater, as most dead cells do not survive intact.

Lymphocyte proliferation assays

Lymphocyte proliferation in response to an antigenic stimulus is used as a measure of the recall response to that antigen and is considered an *in vitro* correlate of the delayed-type hypersensitivity response (DTH). Thus only individuals exposed to a given virus either by natural infection or vaccination would be expected to have a proliferative response to it. However, not everyone who has been exposed to a particular virus will have a detectable proliferative response.

When a lymphocyte is activated through its specific receptor, several immediate activation events occur, including receptor-induced phosphorylation of tyrosine kinases, leading to an influx of calcium, which is induced through the phosphatidyl inositol pathway (Rudd 1994). These initial events lead to the appearance of activation molecules on the cell surface, the release of cytokines and the induction of cell division. Although all of these events can be measured and used as an indicator of lymphocyte activation, the most commonly used technique has been to determine the incorporation of tritiated (^{3}H) thymidine into DNA during the DNA synthesis required for cell division. However, with the availability of commercial ELISA kits, interleukin 2 (IL-2) production is increasingly being used to measure antigenic activation of T cells instead of, or as an adjunct to, a proliferation assay.

The lymphocyte response to viral antigen is T cell dependent, and requires the presence of antigen-presenting cells (APC) in the culture. When using PBL separated on F/H for an assay, monocytes will be present in sufficient numbers to perform this function. However, when using purified T cell subpopulations, one must titrate in sufficient APC to obtain a response. If T cell clones (page 155) are used to investigate the response to a specific antigen, then autologous or HLA-compatible B cell lines transformed with Epstein-Barr virus (EBV-B) can be used as antigen-presenting cells (page 150).

In a clinical situation, proliferative assays can be performed using whole blood (Fletcher 1987). This has the advantage of requiring very little blood. However, for research purposes, separated PBL are preferable since they allow greater control over the actual number of cells in the assay.

Sources of antigen

Many different sources of antigen can be used to stimulate lymphocytes *in vitro*, and the choice for a given virus will depend both on availability and the nature of the research question. Whole inactivated virus is a good stimulus when studying the population response to a virus, so that the responses to all viral proteins are detected. However, purified viral proteins are needed to determine the immunodominant response to the virus. These can be prepared using conventional biochemical techniques or by using recombinant viral proteins. A useful screening technique for viral proteins capable of stimulating a proliferative response involves separating a preparation of whole virus into its constituent parts on a western blot, and using the individual protein bands to stimulate PBL (Lamb et al 1988).

Mapping of immunodominant epitopes within a viral protein requires the use of peptides to stimulate a response. This can be done using a series of overlapping peptides spanning the protein of interest, or by using predictive algorithms to identify potential T cell epitopes (Berzofsky 1993). The former method is more comprehensive, since none of the currently available predictive techniques identifies all empirically determined epitopes. Peptide mapping can be done using PBL from several individuals with different HLA haplotypes, in order to detect as many different epitopes as possible. However, it is often easier to generate a series of T cell clones directed against the protein of interest and use these to determine the MHC restriction of potential epitopes.

Experimental

1. Human AB serum is used for proliferation assays. This can either be obtained commercially or from a blood bank. Sera should be heat-inactivated in a water bath at 56°C before use. Since different lots of sera can potentially have either a stimulatory or a suppressive effect on lymphocyte proliferation, it is advisable to screen several lots separately in a proliferation assay and pool those that have no obvious effect on the responses. This pool can then be frozen in appropriate aliquots and a fresh aliquot used for each experiment.
2. Separate the PBL and resuspend at 10^6 ml^{-1} in RPMI 1640 containing 10% heat-inactivated human AB serum, and supplemented with 2 mM glutamine, 100 U ml^{-1} penicillin and 100 µg ml^{-1} streptomycin (RPMI/AB).
3. Dispense 0.1 ml (10^5 cells) cell suspension into each well of a 96-well round-bottomed microtiter plate.
4. Add 0.1 ml of the appropriate antigen suspension. Assays should be set up with a minimum of three replicates for each antigen concentration. Control wells have 0.1 ml RPMI/AB added to them.
5. Incubate the plate for six days in a humidified incubator at 37°C in 5% CO_2.
6. 18 h prior to harvest, add 0.05 ml of 10 µCi ml^{-1} ^{3}H thymidine to each well (0.5 µCi per well).
7. Harvest the cell cultures onto a glass fiber filter using a semi-automated cell harvester.
8. Transfer filter dots to scintillation vials, add scintillation fluid and count on a β scintillation counter.

Calculation of results

Results can be expressed either as δcpm* or as a stimulation index (SI).

δcpm = stimulated cpm − control cpm

$$SI = \frac{\text{stimulated cpm}}{\text{control cpm}}$$

*cpm = counts per minute

There are advantages and disadvantages to both methods, mainly resulting from the degree to which the control cpm affects the results. If the stimulated counts are high, then δcpm is usually preferred, whereas if the stimulated counts are low, then the SI gives a better indication of a positive response. Frequently, both methods are used to compare different groups under study. Yet another option is to normalize responses (either δcpm or SI) to the response of a standard batch of frozen cells which is run in each assay. Then an individual response is expressed as a percentage of the standard's response. This approach cuts down interassay variation, which can be an important factor in population studies.

Virus-specific cytotoxic T lymphocyte assays

Cytotoxic T lymphocytes (CTL) are considered to be the major line of defense against virally infected cells, and as such, their measurement is an important component of defining the virus-specific immune response. T cell recognition of antigen occurs via the α/β T cell receptor, which recognizes processed viral peptides bound to MHC class I or class II molecules on the target cell. CD8+ CTL are class-I restricted and CD4+ CTL are class-II restricted. The MHC restriction of the CTL is determined by the antigen presentation pathway. Endogenously processed antigen is presented by class I molecules, whereas exogenous antigen, which is taken up into endosomes and subsequently processed by protease digestion, is presented by class II molecules. There are occasional exceptions to this, but in general, these relationships hold.

Since viruses necessarily grow within cells, and since class II molecules have a limited tissue distribution, most viral antigens are endogenously processed and CTL directed against them are CD8+ and class-I restricted. However, there are notable exceptions. In particular, the CTL response in humans to herpes simplex virus 1 (HSV-1) is predominantly class-II restricted (Schmid 1988). Interferon-γ, which is produced by T lymphocytes in response to virus, can induce class II expression on many cells that do not normally express this molecule, and this may play a role in the generation of CD4+ CTL. Class-II restricted CTL have been described more frequently in human systems than in mouse systems.

CTL activity is usually measured using a ^{51}chromium (^{51}Cr) release assay. ^{51}Cr is taken up non-specifically by living cells and released very slowly. Dying cells release it much more rapidly, and the level can conveniently be measured in the supernatant fluid. Since natural killer (NK) cells can kill virally infected cells non-specifically, it is important to either remove them from the CTL population, or to determine the contribution of NK cell activity to the total by assaying killing of a virus-infected, MHC-mismatched target. This can be subtracted from the total CTL activity. Uninfected target cells, or target cells infected with an irrelevant virus should be run as a control in each assay to ensure that the killing observed is virus-specific.

Selection and generation of target cells

There are two considerations in the choice of target cells for a CTL assay. Firstly, the targets must be syngeneic with the effector cells, which in the human system usually means an autologous target cell. Secondly, it must be possible to infect the target with the virus of interest. In practice, the easiest target cell to use is an EBV-B cell line. However, this presupposes that the individual under study is available for repeat blood donations. If this is not possible, then autologous PBL stimulated with phytohemagglutinin (PHA) can be used. These have several disadvantages compared with EBV-B. They do not label well with ^{51}Cr, PHA makes the cells very sticky and therefore hard to separate into a single cell suspension, and the blasts need to be generated 2–3 days before they are required, which usually means that PBL must be frozen and then thawed at the appropriate time to generate targets.

Generation of an EBV-B cell line

1. Isolate PBL on Ficoll/Hypaque. Make up to 10^6 ml^{-1} in RPMI 1640, 20% FCS and 2 µg ml^{-1} cyclosporin A.
2. Add EBV-containing supernatant (from B95.8 marmoset cell line) at a 1:10 dilution and plate cells in 24 well plates at 2 ml per well.
3. Incubate the plates for two weeks at 37°C and 5% CO_2 in a humidified incubator without feeding.
4. After two weeks, the cells should be growing in visible clumps. Transfer to 25 cm^2 flasks and feed with RPMI 1640, supplemented with 20% FCS, 2 mM glutamine, 100 U ml^{-1} penicillin and 100 µg ml^{-1} streptomycin.
5. Expand the line by splitting weekly at 1:5 and freeze down for future use. Cells can be used as targets as soon as there are a sufficient number.

Generation of PHA blasts

1. Using either fresh or frozen PBL, suspend cells in RPMI 1640/AB at 2 × 10^6 ml^{-1}. Add PHA (Gibco) at a final concentration of 1:1000 and transfer to a 25 cm^2 flask.
2. Incubate for 48–72 h at 37°C and 5% CO_2 in a humidified incubator before using as targets.

Cytotoxic T lymphocyte assay

The conditions for generating virus-specific cytotoxic T cells must be determined for each virus to be studied. It is generally necessary to use PBL from an individual who has been exposed to the virus under study, either by contracting the virus naturally, or by receiving a vaccine. This can be determined serologically or by taking an appropriate history. Even if the individual has been recently exposed to the virus, it is usually necessary to restimulate *in vitro* in order to expand the virus-specific population sufficiently to obtain a measurable response. This is true even for latent viruses that are frequently reactivated, such as EBV and herpes simplex. A notable exception is HIV-1, where virus-specific CTL can be detected in fresh PBL from asymptomatic seropositive individuals without further stimulation. Presumably this is a reflection of continuous viral replication providing a continuing antigenic stimulus *in vivo*.

Generation of virus-specific CTL

1. In order to stimulate CTL *in vitro*, cells are incubated with whole virus, soluble viral antigen, virally infected irradiated autologous cells or peptide-pulsed autologous cells for 3–14 days, though approximately seven days is usually optimal. The optimal antigen concentration is determined by titration. If the virus of interest is cytopathic in lymphocytes, then it must be inactivated for use as an antigen. Low levels of recombinant IL-2 (rIL-2) (5–10 IU ml^{-1}) may improve the yield of antigen-specific CTL.
2. To generate virus-specific CTL, isolate PBL and adjust to 2 × 10^6 ml^{-1} in RPMI/AB. Dispense 1 ml into each well of a 24-well plate.
3. Add the predetermined amount of viral antigen in 1 ml RPMI/AB. Control wells receive 1 ml RPMI/AB. Incubate at 37°C and 5% CO_2 in a humidified incubator for seven days (or optimal time for CTL generation).

4. For use in CTL assay, harvest the cells and wash once by centrifugation in HBSS. If necessary, NK cells can be removed at this point by antibody and complement lysis or by magnetic beads. Separation into CD8+ and CD4+ populations for assessment of HLA Class I and Class II restriction can also be performed.

Generation and ^{51}Cr labeling of virus-infected target cells

1. Both EBV-B cells and PHA blasts can be infected overnight with virus to generate CTL targets. The optimal amount of virus must be titrated. This also works for vaccinia constructs containing a particular gene of interest. If the targets are to be pulsed with peptide, this can usually be achieved during the ^{51}Cr labeling step, with a peptide concentration of 10 μg ml^{-1}.
2. To label the target cells, add 200 μCi ^{51}Cr to 10^6 target cells in 0.5 ml RPMI and incubate for 2 h at 37°C.
3. Wash three times with HBSS and count the cells. Resuspend at 10^5 ml^{-1} in RPMI/AB for use.

CTL assay

1. There will be a minimum of two effector cell populations (stimulated and unstimulated), and two target cells (infected and uninfected) in each assay. There may be considerably more if different viral epitopes are being assessed as targets or if HLA restriction analysis is performed.
2. Resuspend stimulated and

unstimulated effector cells at 5 × 10^6 ml^{-1} in RPMI/AB. Distribute 0.2 ml into each well of row A of a 96-well round-bottomed microtiter plate.
3. Make three doubling dilutions of effector cells by adding 0.1 ml RPMI/AB into the next three rows (rows B–D) and using a multi-channel pipetor to transfer cells. This will give four effector to target (E:T) ratios; 50:1, 25:1, 12.5:1 and 6.25:1. Each E:T ratio should be set up in triplicate.
4. Add 10^4 labeled target cells in 0.1 ml to each well containing effector cells and to the wells at the bottom of the plate (rows E–H).
5. Add 0.1 ml RPMI/AB to six wells with target cells only (spontaneous release) and 0.1 ml 1% Triton X to six wells with targets only (maximum release).
6. Incubate for 5–8 h at 37°C and 5% CO_2 in a humidified incubator.
7. To harvest, transfer 0.1 ml supernatant from each well to a plastic tube, taking great care not to disturb the cell pellet.
8. Count tubes on a gamma-counter.

Calculation of results

1. Results are expressed as percentage killing at each effector:target (E:T) ratio.

$$\% \text{ killing} = \frac{\text{specific lysis (cpm)} - \text{spontaneous release (cpm)}}{\text{maximum release (cpm)} - \text{spontaneous release (cpm)}} \times 100\%$$

2. Comparisons between individuals can be made by comparing virus-specific killing at each E:T ratio. Virus-specific killing is calculated by subtracting the percentage killing on uninfected targets (or targets infected with an irrelevant virus) from the percentage killing on infected targets.

Natural killer cell and antibody-dependent cytotoxic cell assays

Natural killer (NK) and antibody-dependent cytotoxic cell (ADCC) activity is mediated by the non-B, non-T fraction of PBL. These cells are large granular lymphocytes (LGL) and are CD56+ and/or CD16+. A small percentage of this population are CD3+ and express the α/β T cell receptor. This is a heterogeneous cell population and it is not yet clear which subpopulations are responsible for the various functional activities associated with it.

NK function was first described as the ability to kill tumor cells non-specifically. It was subsequently found that cells not normally susceptible to NK lysis could be rendered susceptible by viral infection. This ability is greatly enhanced by preincubation of the NK cells with IL-2 to generate lymphokine-activated killer cells (LAK cells). ADCC is mediated through the Fc receptor (CD16) on the effector cell. Virus-specific antibody binds to the infected target, and the cytotoxic cell then interacts with the target via its Fc receptor. NK cell function is usually assayed on a human tumor cell line, while ADCC can be assayed using any NK-resistant cell line that can be infected with the virus of interest. EBV-B cells (page 150) usually work well.

NK cell assay (including LAK cells)

1. Infect and label target cells (tumor cell line K562) as described for cytotoxic T cells. Make up to 10^5 cells ml^{-1} in RPMI/FCS.
2. Make effector cells up to 5×10^6 ml^{-1}

in RPMI/FCS. To assay NK cell activity, use fresh PBL. To generate LAK cells, incubate PBL for 18 h in RPMI/AB with 100 U ml^{-1} rIL-2 and wash twice with HBSS before use.
3. Set up six doubling dilutions of effector cells as described (page 151, step 3), starting at a 50:1 effector:target ratio. Add 10^4 target cells in 0.1 ml to each well. Each effector cell concentration should be set up in triplicate.
4. Set up spontaneous and maximum release for each target as described for cytotoxic T cells (page 151, step 5).
5. Incubate for 4 h at 37°C and 5% CO_2 in a humidified incubator.
6. Harvest and count as described in page 151, step 7.

ADCC assay

1. Infect and label target cells as described for cytotoxic T cells and make up to 10^5 cells ml^{-1} in RPMI/FCS.
2. Dispense 20 µl aliquots of sera to be tested into 96-well round-bottomed microtiter plates. This will give a final concentration of 1:10. For lower concentrations, dilute the sera appropriately in PBS. The sera must first be heat-inactivated to avoid any

possibility of killing due to complement.

3. Add 10^4 target cells in 0.1 ml to each well and incubate plate for 30 min at 37°C and 5% CO_2 in a humidified incubator. This allows antibody to bind to the virally-infected cell. Control wells should contain serum that is antibody-negative for the virus in question.

4. Isolate fresh PBL and make up four cell concentrations in RPMI/FCS; 5×10^6 ml^{-1}, 2.5×10^6 ml^{-1}, 1.25×10^6 ml^{-1} and 0.625×10^6 ml^{-1}. Add 0.1 ml of each cell suspension to the serum/target mixture, setting up triplicate wells for each cell concentration. This will give E:T ratios of 50:1, 25:1, 12.5:1 and 6.25:1.

5. Incubate for 4 h at 37°C and 5% CO_2 in a humidified incubator.

6. Harvest and count as described on page 151.

Calculation of results

1. The percentage killing at each E:T ratio is calculated as described on page 151. For ADCC, the specific killing is calculated by subtracting the percentage killing on virally infected targets incubated with effectors alone from the percentage killing on infected targets incubated with virus-specific antibody.

2. Results from NK assays are often expressed as lytic units (Bryant et al 1992). This method of expressing the results allows data from all E:T ratios to be combined into one number, and if immunophenotyping has been performed on the effector cell population, then the result can be expressed as lytic units per NK cell, which is useful for population studies.

Immunophenotyping

Cell surface markers are used for many purposes in immune analysis. In the assays described in this chapter, the predominant use would be to determine the purity of cell populations after depletion of a specific cell type. However, the monitoring of cell surface markers during the course of an illness can provide useful insights into the disease process. This is seen most clearly in HIV infection, where the number of CD4+ T cells is used as a marker of disease progression. However, in any infectious illness there are characteristic changes in the CD4+ and CD8+ populations, and the appearance of activation markers such as CD38, DR and the IL-2 receptor can also be monitored. In clinical situations, marker analysis is done on whole blood and a complete blood count (CBC) performed in order to express the results as absolute lymphocyte counts. For examining experimental cell populations, separated PBL are used. Three different monoclonal antibodies are routinely used in a single staining procedure, and a standard 2-color panel for clinical use is available from Becton Dickinson.

Experimental

1. Place 0.1 ml whole blood or $2-5 \times 10^6$ separated cells in 0.1 ml in a 12 × 75 mm tube.
2. Add appropriate monoclonal antibody (or antibody mixture) and incubate for 20 min at room temperature.
3. Add 2 ml lysing solution (Becton Dickinson) and incubate 10 min at room temperature.
4. Centrifuge for 3 min at 300 g. Aspirate supernatant without disturbing the cell pellet.
   (Steps 3 and 4 are not necessary for separated cells.)
5. Add 2 ml PBS containing 1% sodium azide and centrifuge for 3 min at 300 g.
6. Add 0.5 ml 1% paraformaldehyde to fix cells and read on a flow cytometer within 24 h. Store cells in the dark until read.

T cell cloning

T cell clones are most valuable for dissecting the fine detail of the immune response to a particular viral protein. A series of clones specific for one protein allows different epitopes to be mapped to different MHC class I or class II molecules. They may also allow the immunodominant epitope for each to be determined. With the description of TH1 and TH2 helper subsets, generating a series of CD4+ clones and determining their cytokine profile may allow one to determine whether a given response is predominantly TH1 or TH2. In general, T cell clones are a tool most useful for studying the detailed mechanics of a lymphocyte/target interaction rather than for elucidating a population response (Feldman et al 1985).

Experimental

1. Stimulate PBL for seven days using conditions known to stimulate a proliferative (T helper) or cytotoxic T cell response to the virus of interest.
2. Prepare feeder cells. Irradiate autologous PBL at 4000 rads and add 10^5 to each well of a 96-well round-bottomed microtiter plate in RPMI/AB with 10 U ml^{-1} rIL-2, and an appropriate concentration of antigen.
3. Plate the antigen-stimulated cells at limiting dilution on the feeder cells. Set up one plate each at 0.3, 1, 3, 10 and 100 cells/well. The final volume in each well should be 0.2 ml.
4. Incubate at 37°C and 5% CO_2 in a humidified incubator.
5. Feed every 4–5 days by replacing 0.05 ml of the culture medium. Clones should be visible at the higher cell concentrations after 7–10 days. The lower concentrations should be grown for 20–30 days.
6. Transfer visible clones to 24-well plates containing 10^4 irradiated feeder cells in 30 U ml^{-1} rIL-2, RPMI/AB and antigen.
7. After seven days, assay clones for activity, either by a proliferation assay or by a CTL assay. Functional assays should be performed 5–7 days after antigen stimulation and at least 48 h after addition of rIL-2 to minimize any non-specific activity. Clones can be further characterized by immunophenotyping and by their cytokine profiles.

Note

T cell cloning is an art. The above is a general protocol from which to begin. All the parameters, including rIL-2 concentration, serum concentration, feeder cell concentration and time between restimulation may be changed to optimize growth of a particular clone. Careful observation of clone growth at each stage is the secret of success.

Cytokines

There are so many cytokines currently described that it is beyond the scope of this chapter to deal with all their different assays. Although historically most cytokines have been detected using a functional assay, the advent of readily available commercial ELISA kits has changed this practice. A biologic assay ensures that only active material is measured. The disadvantage is that so many cytokines have overlapping functions that the only way to be sure that one is measuring the cytokine of interest is to demonstrate that the activity being measured is blocked by an antibody directed against that cytokine. Biologic assays tend to be time-consuming compared with an ELISA. However, there is no certainty that the material measured in an ELISA is biologically active and an ELISA may not be as sensitive as a biologic assay. Both of these concerns can be addressed by careful standardization. If cost is a consideration, it is usually much cheaper to perform a functional assay than to buy ELISA kits.

There are several cytokines of particular interest to virologists. Production of interferon-α, -β and -γ is induced in response to viral infection and can conveniently be measured using their anti-viral activity. Discrimination of the different types of interferon can be performed by using the appropriate antibody to block the assay. Cytokine production is the technique used for discriminating between TH1 and TH2 helper subsets by a given viral protein or peptide. Interferon-γ and TNF-β are used as TH1 cytokines and IL-4, IL-5 and IL-10 are used as TH2 cytokines. Commercial ELISAs are available for all of these. Recently a technique known as ELISPOT has been applied to cytokine detection. This measures the production by individual cells using a monoclonal antibody bound to a membrane. The cells are then washed away and the plate developed like a regular ELISA. This allows each cell's cytokine 'footprint' to be stained and counted, which gives an estimate of the total number of antigen-specific T cells. A generic ELISPOT protocol is given below, which will need to be adapted for the cytokine of interest. The most critical component is the selection of antibody pairs for cytokine capture and detection. A list of appropriate pairs for several cytokines can be found in *Current Protocols in Immunology*, Unit 6.19.

Anti-viral activity of interferon

Preparation of virus

1. Grow Vero cells to confluence in Eagle's minimum essential medium (EMEM) supplemented with 2 mM glutamine, 100 U ml^{-1} penicillin, 100 μg ml^{-1} streptomycin and 10% FCS (EMEM/FCS).
2. Infect monolayers with vesicular stomatitis virus (MOI 0.1–0.01) in minimal volume. Incubate for 45 min at 37°C in 5% CO_2 humidified incubator.
3. Add EMEM/FCS sufficient to cover cells, then incubate for 24 h at 37°C in a 5% CO_2 humidified incubator, or until the monolayer is predominantly destroyed.
4. Collect the supernatants and remove the cell debris by centrifugation (10 min at 50 g).
5. Aliquot the virus on ice in 0.5–1 ml aliquots and store at −170°C. Do NOT store at −120°C, since the virus is unstable at this temperature. Do not refreeze viral aliquots after use.
6. The virus should be titrated in a standard plaque assay to determine its titer.

Interferon assay

1. Any human diploid cell line such as WISH (human amnion), or A549 (human lung carcinoma) should be suitable for this assay.
2. Prepare a single cell suspension in EMEM/FCS from a confluent culture and adjust the concentration to 2×10^6 ml^{-1}.
3. To make dilutions of the samples to be tested, add 50 μl EMEM/FCS to all wells of a 96-well flat-bottomed microtiter plate. Add 0.05 ml of each interferon sample to be tested to one well of row 1 of the plate and 0.05 ml of the reference interferon (NIH, Bethesda) to one well of this row. Thus one plate allows seven samples and the reference to be assayed. Using a multi-channel pipettor, make doubling dilutions through row 10, discarding 0.05 ml from this last row.
4. Add 0.05 ml cell suspension to all wells and mix gently to distribute cells evenly.
5. Add 0.1 ml virus stock diluted in EMEM/FCS to give an MOI of 0.1, to all wells except row 12. Add 0.1 ml EMEM/FCS to this row. This serves as the negative control while row 11 serves as the positive control.
6. Incubate at 37°C in a 5% CO_2 humidified incubator for 24 h, or until the cells in the positive control wells are destroyed (100% CPE).
7. Aspirate the supernatants and wash with cold EMEM/FCS. Add 0.1 ml 0.13% crystal violet in formalin to each well and incubate 10 min at room temperature. Rinse plate with tap water and invert to dry.
8. To read, compare the endpoint for each sample (100% CPE) with the reference standard. Since doubling dilutions are performed, a sample with an endpoint one well less than the standard will have half the amount of interferon, whereas one with an endpoint one well greater will have twice that of the standard.
9. To determine which type of interferon is present, titrate the appropriate reference antibody (NIH, Bethesda), into the interferon sample and measure the reduction in titer.

ELISPOT

Lymphocyte stimulation

1. Before isolating PBL on F/H, remove the plasma and reconstitute blood to its original volume with PBS. Separate PBL and resuspend at 2×10^6 ml^{-1} in RPMI 1640 supplemented with 2 mm glutamine, 100 U ml^{-1} penicillin, 100 μg ml^{-1} streptomycin and 20% autologous plasma (RPMI/aut).
2. Dispense 2 ml cell suspension into 24-well plates and add virus or viral antigen to stimulate. Leave several wells unstimulated as controls.
3. Incubate at 37°C and 5% CO_2 in a humidified incubator for 24 h.
4. Wash stimulated and unstimulated cells by centrifugation three times in PBS.
5. Make cells up to 1×10^6 ml^{-1} in RPMI/aut for use in ELISPOT assay.

Plate preparation

1. Use 96-well microtiter plates with a nylon membrane on the bottom (Biodyne, Silent Monitor type A, 0.45μ).

2. Add 0.1 ml capture antibody diluted in PBS pH 7.2 and incubate overnight at 4°C. Wash the plate three times with PBS.
3. Add 0.1 ml sterile skimmed milk (5% w/v in PBS) to each well and incubate for 1 h at 37°C. Wash the plate three times with PBS before use.

ELISPOT assay

1. Add appropriate dilutions of stimulated and unstimulated PBL to the coated plate. 10^5 cells per well in 0.1 ml is a good number to try for antigen-stimulated PBL. Set up at least three cell dilutions, with duplicate wells for each dilution.
2. Incubate the plate for 48 h at 37°C and 5% CO_2 in a humidified incubator.
3. To develop the plate, wash twice with PBS, followed by two washes with PBS + 0.05% Tween 20 (PBS/Tween).
4. Add 0.1 ml of a different anti-cytokine antibody diluted in PBS/Tween and incubate for 1.5 h at 37°C and 5% CO_2 in a humidified incubator.
5. Wash three times with PBS/Tween 20 and add developing antibody, conjugated to alkaline phosphatase.
6. Incubate 1.5 h at 37°C and 5% CO_2 in a humidified incubator. Wash twice with PBS, followed by two washes with PBS + 0.05% Tween 20 (PBS/Tween).
7. Add substrate (NBT & BCIP), incubate 10–30 min at room temperature, then wash plates with tap water. The optimum time for developing must be determined for each assay.
8. Allow plates to dry, then peel off the nylon membrane and count the spots in individual wells using a dissecting microscope. Results are expressed as number of cytokine-secreting cells per 10^6 input cells.

Addendum

Media

All reagents necessary for making the media used in these protocols can be obtained from: GIBCO BRL, P.O. Box 68, Grand Island, New York 14072–0068.

Cell lines and viruses

All cell lines and viruses used in these protocols can be obtained from:
American Type Culture Collection (ATCC), 12031 Parklawn Drive, Rockville, Maryland 20852, USA or European Cell Culture Collection – (Porton Down, Salisbury, UK).

Radioactive reagents

Sodium ^{51}chromate in saline, 1 mCi ml^{-1}
[methyl-^{3}H]-thymidine, 6.7 Ci mM^{-1} aqueous solution, mCi ml^{-1}
Available from:
DuPont NEN, E.I. Du Pont de Nemours and Co. Inc., Medical Products Department, Biotechnology Division, Wilmington, Delaware 19898, USA.

Stains

Crystal violet is available from:
Sigma Chemical Company, P.O. Box 14508, St Louis, Missouri 63178, USA.
For use: Dissolve 1.3 g crystal violet in 50 ml 95% ethanol. Make up to 700 ml with distilled water and add 300 ml formalin.

NBT/BCIP, *p*-nitroblue tetrazolium chloride (NBT), and 5-bromo-4-chloro-3-indolyl phosphate *p*-toluidine salt (BCIP), are supplied by: BioRad Laboratories, 2000 Alfred Nobel Drive, Hercules, California 94547, USA.

Stock solutions:
Dissolve 250 mg NBT in 3.5 ml dimethyl formamide and 1.5 ml distilled water.
Dissolve 125 mg BCIP in 5 ml dimethyl formamide.
Store at 4°C.

Working dilution:
120 µl BCIP stock solution
120 µl NBT stock solution
20 ml carbonate buffer pH 9.5 (Current Protocols in Immunology, section 10.10).

Generation of EBV-B cell lines

Cyclosporin A is available from:
Sandoz Pharmaceuticals Corporation, East Hanover, New Jersey 07936, USA.
To use, make a stock solution of 2 mg ml^{-1} in 100% ethanol, and store at −20°C. Dilute for use in culture medium.

To generate a stock of infectious EBV, culture B95.8 cells at 10^5 ml^{-1} in RPMI 1640 supplemented with 20% FCS, 2 mM glutamine, 100 U ml^{-1} penicillin and 100 µg ml^{-1} streptomycin, at 37°C and 5% CO_2 in a humidified incubator. Leave for 10–14 days without feeding, then harvest the cell supernatant and aliquot. Store at −70°C. Do not refreeze virus after use.

Cell separation

Ficoll-hypaque lymphocyte separation medium (LSM) is supplied by:
Organon Teknika Corporation, Durham, North Carolina 27704, USA.

Cedarlane rabbit Lo-Tox complement for use

with human cells is supplied by:
Accurate Chemical and Scientific Corporation, 100 Shames Drive, Westbury, New York 11590, USA.

Antibody-conjugated magnetic beads and magnetic particle concentrator are available from:
Dynal Inc., 475 Northern Boulevard, Great Neck, New York 11021, USA.
Advanced Magnetics, Inc., 51 Mooney Street, Cambridge, Massachussets 02138, USA.

Immunophenotyping

A wide range of monoclonal antibodies are available from:
Becton-Dickinson, Immunocytometry Systems, 2350 Qume Drive, San Jose, California 95313, USA.

There are many other companies that supply monoclonal antibodies, and it is generally worth testing several sources to determine the best reagent for a particular purpose.

Cytokines

ELISA kits for cytokine detection and anti-cytokine antibodies for use in the ELISPOT assay are available from:
Genzyme Diagnostics, One Kendall Square, Cambridge, Massachussets 02139, USA.
Bisource International, 950 Flynn Road, Camarillo, California 93012, USA.
R & D Systems, 614 McKinley Place N.E., Minneapolis, Minnesota 55413, USA.

Other suppliers of anti-cytokine antibodies are:
PharMingen, 10975 Torreyana Road, San Diego, California 92121, USA.
Immunotech, Inc., 160B Larrabee Road, Westbrook, Maine 04092, USA.
T Cell Sciences, Inc., 840 Memorial Drive, Cambridge, Massachussets 02139, USA.

Recombinant IL-2 can be obtained from any of the above suppliers.

Reference standards for interferon-γ, -α and -β can be obtained from the National Institute of Allergy and Infectious Diseases, Bethesda, Maryland 20892, USA.

Biodyne Silent Monitor type A (0.45 μ) nylon-backed 96-well microtiter plates for ELISPOT assays are available from:
Pall Corporation, 2200 Northern Boulevard, East Hills, New York 11548, USA.

References

Berzofsky JA (1993) Ann NY Acad Sci 690, 256–264.

Bryant J, Day R, Whiteside TL, Herberman RB (1992) J Immun Meth 146: 91–103.

Coligan JE, Cruisbeek AM, Marguiles DH, Shevach EM, Strober W (Eds.) (1991) Current Protocols in Immunology, John Wiley and Sons, New York.

Feldman M, Lamb JR, Woody JN (1985) Human T cell clones: a new approach to immune regulation. Humana Press, Clifton, Ohio.

Fletcher MA, Baron GC, Ashman MR, Fischl MA and Klimas NG (1987) Diag Clin Immunol 5: 69–81.

Lamb JR, O'Hehir RE, Young DB (1988) J Immunol Meth 110: 1–10.

Mossman TR and Coffman RL (1989) Ann Rev Immunol 7: 145–173.

Rudd CE, Janssen O, Cai Y-C, da Silva AJ, Raab M, Prasad KVS (1994) Immunol Today 15: 225–234.

Schmid DS (1988) J Immunol 140: 3610–3616.

Sher A, Coffman RL (1992) Ann Rev Immunol 10: 385–409.

Section 2

Techniques in Molecular Virology

RNA: transcription, transfection and quantitation

9

J. E. Novak
T. C. Jarvis
K. Kirkegaard

RNA transfection into mammalian cells

When viral infections can be initiated with RNA, RNA transfection can be used to test the phenotype of mutants constructed *in vitro*. If the transfection efficiency is high enough, even the defects of mutations that do not give rise to viable viruses can be studied following transfection (Marc et al 1990). RNA transfection is also useful for starting an infection in cell lines that lack a specific virus receptor (Ball et al 1992), for studying replicating subviral RNAs (Kaplan and Racaniello 1988), for studying the translation of RNAs (Hambidge and Sarnow 1991), and for allowing viral proteins to be expressed. The following methods cover transcribing *in vitro* the RNA to be introduced, checking RNA yield and quality, and three methods for introducing the RNA into cells.

Because RNases are common and exceptionally stable proteins, care must always be taken to prevent RNA degradation. For those not accustomed to working with RNA, a guide for keeping solutions, glassware, etc. free of

RNases can be found in Sambrook et al (1989). Keeping long RNAs intact present special challenges. If RNA molecules 1 kb or longer are to be stored for any length of time, they should be stored in aliquots precipitated in ethanol at −20°C. For short periods, RNAs may be stored in aqueous solution at −70°C. While working with long RNAs, it is best to keep them on ice, in the presence of an RNase inhibitor, or both.

Transcription *in vitro*

The following protocol is designed to give a high yield of RNA, using T7, T3, or SP6 RNA polymerase. A typical yield is 4–10 μg RNA per 100 μl transcription reaction. If quantitation of the transcript is desired, label the RNA with α-^{32}P labeled nucleotide at a low specific activity. The labeling conditions given below, if used to transcribe a 10 kb RNA, would result in only 0.2% of the RNAs containing a

Virology Methods Manual
ISBN 0–12–465330–8

radiolabeled nucleotide, so radioactive decay would not cause significant RNA degradation. For transcription of RNA labeled at high specific activity, as for hybridization probes, see page 174.

Reagents

The following reagents should be RNase-free:

TE: 10 mM Tris-HCl (pH 8.0), 1 mM EDTA

TE with 100 mM NaCl (optional)

DNA to be transcribed (digested with the appropriate restriction enzyme, extracted with phenol, ethanol precipitated, and resuspended in RNase-free TE at 1 mg ml^{-1})

10× transcription buffer:

400 mM Tris-HCl (pH 7.5 at 25°C), 110 mM MgCl$_2$; 20 mM spermidine trihydrochloride (store in aliquots at −20°C)

1M dithiothreitol (DTT; store at −20°C)

Human placental ribonuclease inhibitor

Nucleotide solution: 25 mM each ATP, CTP, GTP, and UTP (adjust pH to 7.0; store in aliquots at −20°C)

Cap analog: m7G(5′)ppp(5′)G, sodium (Pharmacia or Boehringer Mannheim; optional)

[α-^{32}P]UTP, at least 10 mCi mmol^{-1}, diluted to 0.02 mCi ml^{-1} (optional)

T7, T3, or SP6 polymerase

DNase I, RNase-free (Boehringer Mannheim or GIBCO-BRL)

10 M ammonium acetate (optional)

3 M sodium acetate (pH 5.0–5.5) ethanol

RNase-free distilled water

The following reagents need not be RNase-free:

Phenol, equilibrated to pH 7.8–8.0 (either commercially prepared or equilibrated according to Sambrook et al (1989).

Sephadex G-50 spin column (5 Prime–3 Prime Inc.).

Protocol

1. Mix the following, in the order given and at room temperature:
   RNase-free water to 100 µl
   10 µl 10 × transcription buffer
   1 µl 1M DTT
   placental RNase inhibitor, to 0.8 units µl^{-1}
   4 µl nucleotide solution
   4 µl linearized DNA template
   2 µl [α-^{32}P]UTP at 0.02 mCi m^{-1} (optional)
   T7, T3, or SP6 RNA polymerase, 40 units
   If capped RNA is desired, reduce the final concentration of GTP to 0.2 mM and add cap analog to a final concentration of 0.4 µM.

2. Incubate at 37°C, 60–120 min. Remove 1 µl and count in a scintillation counter (optional).

3. It is usually unnecessary to purify the RNA from the DNA template. However, if removal of the DNA template is desired, add RNase-free DNase and incubate according to the vendor's instructions. Save an aliquot before DNase treatment to ensure that the DNase was truly RNase free.

4. If it is not necessary to purify the RNA from the unincorporated nucleotides, phenol extract the sample. Add an equal volume of phenol, vortex, and spin in a microcentrifuge for 3 min at 12,000 g. Aliquot the aqueous phase, then add sodium acetate to 0.3 M and 2.5 volumes of ethanol to precipitate the RNA.

5. If removal of unincorporated nucleotides is desired, either ethanol precipitate with ammonium acetate or use a G50 gel filtration column. The first method is cheaper, the second gives purer RNA.
   (a) Ethanol precipitation with ammonium acetate

Dilute the RNA with TE to 320 µl. Add 320 µl equilibrated phenol and extract. To the aqueous supernatant, add 0.25 volumes of 10 M ammonium acetate, then 2.5 volumes of ethanol. Chill for 5 min on dry ice, then spin at 12,000 g for 10 min. Remove the supernatant, resuspend the pellet in 320 µl TE, and perform the ethanol precipitation twice more. This procedure will remove >95% of the unincorporated nucleotides.

(b) G-50 spin column
Equilibrate the column with TE containing 100 mM NaCl by draining 3 ml through the column. Spin for 4 min at 1000 g at 4°C or according to the manufacturer's instructions. Discard flow-through. Pipette the transcript onto the column and spin for 4 min at 1000 g at 4°C. The transcript will be in the flowthrough. Phenol-extract the flowthrough once, then aliquot the RNA and add 1/10 volume sodium acetate and 2.5 volumes ethanol to precipitate.

Note

Nucleotides bind Mg^{2+} in a 1:1 molar ratio. This transcription reaction contains 11 mM $MgCl_2$ and 4 mM total NTPs, making the free Mg^{2+} concentration 7 mM. If the nucleotide concentration is altered, adjust the $MgCl_2$ concentration to keep the free Mg^{2+} concentration at 7 mM.

Visualization and quantitation of RNA transcripts

Before transfecting, it is often useful to run an agarose gel to check the integrity of the RNA transcript and to quantify the yield of full-length transcript. This protocol calls for aurintricarboxylic acid as an RNase inhibitor (Gonzalez et al 1980).

Reagents

The following should be RNase-free:

TE, dithiothreitol, placental RNase inhibitor, as above
80% ethanol
50% glycerol
RNA markers (e.g. from GIBCO-BRL)

The following need not be made RNase-free:

Agarose
aurintricarboxylic acid (ATA), 50 mM (store at −20°C; use 'aluminon grade', Aldrich, Milwaukee, WI)
ethidium bromide, 1 mg ml^{-1} solution
10× TBE: per liter, 121.1 g Tris base, 61.83 g boric acid, and 7.5 g EDTA, disodium salt
6× DNA loading buffer: 30% glycerol, 0.25% each xylene cyanol and bromophenol blue.
Linearized DNA template
DE-81 paper (Whatman) or other DEAE paper
Glow-in-the-dark face makeup (available from party supply stores).
X-ray film.

Protocol

1. Prepare gel: Melt agarose in 1/2× TBE. Just before pouring the gel, add ATA to 50 µM and ethidium bromide to 0.5 µg ml^{-1}. Also add ATA to 50 µM to the gel running buffer.
2. Prepare RNA: RNA transcripts should be loaded after phenol extraction or both phenol extraction and ethanol precipitation; RNA in untreated transcription reaction will stick in the gel wells. After ethanol precipitation,

rinse the pellet with cold 80% ethanol and dry under vacuum. Resuspend the RNA in a small volume of TE containing 2 mM DTT and 0.8 µg ml^{-1} placental RNase inhibitor. Loading 10% of a 100 µl transcription reaction usually yields a band visible both by ethidium staining and by autoradiography after a few hours exposure.

3. Add glycerol to 10% to each sample. Useful controls to load are RNA markers, the DNA template, and 1× DNA loading buffer.

4. Heat RNAs to 42°C for 2 min before loading the samples. The gel may be run at up to 10 V cm^{-1}.

5. After electrophoresis, visualize the ethidium bromide-stained RNA with ultraviolet light. A rough estimate of RNA yield may be obtained by comparing the fluorescence intensity of the transcript with that of known amounts of RNA markers.

6. For labeled transcripts, dry the gel on a gel dryer using a piece of DE-81 paper as backing. DE-81 paper is preferable to Whatman 3 MM paper because, in unfixed gels, some fraction of nucleic acids pass through Whatman paper, whereas even small nucleic acids remain bound to DE-81 paper.

7. Mark the gel in several places with glow-in-the-dark face makeup. A spot will expose an autoradiograph nicely within 10 min, and even very long exposures will not cause spreading of the spot as would ^{32}P ink. Cover the dried gel with plastic wrap and expose to X-ray film.

8. To quantify RNA transcript, align the gel with the autorad and excise both the desired band and a blank area of the gel for background. Count both in a scintillation counter. To calculate the amount of RNA on the gel:

µg RNA on gel = 1.32 × cpm on gel/ cpm in 1 µl of reaction.

This equation is independent of reaction size and specific activity of the labeled nucleotide added to the reaction, provided it was at least 10 Ci mmol^{-1}. The equation assumes that the transcription reaction contained 1 mM of UTP. If breakdown of UTP in the nucleotide stock solution has caused a significant decrease in the UTP concentration, the RNA yield will be overestimated. The total yield of RNA may be calculated from the fraction of the transcription that was run on the gel.

Transfection methods

Many methods have been developed to transfect DNA into mammalian cells. We present three methods that we have optimized for RNA. Lipofectin transfection and electroporation are useful when only a small quantity of RNA is available. Electroporation is particularly convenient for cells in suspension culture. In our hands, DEAE-dextran has proven useful for studying the replication of transfected RNAs (Novak and Kirkegaard 1994).

Transfection with Lipofectin

This protocol was adapted from Grakoui et al (1989) and JD Pata (University of Colorado, unpublished results).

Reagents

The following should be made or obtained RNase-free:

TE, DTT, and placental RNase inhibitor, as above
RNA to be transfected
Lipofectin (GIBCO-BRL)
PBS: per liter, 8 g NaCl, 1.14 g

anhydrous Na_2HPO_4, 0.2 g KCl, 0.2 g KH_2PO_4, brought to pH 7.0–7.2.

The following need not be RNase-free:

Cells to be transfected (on 60 mm plates; 60–80% confluent)
Culture medium
PBS for rinsing plates.

Protocol

1. Resuspend RNA in TE with 2 mM DTT and 0.8 µg ml^{-1} RNase inhibitor. For each 60 mm plate of cells, use 1–200 ng RNA in a 50 µl volume.
2. Mix 540 µl PBS with 10 µl Lipofectin. Add 50 µl RNA and mix gently. Let sit on ice for 10 min.
3. Remove medium from cells and rinse plates twice with PBS.
4. Add 600 µl transfection mix to each plate. Rock the plates to spread the mix. Let sit at room temperature for 10 min.
5. Remove the transfection mix. Rinse plates once with PBS, and add appropriate medium. Alternatively, a plaque assay for lytic viruses can be performed directly on the transfected cells by adding an agar overlay to the plate after rinsing.

Notes

1. This procedure has been optimized for HeLa cells. In adapting this procedure to other cell lines, check first the concentrations of Lipofectin the cells can tolerate by exposing them to various amounts of Lipofectin in PBS for 10 min. To achieve the best transfection efficiency with a given cell line, amounts of both Lipofectin and RNA should be optimized.
2. Various other liposome transfection reagents are available, including Transfectam (Promega), DOTAP (Boehringer-Mannheim), and Lipofectamine and Lipofectace (GIBCO-BRL). For a given cell line, one reagent may be superior to the others. The protocol given above can be adapted for use of another liposome reagent.

Transfection by electroporation

In electroporation, cells are subjected briefly to high voltage, which creates transient disruptions in the membranes that allow macromolecules to enter. Electroporation devices come in two types: those that generate a square wave and those that use a capacitor discharge to generate an exponentially decaying current pulse. The following protocol is designed for capacitor-discharge machines, which include instruments made by Biorad, GIBCO-BRL, BTX, and International Biotechnologies, Inc.

Reagents

The following should be RNase-free:

TE, DTT, and placental RNase inhibitor, as above
RNA to be transfected
Lipofectin (optional; GIBCO-BRL).

The following need not be RNase-free:

Cells to be transfected (on plates or in suspension culture)
Culture medium
PBS: per liter, 8 g NaCl, 1.14 g anhydrous Na_2HPO_4, 0.2 g KCl, 0.2 g KH_2PO_4, brought to pH 7.0–7.2 (at 25°C) and autoclaved
Electroporation cuvettes, 0.2 or 0.4 cm gap length.

Protocol

1. For each transfection, use 5×10^6 cells. Cells in suspension or adherent

cells that have been removed from plates with trypsin may be used.

2. Wash cells twice with PBS. Resuspend in PBS at 10^7 cells ml^{-1}.

3. Resuspend RNA in TE containing 2 mM DTT and 0.8 μg ml^{-1} RNase inhibitor. RNA for each transfection should be in 50 μl.

4. Add 10 μl Lipofectin to RNA. (Optional; Lipofectin can improve transfection efficiency 10-fold.)

5. Set electroporator capacitance to 25 μF and voltage to 6250 V cm^{-1} cuvette gap length. If a pulse controller is connected, set the resistance to infinite.

6. Mix 500 μl cells with 50 μl RNA. Immediately place in an electroporation cuvette. Pulse twice with the electric current; the second pulse should follow the first as quickly as the electroporator will allow. This process will probably lyse a substantial fraction of the cells.

7. Dilute cells into culture medium and return to growth conditions.

Notes

1. This protocol has been optimized for HeLa cells. A similar procedure has been reported to give efficient DNA transfection in several mammalian cell types (Potter 1988). Many variables are available for optimizing transfection for a given cell line: voltage, capacitance, number of pulses, RNA concentration, and buffer in which cells are electroporated. Conditions for transfecting DNA into the cell line of interest can be used for guidance. DNA transfection protocols for a variety of cell types are available from BioRad.

2. Cells are permeable to some viable dyes such as trypan blue immediately after electroporation, so allow several hours incubation in medium before using dyes to assay the fraction of cells that survive electroporation.

Transfection with DEAE-dextran

Reagents

The following should be made RNase-free:

RNase-free water and placental RNase inhibitor, as above

Buffer A: 10 mM Tris-HCl (pH 8.0), 0.2 mM EDTA, 2 mM DTT, 0.8 U μl^{-1} RNase inhibitor (add DTT and RNase inhibitor just before use).

RNA to be transfected (10 ng–1 μg)

DEAE-dextran, average molecular weight 500,000; dissolved in RNase-free water at 10 mg ml^{-1} and autoclaved

5× TD: per liter, 40 g NaCl, 15 g Tris base, 1.9 g KCl, 0.265 g anhydrous Na_2HPO_4, adjusted to pH 7.4 and autoclaved. (Because Tris-containing solutions cannot be prepared with diethylpyrocarbonate, this solution should be made up with RNase-free chemicals in RNase-free water. To adjust pH, remove small amounts of the solution and check on pH paper. The solution may then be autoclaved or filter-sterilized. Prepare a 5× stock: a 1× solution may not have sufficient buffering capacity for accurate readings with pH paper.)

CaCl$_2$–MgCl$_2$ stock: 10 mg ml^{-1} MgCl$_2$.6H$_2$O, 10 mg ml^{-1} CaCl$_2$.

The following need not be RNase-free

Cells to be transfected (on 60 mm plates; 60–80% confluent) culture medium

TD: per liter, 8 g NaCl, 3.0 g Tris base, 0.38 g KCl, 0.053 g anhydrous Na_2HPO_4, adjusted to pH 7.4 and autoclaved.

Protocol

1. Prepare RNase-free TS (200 µl per plate transfected) by diluting 5× TD into RNase-free water, then adding 1/100 volume $CaCl_2$–$MgCl_2$ stock. Prepare TS for washing cells by mixing TD (not RNase-free) with 1/100 volume $CaCl_2$–$MgCl_2$ stock. TS should be prepared fresh for each experiment.
2. Resuspend RNA in Buffer A; RNA for each transfection should be in 5 µl.
3. Mix together, in this order:
   190 µl RNase-free TS
     5 µl RNA
     10 µl DEAE-dextran solution
   Let sit at room temperature for 10 min.
4. Remove medium from cells and rinse plate once with TS.
5. Add 200 µl transfection mix to each plate. Immediately shake the plate to distribute the solution evenly. Let sit at room temperature for 15 min, shaking the plates occasionally.
6. Remove the transfection mix. Rinse plates once with TS. Add appropriate medium or agar overlay.

Notes

1. This procedure has been optimized for BSC-40 (monkey kidney) and HeLa cells. The optimum concentration of DEAE-dextran may be different for different cell lines.
2. Transfection into some cell types can be improved by a treatment with glycerol or DMSO before adding medium (Lopata et al 1984).
3. When transfecting a large amount of RNA with this method (i.e. around 1 µg per plate) it is important that the RNA be very clean. For RNA transcribed *in vitro*, purification on a G-50 spin column is recommended.

Detection and quantitation of RNA

Several methods are available to quantify specific RNAs in a mixed RNA population: PCR on reverse-transcribed RNA, RNase protection, Northern blots, and dot or slot blots. PCR is the most sensitive, able to detect as few as 10 molecules of RNA (Piatak et al 1993). While PCR is thus the method of choice for detecting very rare RNAs, quantitative PCR often requires substantial effort in designing and executing appropriate controls. RNase protection, though less sensitive, offers more straightforward quantitation. As few as 50,000 molecules can be detected with RNase protection (Novak and Kirkegaard, unpublished results). Northern blots and dot blots are around 10-fold less sensitive than RNase protection, and background from nonspecific hybridization is often higher. These methods are, however, simpler than PCR or RNase protection, and are suitable for some applications. Because Northern and dot blot protocols are widely available (Ausubel et al 1987; Berger and Kimmel 1987; Sambrook et al 1989; commercial suppliers of enzymes and support membranes), they are not included here. Protocols and discussion of applications of RNase protection and PCR are provided, along with protocols for isolating RNA from cells and for preparing RNA probes suitable for RNAse protection and Northern and dot blots.

Extracting RNA from cells

Cytoplasmic RNA

This protocol uses hypotonic buffer and the non-ionic detergent Nonidet P40 to lyse cells. Nuclei are then removed by centrifugation; the RNA is purified by phenol extraction and ethanol precipitation. RNases are inhibited during lysis and subsequent processing by vanadyl ribonucleoside complex (VRC, also called ribonucleoside vanadyl complex). VRC competitively inhibits many RNases by acting as a transition-state analog (Berger and Birkenmeier 1979). Because VRC also inhibits other protein–nucleic acid interactions, removing the VRC can be important. In this protocol, the bulk of the VRC is removed during phenol extraction; the remainder is dissociated with EDTA and removed by ethanol precipitation.

Reagents

The following should be RNase-free:

200 mM EDTA (pH 8.0)
3 M sodium acetate (pH 5–5.5)
ethanol

The following need not be RNase-free:

PBS and equilibrated phenol, as above
Lysis solution: 10 mM Tris-HCl (pH 7.5), 10 mM NaCl, 1% (v/v) Nonidet P40
200 mM VRC
10% sodium dodecyl sulfate (SDS)

Protocol

1. If cells are adherent, remove them from the plate by scraping with a sterile rubber police tool.
2. Pellet the cells by centrifugation; wash twice with PBS.
3. Add VRC to 5 mM to cold lysis buffer; resuspend the cells in 700 µl of this solution. Increase this volume if greater than 10^7 cells are harvested.
4. Freeze the sample, either briefly on dry ice or overnight at −20°C.

5. Thaw the sample and spin at 1500 *g* at 4°C for 10 min to pellet the nuclei.
6. Transfer the supernatant to a fresh tube. Add 35 µl 10% SDS and 700 µl phenol. Vortex vigorously, and spin the sample at 12,000 *g* for 3 min. VRC will turn the phenol layer gray-green.
7. Remove the aqueous phase to a fresh tube. To ensure that no protein present at the interface is transferred, recover no more than 80% of the original volume, and ensure that no whitish material is collected from the interface.
8. Put the sample on ice. Add EDTA to 5 mM. If the solution turns cloudy, spin the tubes briefly before aliquoting the RNA.
9. Aliquot the RNA and add 1/10 volume sodium acetate and 2.5 volumes of ethanol to each tube. Chill to precipitate, either 5 min on dry ice or overnight at −20°C. Store RNAs in ethanol at −20°C until ready to use.

Whole-cell RNA

This procedure is a modification of the method of Chomczynski (Chomczynski and Sacchi 1987). Cells are lysed in the presence of a powerful protein denaturant, guanidinium thiocyanate, to inhibit RNases. By a phenol-chloroform extraction under acidic conditions, protein and DNA are extracted into the interface and the organic layer, while RNA remains in the aqueous layer.

Reagents

The following should be RNase-free:

Isopropanol
80% ethanol

The following need not be RNase-free:

Guanidinium solution: stir together 250 g guanidinium thiocyanate, 17.6 ml 0.75 M sodium citrate (pH 7), 26.4 ml 10% *N*-lauroylsarcosine (Sarkosyl), and 293 ml distilled water. Heating to 65°C may help to dissolve the guanidinium. Store at room temperature for up to 3 months.
Denaturing solution: guanidinium solution with 0.1 M 2-mercaptoethanol (360 µl per 50 ml guanidinium solution). Store at room temperature for up to 1 month.
2 M sodium acetate, pH 4: dissolve 16.4 g sodium acetate in 35 ml glacial acetic acid; adjust pH to 4 with acetic acid, then add water to 100 ml.
Phenol, water saturated (do not use phenol equilibrated with buffer).
Chloroform-isoamyl alcohol, 49:1 (v/v).

Protocol

1. Remove medium from cells. Adherent cells maybe lysed directly on plates. To lyse, add 500 µl of denaturing solution per 5 × 10⁶ cells. (Volumes are given for 5 × 10⁶ cells; if more or fewer cells are used, change the volumes in proportion to cell number.) Pipette the mixture up and down several times with a micropipettor as the cells lyse to shear their DNA.
2. Transfer the lysate to an Eppendorf or Corex tube. Add 50 µl 2 M sodium acetate; mix well by inverting the tube.
3. Add 500 µl phenol; mix well, then add 100 µl chloroform/isoamyl alcohol and mix by vortexing. Place on ice for 15 min.
4. Centrifuge at 10,000 *g* for 20 min at 4°C. Aqueous and organic layers should be about equal in volume. If the volume of the aqueous phase is low, add slightly more chloroform/isoamyl alcohol and repeat the centrifugation.
5. Transfer the aqueous phase to a fresh

tube. Do not transfer any of the loose material at the interface.

6. Add 1 volume isopropanol and chill at −20°C for 30 min to overnight to precipitate the RNA.

7. Centrifuge at 10,000 g at 4°C for 20 min. Discard the supernatant.

8. Resuspend the pellet in 150 µl denaturing buffer. If it is not already in one, transfer sample to an Eppendorf tube.

9. *Optional*: if steps 5 and 6 did not cleanly separate the aqueous layer from the interface, add 15 µl 2 M sodium acetate, 150 µl phenol, and 30 µl chloroform-isoamyl alcohol, mixing after each addition. Spin at 12,000 g in a microcentrifuge and remove the aqueous phase to a fresh tube.

10. Add 150 µl isopropanol or 300 µl ethanol; store the RNA at −20°C.

Notes

1. This procedure should produce RNA clean enough for most applications, including RNase protection, Northern blots, and cDNA synthesis.

2. If the RNA is to be used in PCR analysis and was prepared from cells containing homologous DNA, RNase-free DNase treatment is recommended following the second alcohol precipitation.

Transcription of RNA probes

This procedure is designed for transcription of RNA labeled with ^{32}P at high specific activity. It is similar to the transcription protocol on p 165–166, except the total nucleotide concentration is reduced, and the specific activity can be varied according to the application.

The lifetime of RNA labeled at high specific activity is limited by radioactive decay of ^{32}P to sulphur, which causes strand breakage. For some applications, such as Northern or dot blotting, some RNA degradation presents no problem; for RNase protection, however, the majority of the probe must remain intact throughout the experiment. To obtain intact probe, a good strategy is to use a specific activity that results in an average of one or less ^{32}P atoms per molecule RNA. Thus, RNAs that are degraded by radioactive decay will also lose their label, and will not contribute to the signal. If a higher specific activity is used, it is essential to use the probe quickly. To illustrate, if an RNA probe averages two ^{32}P atoms per molecule, then 30 h after transcription, 11% of the counts will be in degraded RNA.

In calculating how many labeled atoms per molecule a given specific activity will yield, the following numbers may be useful. The specific activity of pure ^{32}P nucleotide is 9100 Ci mmol^{-1}; typical specific activities of commercially available labeled nucleotides are 800 and 3000 Ci mmol^{-1}. If a 200 nucleotide RNA molecule contains 50 uridine residues, it is necessary to dilute the ^{32}P-UTP with cold UTP to 182 Ci mmol^{-1} so that only 1/50 of the UTP in the transcription reaction is ^{32}P labeled. In the reaction conditions given below, labeled UTP at 800 Ci mmol^{-1} would contribute 3 µM UTP to the reaction; UTP at 3000 Ci mmol^{-1} would contribute 0.8 µM UTP.

Requirements for specific activity and quantity of the probe depend on the application and the concentration of the RNA being probed. To detect a fairly abundant viral RNA by dot or Northern blot, the probe specific activity should be around 200 Ci mmol^{-1} UTP. For rare RNAs, the specific activity can be increased to as much as 3000 Ci mmol^{-1} UTP, as long as the background levels are acceptable. The RNA transcribed in one 20 µl reaction is usually enough for several blots. For RNase protection to detect fairly rare RNAs, start with 2 fmol probe per sample, with the probe transcribed at 300 Ci mmol^{-1} UTP. For more abundant viral RNAs, try 20 fmol probe at 30 Ci mmol^{-1} UTP. For ribosomal RNA, try 2 pmol probe at a specific activity of 0.2 Ci mmol^{-1} UTP.

Glow-in-the-dark face paint (available from party supply stores)

Reagents

The following reagents should be made RNase-free:

TE: 10 mM Tris-HCl (pH 8.0), 1 mM EDTA
DNA to be transcribed (as on page 166)
10 × transcription buffer (as on page 166)
100 mM dithiothreitol (DTT; as on page 166)
Human placental ribonuclease inhibitor
Nucleotide solution: 2.5 mM each ATP, CTP, GTP (adjust pH to 7.0; store in aliquots at −20°C)
100 μM UTP (store in aliquots at −20°C)
[α-^{32}P]UTP, 10 Ci ml^{-1}, ≥800 mCi mmol^{-1}
T7, T3, or SP6 polymerase
10 M ammonium acetate (optional)
Ethanol
Distilled water

For optional gel purification:

80% ethanol
KB: 300 mM sodium acetate (pH 5–5.5), 20 mM Tris–HCl (pH 8.5 at 25°C), 1 mM EDTA
1 mg ml^{-1} tRNA (store at −20°C)

The following reagents need not be prepared RNase-free:

Equilibrated phenol

For optional gel purification:

Formamide loading buffer: 90% (v/v) deionized formamide, 0.01% xylene cyanol, 0.01% bromophenol blue, 0.1 × TBE (store at −20°C for up to a month, at −70°C for longer periods; see page 167 for 10× TBE recipe)
Denaturing polyacrylamide gel

Protocol

1. Mix the following, in the order given and at room temperature:
   RNase-free water to 20 μl
   2 μl 10× transcription buffer
   2 μl DTT, 100 mM solution
   Placental RNase inhibitor, to 0.8 units μl^{-1}
   UTP, to desired concentration
   4 μl nucleotide solution: 2.5 mM each ATP, CTP, GTP
   1 μl linearized DNA template, 1 mg ml^{-1}
   5 μl [α-^{32}P]UTP at 10 mCi ml^{-1}
   T7, T3, or SP6 RNA polymerase, 10 units
   Incubate at 37°C, 60–120 min.
2. If removal of the DNA template is desired, add RNase-free DNase and incubate according to the vendor's instructions. Removal of the DNA is not necessary if the probe is to be used for dot blots or Northern blots, or if the probe is to be gel purified. It is, however, essential for RNase protection probes used without gel purification.
3. Dilute the reaction with TE to 320 μl. Remove 1 μl and count in a scintillation counter. Add 320 μl equilibrated phenol, vortex, and centrifuge in a microcentrifuge at 12,000 g for 3 min at room temperature.
4. Remove the aqueous supernatant to a fresh tube. Add 0.25 volumes of 10 M ammonium acetate, then 2.5 volumes of ethanol. Chill briefly on dry ice to precipitate the RNA. Pellet the RNA in a microcentrifuge at 12,000 g for 10 min and remove the supernatant.
5. If the probe is not to be gel purified, resuspend the RNA pellet in 320 μl TE, then perform the ethanol precipitation with ammonium acetate twice more. This procedure will remove >95% of

the unincorporated nucleotides. When the probe is resuspended for use, an aliquot can be counted to find the amount of radioactivity incorporated into RNA; this allows calculating the probe yield as described in step 7.

6. *Optional gel purification*: (a) Rinse the RNA pellet with cold 80% ethanol, then dry the pellet under vacuum. Resuspend in 20 µl formamide loading buffer. Heat to 95°C for 3 min, then load onto a polyacrylamide-8 M urea gel. For efficient elution, choose the lowest percentage of acrylamide that will resolve nucleic acid of the relevant size (Sambrook et al 1989). Gels of 4% or less are slimy enough that handling gel slices is difficult. The capacity of polyacrylamide gels for RNA is large; the RNA may be loaded onto a gel as thin as 0.4 mm in a well 1–2 cm wide.

(b) After electrophoresis, mark the gel with several spots of glow-in-the-dark face paint and expose briefly to X-ray film. Align the gel with the autorad and excise the band representing full-length probe.

(c) If the gel was more than 0.5 mm thick, crush the gel slice by passing it through a disposable 3 ml syringe with no needle. Place the gel slice in an Eppendorf tube and freeze on dry ice. Thaw and add 600 µl KB, 3 µg tRNA and 600 µl phenol. Vortex to mix, then incubate at 4°C for 2–16 hours.

(d) Vortex the probe, then spin in a microcentrifuge at 12,000 *g* for 5 min. The gel material will be found at the interface. Remove the aqueous phase to a fresh tube. Add 200 µl KB to the original tube, vortex, and spin again. Pool the aqueous phases and phenol extract again. Note the volume of the aqueous phase; remove and count 1 µl in a scintillation counter to allow calculation of probe yield.

(e) Precipitate the RNA by adding 2.5 volumes of ethanol; freeze on dry ice or overnight at −20°C. This procedure should elute 90–95% of the RNA from the gel slice.

7. To calculate probe yield, find the fraction of radioactivity incorporated into RNA (F) and the µM concentration of UTP in the transcription reaction, including labeled UTP. RNA yield in fmol is then calculated using:

$$\text{RNA yield} = 4F \times (\mu\text{l reaction volume}) \times [\text{UTP}]/(\text{probe length, nt})$$

The accuracy of this calculation requires that the UTP concentration is accurate and that the uridine residues compose 25% of the RNA sequence.

RNase protection

For RNase protection, a labeled RNA probe is hybridized to the RNA of interest (Zinn et al 1983). RNase digestion eliminates the single-stranded probe that is not hybridized; labeled probe protected by the RNA of interest is then displayed on a polyacrylamide gel. RNase protection can be used to detect as little as 10^{-19} moles of RNA (Novak and Kirkegaard, unpublished results), making it more sensitive than dot blots or Northern blots.

Quantitation

For quantitative RNase protection, a standard curve is needed to ensure that the signal is responsive to differences in RNA concentration. A standard curve (cpm probe protected versus amount of specific RNA) for a series of RNA standards allows one to find the linear range of the assay. Samples in which the probe is in moderate molar excess (greater than 4-fold) over the specific RNA being probed are usually in the linear range, but even if the standards show that the signal is not directly proportional to RNA concentration, the relative amount of specific RNA in the experimental samples can be determined by interpolating from the standard curve. Finding the absolute concentrations of the specific RNA is possible if a known amount of specific RNA is used in the standards. Otherwise, a rough estimate can be obtained based on the amount of probe used and the fraction of probe protected in a given sample.

For most virology applications, the standards may consist of serial dilutions of RNA from infected cells. Either RNA from uninfected cells or tRNA should be added to the dilutions to make the total RNA concentration in each the same, so that the RNase digestion conditions are directly comparable. Preparing many aliquots of each dilution of the RNA standards allows the same standards to be used in multiple experiments.

Including an internal control often improves the accuracy of quantitation by correcting for sample loss or gel loading inaccuracies. A mixture of two probes can be used, one for the RNA of interest, and one for a cellular RNA whose concentration is expected to be the same in all the experimental samples. Any cellular RNA may be used that is abundant enough to give a strong signal and will not vary in intracellular concentration under the experimental conditions. Ribosomal RNA is often useful as an internal control. Because it has a long half-life in the cell, its abundance is less likely to be affected by any alterations in transcription caused by infection. The probes for the experimental and internal control RNAs must result in protected fragments of different length so that they can be separated by electrophoresis. Probe lengths and specific activities should be adjusted so that the protected band that tends to contain more radioactivity will migrate lower on the gel. Both bands will generate a fainter smear of degraded RNAs beneath them (Fig. 9.1), and quantitation is easier if the fainter band is not positioned in the smear below the darker one. When using a cellular RNA as an internal control, add tRNA, not cellular RNA, to equalize the amount of total RNA in the dilutions that generate the RNA standards.

If the complement of the RNA of interest is

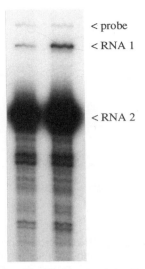

Figure 9.1. Simultaneous detection of two RNAs present in one sample by RNase protection. In this example, RNA 1 and RNA 2 were detected with the same probe; RNA 2 was approximately 100-fold more abundant than RNA 1. Quantitation of RNA 1 was possible only because the band protected by RNA 1 migrates higher in the gel than that protected by RNA 2. The highest band is probe that escaped RNase digestion.

also present in the cell, and the complement is more abundant than the RNA of interest, quantitation by conventional RNase protection works poorly. Two-cycle RNase protection, described below, should be used for detection and quantitation of an RNA in the presence of an excess of its complement.

Distinguishing related RNAs

RNase protection can be used to quantify two related RNAs separately, or to distinguish transcripts with different endpoints or processing characteristics. RNAs that differ by an insertion, deletion, or cluster of point changes can be distinguished easily if the difference is at least seven nucleotides; quantitative distinction of RNAs with smaller differences may require optimizing RNase digestion conditions. In all such experiments, the probe must be designed so that some part is cut when hybridized to one RNA but not the other.

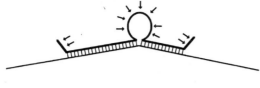

(A) Effective probe design

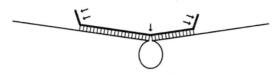

(B) Ineffective probe design

Figure 9.2. Design of RNase protection probe to distinguish an RNA bearing an insertion relative to another RNA. (A) An RNA probe complementary to the insertion variant is shown hybridized to the variant lacking the insertion. The region of the RNA probe that is looped out provides a good target for RNase digestion, symbolized by arrows. (B) An RNA probe complementary to the RNA lacking the insertion is shown hybridized to the RNA containing the insertion. Distinguishing the inserted RNA depends on cutting the probe opposite the loop, which may not be efficient.

Three considerations apply when designing such a probe.

1. When quantifying two RNAs, one of which bears an insertion relative to the other, the probe should be complementary to the inserted RNA, not to the RNA lacking the insertion (Fig. 9.2). When the probe is complementary to the inserted RNA, a single-stranded loop that provides a good RNase target is generated during hybridization. When the probe is complementary to the RNA lacking the insertion, it hybridizes completely to both RNAs, and distinguishing the RNAs would require cutting the probe opposite the insertion loop. While this cutting can occur under normal RNase protection conditions, it usually is not complete. If the probe must match the RNA lacking the insertion, it may be necessary to adjust RNase digestion conditions to those of lower salt, higher temperature, or more RNase.

2. The specificity of the RNases should be considered. Most RNase protection protocols use RNase A and RNase T1, allowing cutting after Cs, Gs, and Us. Therefore, if distinguishing RNAs depends on cutting within a small region of the probe, that region should contain several nucleotides that are not As. If this is not possible, RNase ONE (Promega) can be used, though it is more expensive and sensitive to inhibitors than RNase A and RNase T1.

3. The less prevalent RNA should protect a band that migrates higher in the gel. RNase protection bands are always associated with a fainter smear extending beneath them on the gel (Fig. 9.1) which can be reduced, but not completely eliminated by gel purifying the probe. Thus, an RNA that is much less prevalent can be completely obscured if its protected band is located beneath that of the other RNA.

Mapping the location of mutations

RNase protection can be used to map the position of mutations within an RNA genome. Deletions are the most foolproof (Kirkegaard and Nelsen 1990), but some point mutations, insertions, and crossover sites for RNA recombination can also be mapped (Myers et al 1985; Lopez-Galindez et al 1988; Kirkegaard and Baltimore 1986). This method requires a series of long RNase protection probes to span the genome. For many mutations, hybridization of a wild-type probe to an RNA mutant in that region will result in cutting of the probe at the location of the mutation. The probe need not be completely cut at this site, simply recognizably cut compared to probe hybridized to a wild-type RNA control. This test will show which probe covers the mutation and how far from an end of the probe the mutation lies. Using a probe with slightly different endpoints will then serve to locate the site uniquely.

Reagents

The following should be RNase-free:

Ethanol
1 mg/ml tRNA (store in aliquots at
  −20°C)
3 M sodium acetate pH 5.0–5.5
Radiolabeled probe, precipitated in
  ethanol
RNAs to be probed, precipitated in
  ethanol or isopropanol

The following need not be RNase-free:

Hybridization buffer: 80% (v/v)
  deionized formamide, 40 mM PIPES
  (pH 6.4 at 25°C), 400 mM NaCl, 1 mM
  EDTA (store at −20°C for up to a
  month, at −70°C for longer periods)
RNase cocktail: 300 mM NaCl, 10 mM
  Tris (pH 7.5), 5 mM EDTA, 15 μg ml^{-1}
  RNase A, 1 μg ml^{-1} (or
  350 units ml^{-1}) RNase T1 (store at
  4°C; stable for 3–4 months; do not use
  RNase T1 supplied as an ammonium
  sulfate suspension)
10% SDS
1 mg ml^{-1} proteinase K (store at
  −20°C)
Formamide loading buffer: (see page
  175)
DE81 paper (Whatman; optional)

Protocol

1. Prepare probe: pellet the labeled RNA
   probe, remove the supernatant, and
   rinse the pellet with cold 80% ethanol.
   Dry the pellet under vaccuum.
   Resuspend in hybridization buffer by
   heating to 37°C for 5 min and
   vortexing vigorously. Each sample will
   require 30 μl of probe.
2. If the amount of probe has not already
   been quantified, count 1 μl of
   resuspended probe in a scintillation
   counter; calculate as described
   above. If necessary, add more

hybridization buffer so that the
desired amount of probe is in a
volume of 30 μl.

3. Prepare the samples to be probed by
   pelleting, rinsing, and drying the
   RNAs. Useful controls may be tRNA,
   RNA prepared from cells lacking the
   specific RNA, and an RNA dilution
   series for constructing a standard
   curve. If two RNAs are being probed
   together in the experimental
   samples, it is useful to have controls
   in which each is probed separately.
4. Add 30 μl probe to each sample.
   Resuspend the RNA by heating to
   37°C and vortexing vigorously. If
   20 μg or more of RNA is in a sample,
   it may be necessary to pipet the RNA
   repeatedly to resuspend it. Save
   some probe for gel loading; this will
   probably have to be diluted with
   loading buffer by as much as 1:10 or
   1:100 to yield a signal comparable to
   that obtained from the protected
   samples.
5. Heat the samples to 85°C for 5 min to
   denature the RNA.
6. Incubate at 60°C for 12–20 hours.
   The tubes must be closed tightly to
   prevent water condensing around the
   top of the tube from seeping in.
7. Digest unhybridized probe by adding
   300 μl of RNase cocktail. For most
   applications, incubate either for
   15 min at 37°C or one hour at room
   temperature.
8. Digest the RNases by adding 10 μl
   SDS and 10 μl proteinase K.
   Incubate at 37°C for 15 min.
9. Add 350 μl phenol and vortex. Spin
   for 3 min at 12,000 g, then remove
   270 μl of aqueous supernatant from
   each sample to a fresh tube.
   Removing more supernatant can
   result in contamination of the sample
   with RNases present at the interface.
10. Add 1 μg tRNA, 30 μl sodium acetate,
    and 750 μl ethanol to each sample.
    Chill for 5 min on dry ice, or overnight
    at −20°C to precipitate the RNA.

11. Pellet the RNA, then rinse the pellet with 80% ethanol and dry it. Resuspend in 10 µl formamide loading buffer.
12. Denature the RNAs by heating to 95°C for 3 min. Immediately load onto a denaturing polyacrylamide gel. Also denature and load a sample of probe diluted into loading buffer and labeled RNA or DNA markers; on a denaturing gel, DNA and RNA will have similar, though not identical, mobilities.
13. After electrophoresis, dry the gel. To prevent RNA from leaching out of the gel during drying, it should be either dried on a backing of DE-81 paper, or fixed and dried on Whatman 3 MM or other backing paper. To fix, soak the gel in 7% acetic acid for 10 min, then rinse with distilled water.
14. Expose the gel to X-ray film. Quantitation of the RNase protection signal may be done by densitometry of the autoradiograph (which can be nonlinear), by radioanalytic scanning (AMBIS Systems) or by phosphorimaging analysis (Molecular Dynamics, Fuji or Packard Instruments).

Notes

1. Probes should contain some sequences not complementary to the RNA of interest on one or both ends. Often a small fraction of the probe is not digested by RNases; therefore, noncomplementary sequences are needed to distinguish undigested probe from probe protected by the RNA of interest.
2. Probes 100–600 nucleotide long are desirable. Longer probes are acceptable as long as they are not excessively degraded. Shorter or AU-rich probes may require lowering the hybridization temperature for optimal signal.
3. Gel purification of the probe is recommended for demanding applications, such as detecting very rare RNAs or quantifying two RNAs of very different abundances. For any application, using gel-purified probe often reduces the abundance of spurious bands in the RNase protection pattern.
4. RNase digestion conditions and hybridization conditions can be altered. RNase A and RNase T1 work well and are specific for single-stranded RNA in digests carried out at 4–40°C and with 50–500 mM NaCl. Protection of A·U hybrids, for example, can be carried out at 7°C in 500 mM NaCl with a 3-fold reduction in RNase A concentration.

Troubleshooting

Extra bands, both in experimental samples and in negative control

1. Hybridization may not be stringent enough. Increase hybridization temperature or use a longer probe.
2. RNase digestion may be working poorly. Replace RNase cocktail or increase RNase concentration. If it is suspected that the RNA samples contain contaminants that inhibit RNase, add an extra ethanol precipitation to the RNA preparation procedure.
3. A large amount of probe may be protected by its DNA template. Gel purify the probe or optimize DNase digestion after transcription.
4. The probe may be self-complementary. Check probe sequence using an RNA structure-prediction program; if stable secondary structure is predicted, use higher hybridization and RNase digestion temperatures or redesign probe.
5. The probe may be contaminated with complementary RNA transcribed from

a cryptic promoter. Gel purify or redesign probe.

Extra bands in experimental samples, not in negative control

1. The samples may be overdigested. Lower RNase concentration, lower digestion temperature or increase salt concentration in the RNase cocktail.
2. The sample RNAs may be degraded. Check solutions for RNase contamination or add extra phenol extraction in RNA preparation procedure.
3. The probe may be degraded. Check solutions for RNase contamination or gel purify probe.
4. Premature transcriptional stops may have yielded a heterogeneous probe. Gel purify probe or redesign probe to exclude the sequence generating the stop.
5. Longer RNA may contaminate the probe. Optimize restriction digestion of template to linearize completely, or gel purify template or probe.

No signal

1. The hybridization temperature may be too high. Use a lower incubation temperature or a longer probe.
2. The probe specific activity may be too low. Increase the probe specific activity; see suggestions on page 174.

RNA remains in gel wells

1. Protein may not be completely removed. Extract with phenol carefully after proteinase K digestion.
2. The formamide in the hybridization and loading buffers may be impure. See Sambrook et al (1989) for instructions on deionizing formamide.
3. Ammonium sulfate may have been introduced with RNases. Check enzyme specification sheets.

Two-cycle RNase protection

During viral infection, complementary strands of RNA are often present in the same cell. The probe and the endogenous complementary RNA will then compete for hybridization to the RNA of interest, and the shorter of the two, usually the probe, will have a slower on-rate and a faster off-rate of duplex formation (Bloomfield et al 1974). Polio virus negative-strand RNA, for example, is found in infected cells with a 50-fold excess of positive strands (Novak and Kirkegaard 1991). Poliovirus negative-strand RNA is nearly undetectable by dot blot. Conventional RNase protection yielded a low signal that varied erratically with viral RNA concentration (Novak and Kirkegaard 1991). Northern blots may avoid this problem, assuming that the positive- and negative-strand RNAs migrate differently in the gel system used.

Two-cycle RNase protection (Novak and Kirkegaard 1991) can be used to quantify any RNA in the presence of a greater amount of its complement. The sample RNAs are subjected to hybridization in the absence of probe, leaving the RNA of interest completely hybridized to its complement. RNase digestion then removes the excess complementary RNA. With competition for hybridization to the RNA of interest thus reduced, the probe is added, and the samples are subjected to a second round of hybridization and RNase digestion. Poliovirus negative-strand RNA probed by this method gave a signal more than 100-fold higher than the signal from conventional RNase protection. More importantly, the signal from two-cycle RNase protection was responsive to the amounts of negative-strand RNA in the samples and could be used to quantify these amounts (Novak and Kirkegaard 1991).

Reagents

Same as on page 179.

Protocol

1. Precipitate the RNA samples to be probed by spinning in a microcentrifuge at 12,000 g for 10 min. Remove the supernatants, rinse the pellets with cold 80% ethanol, and dry under vacuum.
2. Add 30 µl hybridization buffer to each RNA sample and vortex to resuspend. Do not add probe at this step.
3. Hybridize the RNAs by incubating at 60°C for 12–20 hours. If the complementary RNAs are shorter than 100 nt, reduce the hybridization temperature to 45–55°C.
4. Subject the RNAs to RNase digestion, proteinase K treatment and phenol extraction as described in steps 7–9 of protocol IIB.
5. Add 5 µg tRNA, 30 µl sodium acetate, and 750 µl ethanol to each sample. Chill for 5 min on dry ice or overnight at −20°C to precipitate the RNA. The samples are now ready to be subjected to the second round of RNase protection, identical to the standard RNase protection procedure. Follow the protocol on page 179, steps 1–14.

Quantitative RT-PCR (reverse transcription of RNA and amplification by polymerase chain reaction)

The legendary sensitivity of PCR, combined with its ability to amplify specific sequences when specifically designed deoxyoligonucleotide primers are used, make it an attractive technique with which to detect viral RNAs.

Synthesis of cDNA from specific viral RNAs can be accomplished by the use of reverse transcriptase (RT) and specific primers; for example, positive strands, negative strands or subsets of viral RNAs can be selectively converted to cDNA. Once the cDNA is made, the combination of primers used for PCR amplification can be used, for example, either to amplify the entire cDNA population or to dictate which of any different RNAs present in the cDNA population will be amplified. The sensitivity of PCR can allow the detection of variant RNAs that might otherwise be present at too low a level for detection, either because of their low concentration in the cell or because of the background from wild-type RNA molecules.

Primers can be designed so that RNAs or DNAs that differ by as little as a single nucleotide can be selectively copied by reverse transcription and PCR (Kwok et al 1990). However, the presence of at least two nucleotide differences between the RNAs to be distinguished greatly increases the specificity (Jarvis and Kirkegaard 1992). The primers, either for cDNA synthesis, PCR or both, should be designed so that the extreme 3′ end of the primer opposes the polymorphic nucleotides (Jarvis and Kirkegaard 1992).

To measure the final amount of DNA product made by PCR, one can either include radiolabeled dNTPs among those to be incorporated during amplification, or end-label one of the PCR primers with [32]P. Following gel electrophoresis to display the products of the PCR reactions, the amount of label in the bands of interest is then determined by excising the bands and scintillation counting, by using a radioanalytic scanner or by phosphorimaging. Use of an end-labeled primer has several advantages over body-labeling the PCR products. First, the pattern on the ensuing gel is often less plagued by background bands, because only those DNAs that include the radioactive primer will be labeled. Second, the relative amounts of radioactivity in bands of different sizes will directly reflect their stoichiometry. Finally, the presence of the labeled primer on the gel following electrophoresis allows one to express the amount of PCR

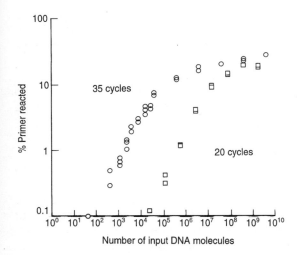

Figure 9.3. PCR signal is displayed as a function of initial DNA template concentration. The PCR signal shown is the percentage of ^{32}P-labeled PCR primer converted into full-length PCR product. The template for the PCR reactions was linearized plasmid DNA containing poliovirus cDNA sequences. The DNA template concentration is provided as the number of DNA molecules per 20 μl reaction. The amplification conditions were as described in the text for 20 or 35 cycles. Reproduced from Jarvis and Kirkegaard (1992) with permission from the publisher.

product formed as a percentage of the primer converted into product, as shown in Fig. 9.3. This not only facilitates determination of the quantitative range of the assay, but provides an internal control for the amount of each reaction loaded on the gel.

The exponential amplification of DNA molecules, although it accounts for the sensitivity of PCR, can also lead to wide variations in signal that depend on variables that are difficult to control rigorously. To ensure that variations in, for example, the temperature of different slots in the PCR machine do not unduly influence the results, duplicate reactions can be a great help. An additional problem with quantitation of PCR signals is illustrated in the experiment shown in Fig. 9.3. At low cDNA concentrations, the amount of product increased linearly with the amount of DNA originally present in the reaction. However, at higher cDNA concentrations or larger numbers of amplification cycles, the amount of product

made by PCR became much less sensitive to the amount of input DNA. Regardless of the number of cycles, the amount of product DNA plateaued when approximately 20–30% of the primers had been incorporated at the polymerase concentration used. Only when 2% or less of the primers had been incorporated was the signal linearly responsive to the amount of input DNA.

Thus, to quantify the amount of RNA originally present in a reaction mixture, two conditions must be met. First, the amount of cDNA synthesized from the RNA must be reproducible or internally controlled so that sample-to-sample variations in the amount of cDNA synthesis will not influence the final measurement. Second, the amount of PCR product synthesized from the cDNA must be within the sensitive range of the assay.

Three different approaches to making RT-PCR a quantitative procedure have been outlined in an excellent review (Foley et al 1993) and are discussed below. Then a detailed protocol for an application of one of these approaches, taken from our own work (Jarvis and Kirkegaard 1992), is provided.

Semi-quantitative RT-PCR

To determine the approximate amount of a specific RNA in a sample, a simple method is to compare the RT-PCR signal obtained from that sample with that of a standard curve. The standards can be generated by transcribing the RNA of interest *in vitro* and making serial dilutions into a preparation of RNA from uninfected cells. Reverse transcriptase reactions on the experimental samples and the standards should be performed in parallel using the same deoxyoligonucleotide primer, nucleotide, buffer and enzyme mixes. Then, PCR should be performed using common primer, nucleotide, buffer and enzyme mixes. Analysis of the amount of PCR product in the standards will identify the sensitive range of the assay and the approximate amount of RNA in the experimental samples that fall within this region can be determined by interpolation.

This kind of assay is only semi-quantitative because it does not take into account possible variations in the yield of RNA in different preparations, the efficiency of cDNA synthesis between different reactions, or variations in sample loading. If, for example, an inhibitor of reverse transcriptase were present in the RNA samples from infected but not uninfected cells, the amount of RNA measured in the infected samples would be erroneously low. Given these caveats, however, this approach is suitable for many applications.

Quantitative determination of relative amounts of RNAs

If an RNA species that does not vary in amount from sample to sample can be identified, it can serve as an internal control for reverse transcriptase activity, RNA yield and gel loading. For virologists, candidate cellular RNAs are stable RNAs whose abundance does not change substantially during viral infection, as is often the case for ribosomal RNAs and mRNAs for ribosomal proteins; other potential internal controls may be known or established empirically. Useful primers for selected ribosomal protein mRNAs from humans, mice, chickens, and *Drosophila* can be found in the review by Foley et al (1993).

Synthesis of cDNA from both the experimental and internal control RNAs, using primers specific for each RNA, should be performed in parallel using the same nucleotide, primer, buffer and enzyme mixes. Although cDNA synthesis from the two RNA species will differ in priming and elongation efficiency, these differences will presumably be the same in every sample and should not detract from the quantitation. The cDNA preparations are serially diluted and the PCR reactions performed under some standard condition for each of the two primer pairs. The difference in dilution required to give the same yield of PCR product for the experimental and control RNAs will provide a relative experimental ratio of the experimental and control RNAs in that sample. Differences in

the experimental ratios of these two products in different RNA preparations will reflect quantitatively the differences in the ratios of these RNAs in the original RNA preparation. Determining the sensitive range for both PCR products by diluting the cDNAs is preferable to comparing them to standard curves because the dilution experiments are internally controlled for the efficiency of cDNA synthesis and RNA extraction.

To obtain the absolute amount of viral RNA from these ratios, one can spike a preparation of RNA from uninfected cells that contain the internal control RNA with known amounts of the viral RNA of interest, transcribed *in vitro*. The experimental ratio of the PCR signals can then be used to generate a standard curve.

When cDNAs from the experimental and control RNAs can be made from the same cDNA primer, assuming the efficiency of their cDNA synthesis is the same, one can determine their absolute ratios by subsequent PCR analysis. This was the approach used by our laboratory (Jarvis and Kirkegaard 1992) to determine the ratio of recombinant to parental RNA present under different conditions in poliovirus-infected cells. This approach is applicable to any two RNAs that share a cDNA primer-binding site but differ sufficiently that the resulting cDNAs can be differently amplified by PCR. In addition to measuring the percentage of viral recombinants or variants in a population, this method could be useful to quantify the products of alternative splicing or to measure the relative accumulation of mutant and wild-type genomes during coinfections.

To use an RNA synthesized from the same cDNA primer as an internal control, the reverse transcriptase reactions for all the samples to be compared are run in parallel, using the same mix of nucleotides, primer, buffer and enzyme. Serial dilutions of the resulting cDNAs are subjected to separate PCR reactions with the two RNA-specific primer pairs of interest. The amounts of PCR product, when plotted as a function of the amount of cDNA dilution, should reveal the linear range for each primer pair (Fig. 9.3). The difference in dilution required to give an identical signal for the two

PCR products gives the experimental ratio of the two cDNAs in the sample. To determine the absolute ratio of these two cDNAs, their relative PCR amplification efficiencies must be independently measured. Differences in amplification efficiency of the two cDNAs could result from differences in annealing of the specific primers, sequence-dependent variation in elongation by the thermostable polymerase, or different lengths of the PCR product. Relative amplification efficiencies can be measured by mixing together known ratios of the two cDNAs, presumably available from DNA plasmids in the laboratory. Then, the relative amplification efficiencies can be used to correct the measured experimental ratio to an absolute ratio.

In the determination of recombination frequencies, the formation of PHLOP products (primer halt-mediated linkage of primers (Frohman and Martin 1990)) can artificially cause the appearance of recombinant cDNAs or PCR products. For a discussion of this problem and its experimental solution, see Jarvis and Kirkegaard (1992).

Quantitative determination of absolute amounts of RNA

This approach requires the addition to the RNA samples of control RNA molecules that contain binding sites for both the cDNA primer and the PCR primers that will be used to detect the RNA of experimental interest. The added RNA should be designed so that the PCR product made from its cDNA will be distinguishable from the RNA of interest. Ideally, the two products will differ only slightly in size, so that their length difference will not cause a substantial difference in their PCR amplification efficiencies.

First, various dilutions of a known amount of the external control RNA are added to aliquots of each RNA sample. Reverse transcription using a common primer will result in the synthesis of cDNA from both experimental and control RNAs. Subsequent PCR reactions under a fixed set of conditions will amplify both cDNAs. The condition at which equal amounts of the two PCR products are synthesized is the condition at which the concentrations of external control RNA and experimental RNA are identical (Wang et al 1989). Actually, the accuracy of this latter statement requires that the efficiencies of cDNA priming and PCR amplification are identical for these two related RNAs. This assumption can be explicitly tested by mixing experiments with known amounts of the two RNAs, synthesized in vitro.

This method is somewhat erroneously termed 'competitive RT-PCR'. The added exogenous control may or may not compete with the RNA of interest for primer and enzyme binding. Within the linear range of the RT and PCR assays, there will be no competition between these two RNAs or their products. Nonetheless, this method can be used to determine absolute concentrations of RNA molecules of interest both in the linear range of the PCR assay and at higher extents of amplification as well (Becker-Andre and Hahlbrock 1989; Gilliland et al 1990).

Reagents

The following should be made or purchased RNase-free:

Deoxyoligonucleotides for cDNA synthesis and PCR analysis (resuspended in water at 2.0 μM)
5× cDNA buffer: 250 mM Tris-HCl (pH 8.3), 375 mM KCl, 15 mM $MgCl_2$, 50 mM DTT
human placental ribonuclease inhibitor
reverse transcriptase from Moloney murine leukemia virus (Superscript RNase H$^-$; GIBCO-BRL)
dNTP mix: 20 mM each dATP, dTTP, dCTP and dGTP
8 M urea
TE buffer: 10 mM Tris-HCl (pH 8.0); 1 mM EDTA
Centricon-100 microfiltration units (Amicon)

The following need not be RNase-free:

T4 polynucleotide kinase
DNase-free RNase (Boehringer-
 Mannheim)
10× kinase buffer: 500 mM Tris-HCl
 (pH 7.6), 100 mM MgCl$_2$, 50 mM DTT,
 1 mM spermidine trihydrochloride,
 1 mM EDTA
[γ-^{32}P]ATP (approx. 3000 Ci mmol^{-1})
2 M potassium glutamate
1 M HEPES (pH 8.4)
100 mM MgCl$_2$
Acetylated BSA
dNTP mix (20 mM each dATP, dTTP,
 dCTP, dGTP)
Amplitaq DNA polymerase (Perkin
 Elmer-Cetus)
light mineral oil (Sigma)
0.025 μM filters, 13 mm diameter
 (Millipore VSWP)
formamide loading buffer (96%
 deionized formamide, 10 mM EDTA)
formamide loading buffer with dyes
 (90% deionized formamide, 0.01%
 xylene cyanol, 0.01% bromophenol
 blue, 10 mM EDTA)
Petri dish
Whatman DE-81 paper

Protocol

cDNA synthesis

1. Prepare 15 μl samples of each desired
   RNA sample. Prewarm to 47°C.
2. Prepare enzyme/primer mix. For 9–10
   reactions, mix in the order given:
   H$_2$O to final volume of 350 μl
   100 μl 5× cDNA buffer
   400 units placental ribonuclease
    inhibitor
   37.5 μl dNTP mix
   2.5 μl deoxyoligonucleotide primer
   400–2000 units reverse transcriptase
    (to optimize specificity, the amount
    should be determined for each RNA/
    primer pair and batch of enzyme)
   Prewarm the solution to 47°C.

3. Add 35 μl enzyme/primer mix to each
   RNA sample. Incubate for 1 h at 47°C.
4. Add 50 μl 8 M urea, then 1 unit DNase-
   free RNase to each sample. Incubate
   1 h at 60°C.
5. Add 400 μl TE to each sample. Place
   in Centricon-100 microfiltration unit,
   spin at 900 g for 15 min. Add 1 ml TE
   to each unit and respin for 35 min at
   900 g. This procedure will remove
   nucleotides, primers, and small RNA
   molecules. Store the remaining
   volume (about 50 μl), at −70°C until
   ready for further analysis.

Labeling PCR primers

1. Mix together in the order indicated:
   H$_2$O to 50 μl
   10 μl 2.0 μM primer (enough for 20
    PCR reactions)
   40 μCi [γ-^{32}P]ATP
   5 μl 10× kinase buffer
   5–10 units polynucleotide kinase.
   Incubate at 37°C for 30 min.
2. To remove ATP and kinase buffer,
   'drop-dialyze' (Berger and Kimmel
   1987) the sample. Float the Millipore
   filter, shiny side up, in a Petri dish filled
   with 5–10 ml of TE. Carefully add the
   50 μl sample to the center of the
   floating filter. After 2–3 hours, remove
   the sample from the center of the filter;
   sample loss should be less than 10%
   (Marusyk 1980).
3. The specific activity of the recovered
   deoxyoligonucleotide primer should
   be approximately 1 μCi pmol^{-1}. Store
   the labeled primer at −20°C for no
   more than 1–2 days.

PCR amplification

1. For each pair of PCR primers, prepare
   a mix containing the primers, dNTPs,
   buffers and enzymes. The following
   mix is sufficient for 19–20 samples.
   H$_2$O to 300 μl
   10 μl 2 M potassium glutamate
   10 μl 1 M potassium HEPES (pH 8.4)

13.2 µl 1 M $MgCl_2$

40 µg acetylated BSA

10 µl solution of 20 mM each dNTP

100 µl 2.0 µM cold PCR primer

50 µl ^{32}P-labeled PCR primer (now approximately 0.4 µM; see protocol above)

40 units Amplitaq DNA polymerase

For each PCR reaction, transfer 15 µl of this mix to a 0.5 ml tube on ice.

2. Set up DNA template samples; make serial dilutions of cDNA samples and plasmid controls in TE. Add 5 µl of each desired DNA sample to one of the 15 µl aliquots of primer/enzyme mix. Then add 25 µl light mineral oil to the top of each sample.

3. Subject samples to thermocycling in a programmable thermal cycler. The samples in Fig. 9.4 were subjected to a temperature profile of 1 min at 94°C, 1 min at 60°C and 2 min at 72°C for 20–35 cycles.

4. Remove 5 µl from the bottom of each tube and transfer to a new tube. Add 15 µl of formamide loading buffer without dyes. Immediately before electrophoresis, heat samples at 95°C for 1 min, then chill on ice before loading.

5. Electrophorese samples in a denaturing polyacrylamide gel. Include a lane of labeled DNA markers of appropriate sizes, and a lane of formamide loading buffer that contains dyes so that the progress of electrophoresis can be monitored. Choose a gel percentage and electrophoresis conditions so that the labeled primer does not electrophorese off the bottom of the gel.

6. Dry the gel onto DE-81 paper. Quantify the amount of radioactivity in the product and primer bands by radioanalytic scanning, phosphorimaging analysis, or by excising the bands and scintillation counting.

List of Suppliers

5 Prime → 3 Prime, Inc.	5603 Arapahoe Avenue, Boulder, CO 80303, USA.	800–533–5703
AMBIS Systems	3939 Ruffin Road, San Diego, CA 92123, USA.	800–882–6247
Amicon	17 Cherry Hill Drive, Danvers, MA 01923, USA.	800–343–0696
Bio-Rad	3300 Regatta Boulevard, Richmond, CA 94804, USA.	800–227–5589
Boehringer Mannheim Corporation	9115 Hagne Road, Indianapolis, IN 46250–0414, USA.	800–262–1640
BTX, Inc.	3742 Jewell Street, San Diego, CA 92109, USA.	619–597–6006
Fuji Medical Systems U.S.A., Inc.	333 Ludlow Street, Stamford, CT 06912–0035, USA.	800–431–1850
International Biotechnologies, Inc.	25 Science Park, New Haven, CT 06535, USA.	800–243–2555
Life Technologies, Inc. d.b.a. Gibco BRL	3175 Staley Road, Grand Island, NY 14072, USA.	800–828–6686
Molecular Dynamics	928 East Arques Avenue, Sunnyvale, CA 94086, USA.	800–333–5703
Packard Instrument Company, Inc.	2200 Warrenville Road, Downers Grove, IL 60515, USA.	312–969–6000
Perkin-Elmer/Cetus	761 Main Avenue, Norwalk, CT 06859–0156, USA.	800–762–4002
Pharmacia LKB	800 Centennial Avenue, Piscataway, NJ 08854, USA.	800–526–3593
Promega	2800 Woods Hollow Road, Madison, WI 53711–5399, USA.	800–356–9526
Sigma Chemical Company	P.O. Box 14508, St. Louis, MO 63178, USA.	800–325–3010

References

Ausubel FM, Brent R, Kingston RE, Moore DD, Seidman JG, Smith JA, Struhl K (1987) Current Protocols in Molecular Biology. Greene Publishing Associates and John Wiley & Sons, Brooklyn, New York.

Ball LA, Amann JM, Garrett BK (1992) J Virol 66: 2326–2324.

Becker-Andre M, Hahlbrock K (1989) Nucl Acids Res 17: 9437–9446.

Berger SL, Birkenmeier CS (1979) Biochemistry 18: 5143–5149.

Berger SL, Kimmel AR (1987) Guide to molecular cloning techniques. Academic Press, Orlando.

Bloomfield VA, Crothers DM, Tinoco I (1974) Physical chemistry of nucleic acids. Harper & Row Publishers, Inc., New York.

Chomczynski P, Sacchi N (1987) Anal Biochem 162: 156–159.

Foley KP, Leonard MW, Engel JD (1993) Trends in Genetics 9: 380–384.

Frohman MA, Martin GR (1990) In: PCR Protocols. Innis MA (Ed.) Academic Press, New York, pp 228–236.

Gilliland G, Perrin S, Blanchard K, Bunn HF (1990) Proc Natl Acad Sci USA 87: 2725–2729.

Gonzalez RG, Haxo RS, Schleich T (1980) Biochemistry 19: 4299–4303.

Grakoui A, Levis R, Raju R, Huang HV, Rice CM (1989) J Virol 63: 5216–5227.

Hambidge SJ, Sarnow P (1991) J Virol 65: 6312–6315.

Jarvis TC, Kirkegaard K (1992) EMBO J 11: 3135–3145.

Kaplan G, Racaniello VR (1988) J Virol 62: 1687–1696.

Kirkegaard K, Baltimore D (1986) Cell 47: 433–443.

Kirkegaard K, Nelsen B (1990) J Virol 64: 185–194.

Kwok S, Kellogg DE, McKinney N, Spasic D, Goda L, Levenson C, Sninsky JJ (1990) Nucl Acids Res 18: 999–1005.

Lopata MA, Cleveland DW, Sollner WB (1984) Nucl Acids Res 12: 5707–17.

Lopez-Galindez C, Lopez JA, Melero JA, de la Fuente L, Martinez C, Ortin J, Perucho M (1988) Proc Natl Acad Sci USA 85: 3522–3526.

Marc D, Masson G, Girard M, van der Werf S (1990) J Virol 64: 4099–4107.

Marusyk R (1980) Anal Biochem 105: 403–411.

Myers RM, Larin A, Maniatis T (1985) Science 230: 1242–1246.

Novak JE, Kirkegaard K (1991) J Virol 65: 3384–3387.

Novak JE, Kirkegaard K (1994) Genes Dev 8: 1726–1737.

Piatak M, Luk K-C, Williams B, Lifson JD (1993) BioTechniques 14: 70–81.

Potter H (1988) Anal Biochem 174: 361–373.

Sambrook J, Fritsch EF, Maniatis T (1989) Molecular Cloning: A Laboratory Manual. Cold Spring Harbor Laboratory Press, Cold Spring Harbor.

Wang AM, Doyle MV, Mark DF (1989) Proc Natl Acad Sci USA 86: 9717–9721.

Zinn K, Di Maio D, Maniatis T (1983) Cell 34: 865–879.

DNA viruses:
DNA extraction,
purification and
characterization

10

D. J. McCance

This chapter will deal with various techniques used when working with DNA viruses and in particular, viruses containing small molecular weight DNA, such as those contained within the papovavirus family. However, many of the techniques can be applied to the herpes and adenovirus families, in particular when working with subgenomic fragments of these larger viruses. In general the problems working with DNA are not so great as those with RNA, since the double-stranded species is less easily denatured. However, for many of the experiments to be carried out with DNA, the preparation of pure, clean DNA is essential.

Virology Methods Manual
ISBN 0–12–465330–8

Extraction of viral DNA

With viruses that can be propagated in tissue culture DNA can be extracted from virus particles which have been purified as described in chapter 4. However, for papillomaviruses, which cannot be propagated in cell culture, or for viruses with low molecular weight DNA, their genomes can be extracted directly from cells, without contaminating high molecular weight DNA, i.e. chromosomal DNA. In addition viral genomes, which may integrate into chromosomal DNA, can be detected by methods which extract chromosomal DNA.

Low molecular weight viral DNA

There are two methods of extraction, which have been used equally successfully to isolate small molecular weight viral DNA. The first is a method described by Hirt (1967) and the second is a method adapted from the extraction of plasmid DNA from bacterial cultures by an alkaline lysis protocol (Sambrook et al 1989).

Method 1

1. Cells in 100 mm petri dishes are washed in PBSA before adding 2 ml of Hirt mixture (Table 10.1).

2. This is left at room temperature for 15 min before adding 0.5 ml 5 M NaCl and scraping the cells into a 15 ml polystyrene centrifuge tube.

3. After incubation for at least 2 h (it can be left overnight) at 4°C, high molecular weight DNA and cell debris are pelleted by centrifugation at approximately 3000 g for 15 min.

4. The supernatant is transferred to microcentrifuge tubes and extracted sequentially using phenol (saturated with 10 mM Tris, pH 8; 1 mM EDTA [TE]) and phenol and chloroform (1:1 ratio) and finally chloroform alone. Chloroform is always used as a mixture of chloroform:isoamyl alcohol (24:1).

5. The DNA is precipitated by addition of a 0.6 volume of isopropanol and recovered by centrifugation in an Eppendorf microcentrifuge for 20 min at 4°C.

6. The precipitate of DNA is washed in 70% ethanol and redissolved in TE or water.

Note

For long term storage it is best to redissolve in TE as DNA will denature over time in water.

Table 10.1. Buffers for extraction of DNA from cells and tissue.

Reagents	A	B	Hirt	Solution I	Solution II	STE
Tris-HCl, pH 8	10	50	50 (pH 7.5)	–	–	10
EDTA*	10	10	10	–	–	1
NaCl	10	10	130	130	–	100
SDS#	0.5%¶	10	0.67%	0.67%	–	–
Potassium Acetate§	–	–	–	–	3000	–

* EDTA, ethylene diamine tetra acetic acid is made up as a 500 mM solution adjusted to pH 7.5 with NaOH.
\# sodium dodecyl sulphate.
¶ % expressed as w/v.
§ 60 ml of 5 M potassium acetate and 11.5 ml of acetic acid made to 100 ml with water.

Method 2

1. 100 mm Petri dishes containing cells are washed in PBS and then 0.6 ml of solution I (Table 10.1) added and the lysates scraped into Eppendorf tubes.
2. The contents are mixed with 0.3 ml of solution II (Table 10.1) and high molecular DNA precipitated by centrifugation at 10,000 g for 5 min.
3. The supernatant is removed and DNA precipitated with 0.6 volume of isopropanol and the DNA recovered by centrifugation for 20 min at 10,000 g at 4°C.
4. The DNA is dissolved in 20–30 μl of TE (pH 7.5) and treated with an equal volume of 5 M lithium chloride (LiCl) on ice for 5 min, spun for 10 min and the supernatant containing low molecular weight DNA removed. The pellet contains high molecular weight DNA and RNA precipitated by LiCl.
5. The DNA in the supernatant is precipitated as above in method 1, step 5, washed in 70% ethanol and resuspended in water or TE.

Note

The DNA recovered by this method is more pure than method 1, however, in both cases it may be necessary to remove some contaminating small molecular weight RNA using DNAse-free RNAse (20 μg ml^{-1}, for 1 h at room temperature) followed by proteinase K (100 μg ml^{-1}, with addition of SDS to 0.5% and incubation at 37°C for 1 h) and then extraction with phenol and phenol:chloroform as described above.

The DNA is ready to digest with restriction enzymes or for subcloning.

High molecular weight DNA

High molecular weight DNA can be extracted from cell culture and tissue by the same general method and is adapted from Gross-Bellard et al (1973). The buffers to be used are described in Table 10.1.

1. Cells are washed in PBS and then 5 ml of buffer A per 100 mm plate plus 100 μg ml^{-1} of proteinase K is added, the cells scraped from the plate and incubated for 1 h at 37°C.
2. In the case of tissues, they are finely minced with scissors then homogenized in 5 ml of buffer A containing 100 μg ml^{-1} of proteinase K in a tissue homogenizer and incubated overnight at 37°C. This incubation time ensures that the tissue will be completely solubilized in the buffer.
3. After the incubation period for cells or tissue, the homogenates are extracted with TE saturated phenol, followed by phenol:chloroform (1:1) and then chloroform alone and in each case, the aqueous phase is separated by centrifugation at 10,000 g for 15 min at room temperature. At this stage the aqueous phase will be quite viscous and care has to be taken not to take off the white protein interphase between the aqueous and organic phases. In addition, to ensure that the DNA is not sheared, wide mouthed pipettes should be used to remove the aqueous phase. Wide mouthed Pasteur pipettes can be made using a diamond point pencil to remove part of the tip.
4. The aqueous phase is then treated at room temperature with RNase (20 μg ml^{-1}) for 1 h, followed by proteinase K (100 μg ml^{-1}) plus SDS to 0.5%, for 1 h at 37°C.

5. The proteins are then extracted with phenol, phenol:chloroform and finally chloroform alone. Again it is important to use wide mouthed pipettes to prevent shearing of the high molecular weight DNA.

6. To precipitate the DNA, 0.6 volume of isopropanol and 1/10 volume of 5 M ammonium acetate is added and the contents of the tube mixed very gently. At this stage, even at room temperature, chromosomal DNA will precipitate and will be seen as white fluffy strands.

7. These strands can be removed with a wide mouthed pipette and washed in 70% ethanol and then dissolved in TE or water. Lower molecular weight DNA can be precipitated from the remaining extraction by placing the tube at $-20°C$ for 1 h and spinning the DNA out at 10,000 g for 15 min at 4°C.

Extraction of DNA from viral particles

DNA can be extracted from virus particles by lysis of the virions and purification of the genome by techniques described above. In some cases where the virus is very cell associated, such as varicella zoster, or some strains of human herpes virus type 6 (HHV-6), it may be necessary to extract the DNA from the cells. The following method has been used very successfully to extract DNA from HHV-6 (Dewhurst et al 1992):

1. Tissue culture cells (30–50 $\times$ 10^6 cord blood mononuclear cells) are harvested at maximal cytopathic effect and the cells spun out at 1000 g for 15 min at 4°C. When using this technique for herpes simplex fewer cells will still give you workable levels of DNA.

2. The supernatant containing the virions is removed and transferred to a 40 ml Oak Ridge tube and centrifuged at 25,000 for 2 h. Any tube of approximately 40–50 ml will do, as long as it will withstand the centrifugal forces.

3. All of the media apart from approximately 1 ml is removed and the virions are resuspended in this volume and then transferred to a 1.5 ml Eppendorf tube.

4. The virions are briefly pelleted for 1 min at room temperature in a microfuge, the medium aspirated and the virion DNA extracted by adding approximately 600 µl of STE (Table 10.1) with 1% sarkosyl and RNAse (100 µg ml^{-1}) and proteinase K (200 µg ml^{-1}) and incubating the mixture at 56°C overnight. It may appear strange to have both proteinase K and RNAse in together, but the RNAse activity is so efficient it will digest any RNA present.

5. Next day the DNA is extracted twice with phenol:chloroform (1:1) and once with chloroform before a 1/10 volume of 5 M NaCl is added and the tube is topped up with cold isopropanol and the DNA precipitated at $-70°C$ for 15 min.

6. The DNA is spun out in an Eppendorf centrifuge for 20 min, washed in 70% ethanol, dried and resuspended in 0.2 ml of TE. This method gives 0.1 to 1 µg ml^{-1} of HHV-6 DNA.

Quantitation of DNA preparations

The concentration of DNA can be measured spectrophotometrically at 260 nm using the formula that 1 OD unit = 50 µg ml^{-1} (40 µg ml^{-1} for single-stranded DNA and RNA). The purity can be estimated by also measuring the OD at 280 nm and the 260/280 ratio should be 1.8 if the DNA is not contaminated with phenol or protein.

Sizing and analysis

Gel electrophoresis

The most direct way to determine the size of the isolated DNA is to run the preparation on an agarose gel containing ethidium bromide (0.5 µg ml^{-1}), which will bind to the DNA and will enable its visualization after exposure of the gel to ultra violet light. An alternative to running the gel with ethidium bromide, is to soak the gel in an ethidium bromide solution (2 µg ml^{-1}) for 30 min after electrophoresis. Ethidium bromide is carcinogenic, so care must be taken to reduce exposure of laboratory personnel to this substance. The test DNA is run along with marker DNA of known size. This technique is used mainly for double-stranded DNA, which runs at distances proportional to size. For double-stranded DNA neutral buffers like Tris-acetate (Table 10.2) can be used to make the gel and for running buffer. For single-stranded DNA, alkaline gels and buffers are used to minimize the secondary structures, which may cause the DNA to run abnormally. Typically for alkaline gels, agarose is dissolved in water by boiling, then cooled to around 60°C and NaOH added to a final concentration of 50 mM and EDTA to 1 mM. The gel is poured and run in alkaline buffer (Table 10.2). Ethidium bromide does bind to single-stranded DNA as well as to double-stranded DNA and will not bind in the alkaline gels. Therefore the gels must be neutralized with a solution of 1 M Tris (pH 7.6), and 1.5 M NaCl for 1 h after electrophoresis, and then can be treated with ethidium bromide.

Agarose gels are used to separate DNA bands of 0.5 to 10 kb in size. For analysis of smaller band sizes, then polyacrylamide gels are used. Polyacrylamide is usually used for protein separations, but is also used to separate DNA fragments of 10–500 bases, and can be used for band sizes up to 1000–2000. Nondenaturing gels, i.e. without SDS, are used and are run in a Tris borate buffer (Table 10.2). Usually 10–12% gels are used. For 10% gels:

> 30% acrylamide (stock is 33.3 g of acrylamide and 0.87 g of bis [N-methylene bisacrylamide] made up to 110 ml in distilled water) (10.6 ml)
> Tris buffer (pH 8.8) (18.5 g of Tris base to 100 ml; adjust pH to 8.8 with HCl) (8 ml) distilled water (13.1 ml)
> 10% ammonium persulfate (0.16 ml)
> TEMED (N,N,N$_1$,N$_1$-Tetramethylethylenediamine) (0.015 ml)

Restriction endonuclease analysis

Restriction endonuclease analysis is a way to determine if the DNA isolated is the same as prototypical viral DNA. For instance, the human papillomaviruses type 16 (HPV-16) is cut six times by the restriction endonuclease *Pst* I. Therefore, after isolation of the genome from biopsy material, testing with this and

Table 10.2. Electrophoresis buffers.

Buffer	Concentration per liter*
1× Tris-acetate	4.8 g Tris base + 1.1 ml glacial acetic acid + 2 ml 1 mM EDTA (pH 8.0)
0.5× Tris-borate	10.8 g Tris base + 5.5 g boric acid + 4 ml 1 mM EDTA (pH 8.0)
1× alkaline	5 ml NaOH + 2 ml 1mM EDTA (pH 8.0)

* It is possible to make Tris-acetate at 10× and Tris-borate at 5×.

other enzymes will indicate if the viral DNA isolated is HPV-16. Other larger DNA viruses, such as herpes simplex types 1 and 2 can be differentiated by restriction endonuclease analysis using, for instance, the *Kpn* I enzyme. In addition, HSV-1 types isolated from different individuals can exhibit different restriction patterns. The buffers used for restriction digests come with the enzyme from the manufacture, so these do not need to be prepared. However, several enzymes work best in different salt concentrations, and on some occasions it is desirable to digest with two enzymes at the same time.

There is a buffer, called KGB (Sambrook et al 1989), which allows two enzymes with different salt concentration optima to function at 75–100% of activity in their respective optimum buffers. The make-up is 100 mM potassium acetate; 25 mM Tris-acetate, pH 7.5; 10 mM magnesium acetate; 50 μg ml^{-1} bovine serum albumin; 0.5 mM β-mercaptoethanol. Note, this can be made 2× concentration. KGB works for 60–80 of the commonly used enzymes.

Extraction of DNA bands from gels

There are a number of ways of extracting bands from gels for use in cloning or labeling the fragment for hybridization studies. Once the band is visualized using ethidium bromide, it can be cut out from the gel using a sterile scalpel or razor blade. It is best to remove the band with as little extra gel as possible surrounding the DNA, since some agarose preparations contain inhibitory sulfated polysaccharides, which may inhibit enzymes used for cloning and labeling. Ultrapure preparations and low melting agarose, usually labeled for use with DNA are best if the bands are going to be used for subse-

quent cloning or as radiolabeled DNA probes. Once the gel piece containing the band is removed, then the DNA can be extracted by the method of personal choice.

Electroelution

A common, simple, but time consuming technique is to place the gel piece in dialysis tubing along with a small amount of electrophoresis buffer, and place the bag at right angles to the direction of the current and keep it in place with a glass plate. The DNA is then electrophoresed from the gel into the surrounding buffer in the dialysis bag, at 100 V for 2–3 hours. Just before removing the bag from the electrophoresis tank, reverse the current for 2–3 min to remove DNA adhering to the insides of the dialysis bag. The buffer is then extracted with phenol, phenol/chloroform and finally chloroform and precipitated with salt and ethanol before being dissolved in an appropriate buffer for the next stage.

Freeze/thaw method

A quicker method is to take the gel slice and cut it into small pieces and place in an Eppendorf tube. The tube is frozen in liquid nitrogen, or an ethanol/dry ice bath and thawed three times. The tube is then spun in a microcentrifuge for 5 min and the buffer containing DNA placed in a fresh tube. The gel fragments are removed and placed in a 0.5 ml Eppendorf tube which has a small hole made in the bottom with a syringe needle, and a small plug of glass wool. The glass wool should be siliconized prior to use. This is done by soaking the wool in Sigmacote (Sigma) for a few minutes, then rinsing in distilled water, drying and autoclaving. This 0.5 ml tube is placed inside a 1.5 ml tube and the tubes spun for 5 min in the microfuge. The remaining liquid in the gel is spun into the lower 1.5 ml tube and then combined with the original supernatant. The second spinning is important as it may contain up to 30% of the DNA in the gel slice. Extract the combined volume with phenol:chloroform and then with chloroform, precipitate the DNA and wash the pellet twice in 70% ethanol, and resuspend in water or TE. This method is particularly good for smaller fragments of 500–2000 bp. These methods will extract 20–50% of the DNA contained in the gel.

There are a number of kits on the market for the extraction of DNA from gel slices and all claim a good deal of success in extracting over 50% quantities of the DNA fragment. The kits are used to extract DNA from agarose and polyacrylamide gels using solubilizing agents and then usually some bead, column or filter purification system to give clean DNA preparations. If just starting work with DNA, it would be prudent to use a kit for the initial isolation of DNA fragments, plasmids or viral genomes.

Labeling of probes

In this section the methods of labeling viral DNA genomes or fragments will be described and discussed. At present the most sensitive technique for DNA–DNA, or DNA–RNA hybridization is using radiolabeled probes. However, the methods described can also be used to label DNA for non-radioactive detection systems.

Nick translation and random primer labeling

These methods, especially the latter, are the most commonly used methods for DNA labeling and will give labeling of DNA throughout the length of the DNA molecule. Some methods discussed below will only label the ends of DNA.

Nick translation

This method uses DNAse I to nick the DNA probe randomly through the two strands and then, with DNA polymerase I, radiolabeled bases are incorporated at the site of the nicked DNA (Rigby et al 1977). The temperature of the reaction is 14°C since the polymerase activity of the enzyme is faster than the exonuclease activity. The result at 37°C would be a snapback reaction, where the polymerase will snapback and copy the new strand it has just synthesized rather then keep on the original template. The DNase concentration has to be such that the DNA probe is not completely digested and so testing of batches is necessary before starting the test reactions, but around 10 ng ml^{-1} of pancreatic DNase I is a good starting concentration. Stock solutions of the DNase I can be made in 0.15 M NaCl and 50% glycerol. In addition to the concentration of the DNase I, the amount of triphosphates in the reaction mix is important. For radiolabeled probes one of the four triphosphates will be ^{32}P- or ^{35}S-labeled and obtained from Amersham or NEN. The specific activity of the triphosphates sold varies, but for 'hot' probes high specific activity triphosphates are favored. A typical reaction mix would be the following:

Reaction mix

The following are added on ice:

> 10× Nick translation buffer (Table 10.3)
>   (2.5 µl)
> DNA probe (100–500 ng)
> unlabeled dNTPs (20 nmoles of each)
> α-^{32}P dNTP (dCTP ≥ 3000 Ci
>   mmole^{-1}) (5 µl)
> DNase I (1 µl (10 ng ml^{-1}))
> DNA polymerase I (*E. coli*) (2.5 units)
> distilled water (added to total volume of
>   25–50 µl)
> The reaction is left at 14°C for 1 h.

Random priming

This method (Feinberg and Vogelstein 1983, 1984) has largely superseded the nick translation technique and uses the fact that if heterogeneous oligonucleotides are added to a denatured probe DNA, they will form hybrids at regions of homology. The primers can be produced from salmon sperm or calf thymus DNA by DNase I activity, synthesized or more commonly purchased from one of the companies that manufacture random priming kits. Once the primers hybridize then new DNA strands can be synthesized using the klenow fragment of DNA polymerase I since with this method the exonuclease activities of the polymerase are not required. The radiolabeled bases are used as for the nick translation method. A typical reaction mix is:

Reaction mix is made up on ice

Boil the following for 5 min:
  the probe (25–50 ng)
  water to make up volume to 25 µl
Quench on ice and add the following:
  20 mM dithiothreitol (1 µl)
  10× random primer buffer (Table 10.3)
    (2.5 µl)
  dNTPs (0.5 mM) (1 µl of each)
  α-^{32}P dCTP (3000 Ci mmole^{-1}) (5 µl)
  klenow fragment (2.5 units)
The reaction is carried out at 37°C for
30 min.

Note

It is important to denature DNA by
heating to create single-strands so the
primers can hybridize.

End-labeling of DNA probe

Small DNA fragments of oligonucleotides too
small to be efficiently labeled by the above
techniques can be end-labeled using a kinase
enzyme, or if the DNA has overhangs at the
ends, e.g. a restriction site, then the overhang
can be filled in with labeled bases using the
klenow enzyme. End labeling with the kinase
means that only two molecules of ^{32}P are
incorporated per DNA molecule, and γ-^{32}P
dATP has to be used for the transfer of the
labeled phosphate to replace phosphate at
the 5-prime end of each strand of DNA. For
efficient transfer or the phosphate group, the
DNA probe should be dephosphorylated prior
to labeling (see the section on cloning). The
filling in reaction is the same as the random
priming without the primers and addition of
one or more labeled bases that are complementary to one or more bases at the ends of
the fragment. It is possible, using this latter
method, to label only one end of the fragment
by choosing the appropriate base. End-labeling is often used to label markers for gels.

The kinase end-labeling has the following
reaction mix:
  10× kinase buffer (Table 10.3) (5 µl)
  DNA fragment (1–50 pmoles)
  γ-^{32}P dATP[3,000 Ci mmole^{-1}]
    (50 pmoles)
  T4 kinase (10 units)
  distilled water to 50 µl

The reaction is allowed to proceed for 30
to 45 minutes at 37°C.

Table 10.3. Labeling buffers.

Reagent	Nick translation	Random primer	Transcription	End labeling*
		Buffers (× 10)		
Tris-Cl	0.5 M, pH 7.5	–	0.4 M, pH 7.5	0.5 M, pH 7.6
MgSO$_4$	0.1 M	–	–	–
DTT	1 mM	–	–	50 mM
BSA	500 µg ml^{-1}	–	–	–
HEPES	–	0.9 M	–	–
MgCl$_2$	–	0.1 M	60 mM	0.1 M
NaCl	–	–	50 mM	–
Spermidine	–	–	20 mM	1 mM
EDTA	–	–	–	1 mM, pH 8.0

* When using the klenow fragment for filling in overhanging ends then a number of buffers can be used
including restriction buffers.

Labeled RNA from DNA

It is possible to transcribe labeled RNA from a DNA template using RNA polymerase. This is useful for RNA–RNA and RNA–DNA hybridizations, which are more sensitive and with less background than Southern blots using DNA–DNA hybridization. This latter advantage is because the filters can be treated with RNAse, which will digest non-specific RNA bound to the filter leaving the double-stranded hybrid unaffected. The DNA fragment first has to be cloned into a vector containing cloning sites bounded by RNA polymerase promoters so that sense and anti-sense strands can be transcribed. There are a number of these vectors available from Promega, WI, USA. There are a number of polymerases, T3, T4, T7 and SP6 which can be used (Studier and Rosenberg 1981). The other advantage of this system is that since mRNA is often only coded from one strand of the DNA it is possible to make a RNA probe from both strands of a fragment and use one as the test probe, homologous to the sense strand, and the other as a negative control, homologous to the anti-sense strand.

Once the DNA of interest is cloned into the vector then both the sense and anti-sense strands can be transcribed. In the example given in Fig. 10.1, the plasmid should be linearized by *E. Co*RI for T7 transcribed RNA and *Bam* HI for T3 transcribed RNA. Once linearized the DNA is extracted with phenol, phenol:chloroform and finally chloroform to remove the enzyme, and precipitated with ethanol and 3 M Na acetate before being redissolved in RNase-free water. To make RNase-free water, diethyl pyrocarbonate (DEPC) is added to distilled water at a final concentration of 0.1%, the mixture shaken for a few minutes and the bottle left for an hour at 37°C before being autoclaved for 15 min at 15 PSI. It is important that all the tubes and solutions used for the transcription are RNase free. It is therefore best to use plastic disposable tubes and handle only with gloved hands. The order of addition of components to the reaction mix is important and is given here:

RNase free dH$_2$O (up to 20 µl)
10× buffer (Table 10.3) (2 µl)
DNA template (0.4 pmole [equivalent to 0.8 µg of a 3 kb piece of DNA])
100 mM DTT (2 µl)
RNAsin (1 µl)
ATP, GTP and CTP mixture [5 mM each] (2 µl)
α-^{32}P-UTP[3000 Ci mmole^{-1}] (5 µl)
T7 or T3 RNA polymerase (5 units)

Incubate the mixture at 37°C for 1 h.

Incorporation levels

In the above labeling methods the reactions are stopped by adding 5 µl of 0.5 M EDTA, or heating to 65°C for 5 min. Once the reaction is complete incorporation levels can be assessed by loading 1–2 µl of the reaction mix onto two filters (Whatman microfiber GF/A filters), drying and washing one of the filters with 7% TCA and then ethanol. The unwashed filter will indicate the total radioactive count and the washed filter just the radioactivity incorporated into the DNA probe. For counting the filters can be placed in scintillation fluid and counted in the range for ^{32}P.

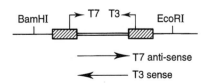

Figure 10.1. RNA polymerase transcription.

Separation of labeled probe from unincorporated bases

If necessary the unincorporated bases are removed from the probe by passing the probe through sephadex G50 equilibrated with STE buffer (10 mM Tris Cl, pH 8.0; 100 mM NaCl and 1 mM EDTA). The high salt prevents the DNA from binding to the column. The labeled DNA comes out with the exclusion volume and if it is labeled with ^{32}P then it can easily be monitored with a geiger counter. Alternatively the free bases can be removed by precipitating the DNA two or three times using ethanol and Na acetate (2 × volume of ethanol and 0.1 volume of 3 M Na acetate, pH 5.2).

The above methods can be used to label DNA with ^{32}P, ^{35}S and biotinylated triphosphates.

Hybridization methods

In this section DNA–DNA, DNA–RNA and RNA–RNA hybridization will be described and will predominantly concentrate on radiolabeled probes since they are the most sensitive detection system, although non-radiolabeled probes can be used in all the situations mentioned below.

Southern blotting

In most situations, hybridization takes place with the target DNA attached to a solid matrix such as nitrocellulose or nylon filters and the probe in solution. Southern (1975) devised a method to transfer the target DNA from an agarose gel to nitrocellulose filters and the method is the same for transfer to nylon filters and can be used to transfer RNA to filters, a process called Northern blotting (see next section).

DNA to be hybridized is run on an agarose gel and, when the dye is near the bottom, the gel is removed from the electrophoresis tank and the DNA is denatured so that it is transferred as single stranded molecules ready to form hybrids with the labeled probe. If the DNA to be transferred is of high molecular weight, especially if looking for integrated sequences in chromosomal DNA, then the gel is first depurinated. This is only necessary if it is known that the bands of interest are ≥ 10 kb. The full process is as follows:

1. Depurination is carried out by soaking the gel in 0.1 N HCl for approximately 15–30 min. A good test of the length of time is to soak for as long as the bromophenol blue dye takes to turn a yellow/amber color. This treatment depurinates the DNA creating strand breaks, so that the DNA is now made up of shorter lengths for ease of transfer. Treatment for too long may produce bands less than 1 kb and decrease efficiency of transfer.

2. The gel is then washed twice in distilled water and then soaked in 1 M Tris-HCl, pH 8.0 plus 0.5 M NaOH for 1 h, and then washed again in distilled water.

3. Finally the gel is soaked in neutralization buffer of 1 M Tris/HCl, pH 8.0 plus 1.5 M NaCl for a further hour. All the soakings should be carried out with the gentle shaking. The gel is now ready for transfer to filters and is placed on a solid support, which straddles a tank containing transfer buffer (Figure 10.2). Across the support is filter paper (Whatman 3MM) which dips into the transfer buffer and acts as a wick for transfer of the buffer up through the gel. On top of the nitrocellulose is the gel and then filter paper, or cheaper paper towels and on top a weight. The weight does not have to be very heavy, but just enough to apply a downward pressure (a 500 ml bottle full of water is quite adequate). The transfer buffer tracts up the paper wick through the gel, carrying the DNA in the flow. While the buffer goes through the filter, the DNA is trapped. Transfer takes 10–15 h, or overnight. After transfer the filter is air dried, placed in a filter paper pocket and baked at 80°C in a vacuum for

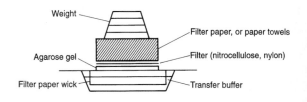

Figure 10.2. Southern and Northern blotting.

15–30 min. The longer the baking time, the more brittle the filter becomes. The filter can now be used for hybridization, or stored under vacuum in a desiccator. Alternatively the DNA can be fixed to the membrane using short wave UV light and a number of types of apparatus are commercially available.

Northern blotting

The agarose gel system used for RNA is different from DNA, and the most commonly used technique is a formaldehyde/formamide method (Kopchik et al 1981). For a 150 ml agarose gel (usually 1% for most purposes) the following is added:
Agarose (1.5 g)
10× MOPS (3-[4-Morpholino] propane sulfonic acid) buffer (15 ml)
200 mM MOPS, pH 7.0; 50 mM Na acetate; 10 mM EDTA, pH 8.0; make up in DEPC treated water and pH with NaOH.
distilled water (115 ml)
Boil to dissolve and cool to approximately 60°C and add 24.5 ml of formaldehyde and pour the gel. It is best to pour the gel in a fume hood as formaldehyde gives off unpleasant and potentially dangerous fumes. Viral RNA can be prepared as described in chapter 9 and then prepared for electrophoresis as follows:
RNA (should be 5–10 μg of poly A RNA or 30 μg of total RNA) (5 μl)
formaldehyde (3.5 μl)
formamide (10 μl)
10× MOPS (2 μl)
This mixture is denatured at 65°C for 10 min, then 1 μl each of ethidium bromide and loading dye are added and the sample loaded and run at 150 V. The

18S and 28S ribosomal RNAs can then be visualized with UV light and the integrity of the RNA preparations judged by the extent of break down of the ribosomal RNAs. If the RNA integrity is high, then the gel can be blotted as for DNA gels. The gel does not need to be treated to denature the contents as the samples were denatured prior to loading. After blotting, the filter is treated the same way as for DNA filters except that it is briefly washed in transfer buffer to remove excess formaldehyde, then dried and baked as above.

Note

While there are other methods for the electrophoresis of RNA, this is the easiest and gives the best results.

Dot blots

Dot blotting does not require electrophoresis of the sample and the DNA, or RNA, is added directly to the filter in a denatured form, dried and the filter baked. There are commercially available manifolds for loading samples onto filters with the aid of a vacuum, but they can be added to filters by hand, drop by drop. When unable to use a manifold and vacuum then volumes should be kept to a minimum, i.e. 20–100 μl.

DNA

Samples of DNA can be loaded onto filters in water or TE, but it needs to be denatured before the filter is baked. Once the DNA sample is added the filters are then laid on a piece of Whatman 3MM filter paper, which is soaked in the denaturation buffer for 10 min, as for Southern blot transfer. The filter is then transferred to filter paper soaked in distilled water for a few minutes and then onto filter paper soaked in neutralization buffer for 10 min. The filter is then placed on distilled water soaked paper, dried and baked at 80°C in a vacuum oven for 15–30 min as for the Southern blots.

RNA

RNA samples are loaded onto the filter already denatured. The denaturation step is the same as for Northern blotting, with the sample of RNA mixed with:
   Formaldehyde (7% final)
   Formamide (50% final)
   20 × SSC (1 × final)
This mixture is heated at 65°C for 10 min, cooled on ice and loaded onto a filter. The filter is dried and baked at 80°C as above.

Hybridization conditions

Filters used for hybridization are either nitrocellulose, nylon or a combination of both. In this section hybridization conditions will be described for nitrocellulose, since there is very little change when using nylon filters, although the latter are more resistant to physical manipulations.

Southern blot hybridization

1. Filters are first wetted in distilled water. Hybridization can be carried out at high temperature or at lower temperatures in the presence of formamide. The temperature, formamide concentration and the salt concentration dictate the stringency of the hybridization reaction. The higher the temperature or formamide concentration and the lower the salt concentration then the higher the stringency of the hybridization. Therefore it is possible to alter the

stringency by changing each of the three conditions. The stringency of hybridization can be worked out from the formula:

$$Tm = 81.5°C - 16.6(\log_{10}[Na^+]) + 0.41(\%G+C) - 0.63(\%formamide).$$

For a viral DNA fragment of 8 kb then the following hybridization mixes are for high stringency, i.e. Tm = −25°C.

Prewash:

	At 68°C:	At 42°C:
SSC	× 3 (or 3 × SSPE)	× 3 (or 3 × SSPE)
Denhardt's	× 10 (or 0.2% BLOTTO)	× 10 (or 0.2% BLOTTO)
SDS	0.5%	0.5%
denatured single-stranded salmon sperm DNA	400 μg ml^{-1}	400 μg ml^{-1}
formamide	none	50%
distilled water	up to 10 to 20 ml	

Denhardt's ×100 is:
   10g Ficoll (Type 400)
   10g polyvinyl-pyrrolidine
   10g bovine serum albunium (Fraction V) to 500ml with distilled water.

(Single-stranded salmon sperm DNA [ssstDNA] is boiled for 5 min. before adding)
   For low stringency hybridization (Tm = −40°C), 5×SSC should be used at 57°C and 5×SSC plus 20% formamide at 42°C

Table 10.4. Hybridization buffers.

Reagents	20× SSC	20× SSPE
NaCl	3 M	3 M
Na citrate	0.3 M	–
NaH$_2$PO$_4$.H$_2$O	–	0.2 M
EDTA	–	0.025 M

Both 20× SSC [3 M Na chloride; 0.3 M Na citrate] and 20× SSPE [3 M Na chloride; 0.2 M NaH$_2$PO$_4$; 0.02 M EDTA] are buffered at pH 7 and pH 7.4 respectively with 10 N Na hydroxide and sterilized by autoclave.

Note

Nylon filters are usually hybridized with formamide present. Blotto is nonfat dried milk and should only be used for DNA–DNA hybridizations. It is a cheaper and easier alternative to Denhardt's. ssstDNA is used to block non-specific binding of the probe to the filter and it has been our experience that 400 $\mu g\ ml^{-1}$ will give very low background at high stringency (Fig. 10.3).

Filters should be prewashed for 2 h in a plastic box or sealable plastic bag in a shaking water bath before addition of the probe.

Hybridization

The DNA probe, usually in 50–100 μl of TE, is boiled for 5 min before addition to hybridization mix. The whole hybridization mix can be replaced or the probe can be added to the prewash mix. If the prewash solution is used it is preferable that the prewash takes place in a sealable plastic bag as small volumes are necessary for the probe to make contact with homologous sequences on the filter in as short a time period as possible. There are now hybridization apparatus which usually use glass tubes and hybridization should be carried out as per manufacturers instruction.

Washing

Hybridization is usually carried out for 12–15 h (or overnight), after which the filters are washed as follows:

1. Twice with 2× SSC plus 0.1% SDS at room temperature for 2–3 min each.
2. Then at least two washes in 0.5× SSC at 68°C for 30 min each.

For low stringency washes the temperature is lower and the salt concentration higher than used above.

The formula given above can be used to tailor the conditions to individual situations.

Note

It is important that the filters are not dry at any stage of the hybridization or washing process otherwise the probe remains permanently on the filters and they cannot be easily reused.

3. Filters are now ready to be exposed to X-ray film. From the final wash the filters should be wrapped in Saran Wrap and placed in a X-ray cassette with intensifying screens to increase efficiency of exposure. Exposure is carried out at −70°C as this again increases the sensitivity of the intensifying screens.

Figure 10.3 shows the hybridization of DNA from a number of cervical biopsies using human papillomavirus type 16 (HPV-16) full length genome at low stringency followed by a low stringency wash (Tm = −40°C, Fig. 10.3A) and exposure to X-ray film. The filter was then washed at high stringency (Tm = −10°C) and re-exposed (Fig. 10.3B). The figure shows that at low stringency the HPV-16 probe hybridizes to HPV-6 and -11 virus DNA and an unknown HPV type (X, Fig. 10.3A), but after the high stringency wash only the homologous HPV-16 DNA is detected in the biopsy DNA.

Note

Before exposing nitrocellulose filters to such low temperatures during exposure to X-ray film they should be soaked in a solution of 50% glycerol and 2× SSC. This will keep the filters from becoming brittle at low temperature, so that they can be stripped of probe and reused for hybridization.

(A)

16 16 6 11 X 16 16 16

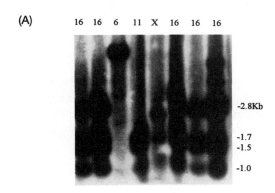

-2.8Kb

-1.7
-1.5

-1.0

(B)

16 16 6 11 X 16 16 16

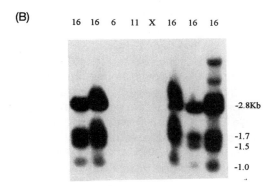

-2.8Kb

-1.7
-1.5

-1.0

Figure 10.3. A Southern blot of DNA extracted from premalignant lesions of the cervix, digested with *Pst* I and probed with ^{32}P-labeled HPV-16 DNA at (A) low stringency (Tm = $-40°C$) and (B) high stringency (Tm = $-10°C$). The numbers above the lanes indicates the HPV type detected with X being a related but unknown type. At low stringency the HPV-16 probe detects HPV-6, -11 and -X, but at high stringency only the homologous HPV-16 genome is detected. The size markers at the right are in kilobases (kb).

At low stringency hybridizations many different human papillomaviruses can be detected using only one probe. Even at high stringency certain probes of human herpes virus (HHV) 6 will detect HHV-7 fragments, so care must be taken to identify the virus by other methods, such as by restriction mapping of the fragment.

Northern blot hybridization

RNA filters can be hybridized with DNA or RNA probes, but the general procedure is similar to Southern filters. It should be remembered that RNA–RNA hybrids are more stable than RNA–DNA hybrids and in turn these are more stable than DNA–DNA hybrids. Therefore the hybridization temperature will need to be higher for stringent conditions. For instance, the Tm in solution of a RNA–RNA hybrid will be approximately 10°C higher than an equivalent DNA–DNA hybrid. It is convenient to keep hybridization conditions similar and then wash at different stringencies for the RNA filters.

Prewash

SSC (3×)
Denhardt's (10×)
dextran sulfate (10%)
SDS (0.5%)
formamide (50%)
salmon sperm (400 µg ml^{-1})
distilled water (to 10 ml)

This is incubated in a plastic bag at 42°C for at least 2 h before addition of the probe.

Hybridization

The probe is added and the bag resealed and incubated overnight at 42°C.

Note

The addition of dextran sulfate is optional, but it decreases the aqueous volume in which the probe is contained as it is excluded from the polymer phase. Therefore the rate of hybridization is increased and so is the efficiency of hybridization over a given time. If it is added, it is best to add the dextran to the water, SSC and Denhardt's and dissolve at 37°C before adding the rest of the components. After the wash the labeled

RNA or denatured DNA is added and hybridization is continued for 10–15 h.

Washing

This is the same for DNA–DNA hybridization, but can be carried out at lower salt concentration, especially for RNA–RNA hybrids. So for the latter, washes with 0.1× SSC and 0.1% SDS at 68°C are appropriate. In addition after the final wash RNA–RNA filters can be soaked in 1 µg ml^{-1} of RNase at room temperature for 15 min. This removes the single-stranded probe, which has bound non-specifically to the filter and therefore cuts down on background or noise to signal ratio. The filters are rinsed and exposed to X-ray film as for DNA–DNA hybridization.

acetone at room temperature gives the least background and gives good penetration of the probe, but does not preserve tissue morphology as well as the methods below. Cells in culture can be fixed with methanol or acetone and morphology is adequate.
2. Fixation of tissues in 4% paraformaldehyde and wax embedding gives very good tissue preservation, but because it is a cross-linking fixative it reduces probe penetration and gives higher background. Therefore the probe and the section need additional treatment to overcome these difficulties.
3. 1% glutaraldehyde fixation has the same advantages and disadvantages as paraformaldehyde treatment.

In situ hybridization

In situ hybridization on tissue sections or tissue culture cells is usually carried out with ^{35}S-radiolabeled or biotin-labeled probes. As above the nucleic acid probe can be DNA or RNA and the same advantages and disadvantages apply. For ^{35}S-labeled RNA probes then a very low noise to signal ratio can be achieved using RNase treatment after hybridization. The background noise will depend on the method of fixation and can be reduced further by other manipulations.

Fixation

Cells or tissue sections are usually fixed by one of three methods, which have their own advantages and disadvantages.

1. Freezing tissue in liquid nitrogen followed by sectioning in a cryostat and fixation in methanol at −20°C, or

Treatment of slides prior to addition of sections

The sections need to be securely fixed to the glass slides since their treatment during the hybridization reactions can very easily cause them to lift off. Slides are usually treated with some kind of positively charged compound so that electrostatic forces will help to keep the section attached throughout the following processes. One of the best methods is to use 3-aminopropyltriethoxysilane (TES, Rentrop et al 1986) for slide preparation as follows:

1. Acid clean slides for 2 h in 0.06 N HCl, rinse in distilled water and dry.
2. Make up 2% TES in dry acetone (new bottle) with constant stirring.
3. Dip slides into the solution for a few seconds, remove and wash twice in acetone followed by distilled water.
4. Dry slides at 42°C and store in a slide box until used. Slides can be stored for several weeks before any noticeable deterioration is observed.

Treatment of sections and *in situ* hybridization

DNA–DNA hybridization

1. Dewax slides with two soakings in xylene for 5 min each.
2. Then take the slides through a series of rinsings in alcohol
   5 min in absolute alcohol (I)
   2 min in absolute alcohol (II)
   2 min in 50% alcohol (III)
   Then into tap water
3. Cover sections with 0.2 N HCl at room temperature for 20 min.
4. Wash in distilled water.
5. Wash in proteinase K buffer (50 mM Tris, pH 7.8; 5 mM EDTA), warm the slides to 37°C and add proteinase K to a final concentration of 2 μg ml^{-1} and incubate for 5 min. (Proteinase treatment is essential for sections fixed with paraformaldehyde or glutaraldehyde in order to digest the tissue and allow penetration of the probe.)
6. Wash well with stop buffer (100 mM Tris, pH 7.8; 100 mM NaCl; 2 mg ml^{-1} glycine).
7. Wash in distilled water dehydrate through the alcohols in the opposite direction to that above.
8. Add approximately 25 μl of the hybridization mix. The amount will depend on the size of the section, but as little as possible should be used:
   20× SSC (10 μl)
   100× Denhardt's (10 μl)
   single-stranded salmon sperm (ssst) DNA (400 μg ml^{-1})
   50% dextran sulphate (20 μl)
   deionized formamide (40 μl)
   1 M DTT (1 μl)
   distilled water (to 100 μl)
9. Place a siliconized cover slip on top of the section and place the slides in a moist box.
10. Heat the slides to 95°C for 10 min to denature DNA and then leave the reaction at 37°C overnight.

Note

Paraformaldehyde or glutaraldehyde fixed tissue do not allow efficient penetration of the probe. Proteinase K as mentioned above is necessary, but using probes of 100–150 base pairs is important (Angerer et al 1987). Small DNA fragments from a large gene can be made with DNase treatment (Collins et al 1988). The concentration of DNase to use to create the desired sizes can be assessed using agarose gels.

Washing slides

1. The coverslip is removed by gently lowering the slide into a jar containing 2× SSC warmed to 37°C.
2. Wash the slides twice at 37°C in 50% formamide and 2× SSC for 15 min each time, then twice in 2× SSC for 15 min at 37°C.
3. Dehydrate sections and in the dark room carry out the following:
   (a) add 5 ml of Kodak liquid emulsion (prewarmed to 42°C) to 5 ml of 10% glycerol and mix gently with a pipette.
   (b) pour the mixture into a small slide box and gently dip slides into the emulsion to cover the section.
   (c) remove slides and dry completely before placing them in a light-tight box with a small bag of desiccant and exposing at 4°C. The time of exposure will depend on the abundance of target and so various times should initially be tested.
   (d) the slide can then be developed by placing in Kodak D19 developer for 4 min followed by washes in distilled water and fixation in

Kodak Hypam fixer for a further 4 min. The slides are washed in distilled water and counter stained with a cell stain such as hematoxylin, dehydrated and mounted in depex.

Figure 10.4 is an example of DNA–DNA hybridization on a section from a premalignant lesion from the cervix when hybridized with ^{35}S-labeled HPV-16 DNA (Fig. 10.4A), while there is no signal detected when hybridized with HPV-6 labeled DNA (Figure 10.4B).

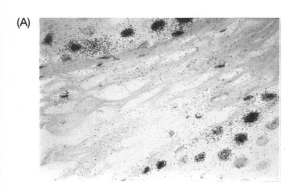

(A)

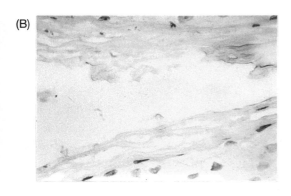

(B)

Figure 10.4. *In situ* hybridization of a biopsy section of a cervical intraepithelial neoplasia probed with either ^{35}S-labeled HPV-16 (A), or ^{35}S-labeled HPV-6 (B) DNA at high stringency, showing the presence of HPV-16 and absence of HPV-6 in the lesion.

RNA–RNA hybridization

1. The sections are dewaxed and rehydrated as above.
2. The slides are then acetylated to reduce background due to electrostatic binding of the probe by neutralizing the positive charge on the section and glass slide. Place 0.25 ml of acetic anhydride in the bottom of a large coplin jar and then put slides into the jar. Then carefully pour in 100 ml of 0.1 M triethanolamine, pH 8.0. Incubate in acetylation solution for 10 min.
3. Wash slides in 2× SSC, and then in proteinase buffer as above.
4. Warm proteinase buffer to 37°C before adding the enzyme to 1 μg ml^{-1}.
5. Wash slides in stop buffer and then distilled water before dehydrating for the hybridization reaction.
6. The labeled RNA probe is precipitated to eliminate unincorporated bases as described above. The precipitated pellet is resuspended in the following hybridization mix:
   50% deionized formamide (25 ml)
   2× SSC (5 ml)
   1× Denhardt's (0.5 ml)
   10% dextran (10 ml)
   100 mM DTT (5 ml)
   ssst DNA (400 μg ml^{-1})
   distilled water (to 50 ml)
   Approximately 25 μl is placed on each section and a siliconized coverslip put on the top and the slide immersed in mineral oil and hybridized overnight at 42°C.
7. After hybridization the oil is washed off with three changes of chloroform. Surface tension will keep the coverslip in place during this procedure.
8. The slides are then immersed in 2× SSC to remove the coverslips and the sections are washed twice for 15 min each in 2× SSC at room temperature.
9. The sections can now be treated with RNAse (20 μg ml^{-1}) in 10 mM Tris, pH 7.8; 0.5 M NaCl and 1 mM EDTA for

30 min at 37°C if desired. It may not always be necessary to treat with RNase.

10. The sections are then washed twice in 0.1× SSC and 10 mM DTT at 45–50°C, and then dehydrated through the alcohols before photographic emulsion is applied as above.

All of the above *in situ* hybridization techniques can be used with non-radiolabeled probe such as biotinylated triphosphates with very little adjustment to the methodology as laid out above. The sensitivity is lower but adequate for many applications. There are a number of kits on the market using these non-radioactive reagents.

Polymerase chain reaction (PCR)

The polymerase chain reaction is a powerful tool to amplify specific regions of DNA using primers which are at either end of the region to be amplified (Fig. 10.5). The two primers 1 and 2 are homologous to two different strands of the duplex at either end of the fragment to be amplified and are in the 5-prime to 3-prime direction of each strand. On denaturation of the double stranded DNA and on the addition of the polymerase enzyme two new double strands are synthesized between the primers. After the first round of amplification two new strands of DNA are made and after the second, four new strands are synthesized. After 30 rounds, or cycles then 1.1×10^9 double strands will be made. If we take SV40 ($M_r = 3.4 \times 10^6$) as an example then 10^{11} molecules are equivalent to approximately 1 µg of DNA, so from one molecule 10 ng of DNA will be synthesized, which is more than sufficient to detect by hybridization techniques and sufficient to clone (see page 213). A review of the procedures can be found in Innis and Gelfard (1990).

The polymerase used in the amplification reactions has to be stable at very high temperatures of around 95°C, because between each cycle the DNA has to be denatured to create single strands so that the primers can form hybrids and initiate the synthesis of two new strands. The DNA polymerase used is called *Taq* polymerase as it was first isolated from *Thermophilus aquaticus*, a bacterium which lives in hot springs. After the denaturation step at 95°C the reaction is cooled to around 55°C for annealing of the primer and then heated to 72°C for the primer extension reaction with the *Taq* polymerase. These temperatures will vary depending on the G-C content of the primers and whether the primer is completely homologous to the target DNA. The reaction mix below is a good starting point for a PCR reaction with homologous primers with 45% G-C content. More information on PCR reactions and techniques can be found in Innis et al (1990).

Reaction mix

Template DNA (10^5 to 10^6 molecules [using SV40 means 1 pg to 10 pg])
Primers (20 pmol of each [this will give around 10^{15} molecules])
Tris-HCl, pH 8.3 (20 mM)
MgCl$_2$ (1.5 mM [can vary for different primers, range 0.5 to 2 mM])
KCl (25 mM)
BSA (100 µg ml^{-1})
dNTP (50 µM of each)
Taq polymerase (2 units)

The reaction mix is covered in mineral oil to prevent evaporation during the high temperature cycles. There are now special PCR tubes which abrogate the use of mineral oil. This is an advantage as some sources of oil can be inhibitory to

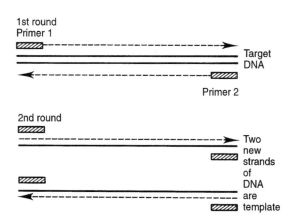

1st round
Primer 1
Target DNA
Primer 2

2nd round
Two new strands of DNA are template

Figure 10.5. PCR amplification.

the enzyme. Cycles are usually around thirty, with each having 1 min at 95°C, then 1 min at 55°C for annealing and 1–2 min at 72°C for elongation. After the final cycle elongation is extended to 5 min. The times and temperatures will vary for different primers, but these conditions would be a starting point for many different applications.

As mentioned above, the sequence of the primer is important and it is best to aim for one with a content of at least 45% G-C. This is not always possible and so it is likely that the annealing temperature will need to be lowered to accommodate a high A-T ratio. Primers can also be used to place restriction sites at either end of the amplified fragment even though they are not part of the original template. After the first cycle these sites will be amplified with the rest of the fragment. The restriction sites are placed at the 5-prime end of the primers and the rest of the primer consists of at least 10 bases which are homologous to the template. This makes the PCR product easy to clone (see page 213).

Basic methods for cloning

Cloning of a desired gene or fragments of DNA is a standard technique, however, the cloning vector that is used will depend on the application to which the DNA will be used. More extensive coverage of cloning techniques can be found in Sambrook et al 1989. If the DNA is to be used for transcription of the gene in mammalian cells then transcription vectors with a variety of promoters are available. If it is to be used to transcript and translate proteins *in vitro* then a vector which will transcribe and translate mRNA *in vitro*, such as the pGEM vectors from Promega should be used. The cloning techniques described will use a generic vector although it will be relevant to specific types of vector. An important point is that, for some vectors, particular bacterial cells may have to be used for successful cloning. In addition, for the cloning of PCR products, the TA Cloning Kit from Invitrogen is extremely useful.

Ligation of insert to vector

Cloning is the ligation of a fragment DNA (insert) of interest into a vector, usually a bacterial plasmid. The ligated DNA plus plasmid can be placed into bacteria and amplified in cultures of a few milliliters up to several liters. For ease of ligation it is preferable to use DNA with restriction sites at either end. All cloning vectors contain a series of restriction sites in a short length of DNA called a polylinker. Restriction enzymes which produce overhang-

ing ends (sticky ends) are the most effective when it comes to joining one piece of DNA to another. Purity of DNA is also a factor in efficiency and the methods of isolating DNA fragments described previously should give good results. Figure 10.6 illustrates the principle of cloning. The polylinker is part of the bacterial plasmid and will contain several commonly used restriction sites making cloning relatively easy. Cloning can be achieved with DNA that is blunt-ended, but this will need more DNA and some altered conditions to optimize efficiency. Some vectors have a built-in detection system to indicate if the fragment has been cloned into the vector. For example, plasmids may contain cloning sites, or a polylinker in the middle of the lacZ gene, which produces a blue color when induced by galactose or an analogue. If a piece of DNA is cloned into the polylinker it will disrupt the gene and white colonies will be produced on induction. Therefore the presence of white colonies is a visual sign of successful cloning. However, it is always necessary to confirm this using Mini-Preps (see page 217).

The DNA to be cloned is isolated and purified as described previously. The bacterial plasmid is also digested with the appropriate restriction enzymes and, to avoid any undigested plasmid remaining, the linear form can be run on an agarose gel, isolated and purified. If the vector is digested with only one enzyme and therefore has homologous sticky ends then it is possible that the plasmid will self ligate and give a large background of plasmids without the required insert. To minimize this the plasmid DNA is dephosphorylated after restriction enzyme digestion and before gel purification. This is done using calf intestine alkaline phosphatase (CIP) enzyme in the following protocol. After

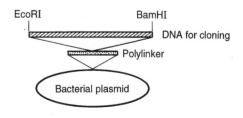

Figure 10.6. DNA cloning.

restriction enzyme digestion the DNA is extracted twice with phenol/chloroform and precipitated as described. The DNA is then dephosphorylated in the following reaction mix:

10× CIP buffer (10 µl)
  10 mм $ZnCl_2$; 10 mм $MgCl_2$; 100 mм Tris Cl; pH 8.3.
DNA (10–20 µg)
CIP enzyme (1 unit $pmol^{-1}$ sticky ends, or 1 unit 2 $pmol^{-1}$ for blunt or recessed ends)

The reaction is incubated at 37°C for 30 min and the enzyme is then inactivated at 75°C for 15 min in the presence of 5 mм EDTA followed by two extractions with phenol/chloroform and precipitated as above. The DNA can now be run on a gel, isolated and purified.

Cloning of sticky-ends

The two DNAs can now be ligated as follows:

DNA fragment (100–200 ng [For sticky end ligation a ratio of insert to vector of 2:1 is usual])
Plasmid DNA (50–100 ng)
10× ligation buffer (1 µl)
Ligase enzyme (T4 ligase) (0.1–0.5 Weiss units)
  500 mм Tris Cl, pH 7.0; 100 mм $MgCl_2$; 100 mм DTT; 10 mм ATP; 500 µg ml^{-1} BSA.

Cloning of blunt-ends

Since blunt end ligation is much less efficient than for sticky ends, some alteration of the ligation conditions is necessary:

1. Lower levels of ATP to a maximum of 0.5 mм.
2. To increase the concentration of blunt-ended DNA, polyethylene glycol (PEG) is added to a maximum of 15% to increase the macromolecular crowding without increase of actual numbers of molecules.

3. More enzyme is required, up to 50 Weiss units.

Ligations can be incubated at a number of temperatures for different times, e.g. overnight at 14°C (10–15 h); 4–5 h at room temperature, or 1 h at 37°C. The control reaction is to ligate just the vector to test the efficiency of the dephosphorylation reaction. After transformation of bacteria very few colonies should be seen with the vector alone.

Cloning of PCR products

If PCR products are produced with enzyme sites at the ends then the fragments can be isolated on gels, purified and digested with the appropriate enzyme(s) and cloned as for sticky-end fragments. However, situations arise when this is not possible. The most convenient way to clone PCR products in this case is to use the TA Cloning Kit from Invitrogen*. This kit takes advantage of the fact that the *Taq* polymerase (not other high temperature resistant polymerases used in PCR) adds an extra deoxyadenosine to the end of the fragments which is not template dependent. The kit provides a linear vector with an extra deoxythymidine at the ends to act as a complementary sticky-end. So any PCR product can be cloned into this vector and once amplified in bacteria can be removed from any of a number of cloning sites which straddle the original A-T cloning position, and cloned into the vector of choice. While the purchase of the vector can be costly ($12.5 per reaction) over time, it is extremely easy to clone PCR products which, because they are often small, reduces efficiency. We have found that the time saved makes up for the expense.

After ligation the plasmids are transformed into bacteria. To select for bacterial cells containing the plasmid the vector carries an antibiotic resistance gene, which commonly will confer resistance to either ampicillin, tetracycline, or kanamycin.

One common feature of cloning is that the bacteria have to be made competent for transformation of the ligated plasmid. There are basically two methods used to transform bacteria – chemically and by electroporation.

Production of competent bacteria

Many companies such as Gibco-BRL sell competent bacteria, but only strains that are commonly used such as DH-5 and HB101. If it is necessary to use a specialized bacterial strain then the following methods can be used.

Competent bacteria for electroporation

Electroporation is the most efficient method for transformation of bacteria (Dower et al 1988; Taketo 1988), but it does necessitate the purchase of an electroporator, or Gene Pulser. This instrument passes an electric current through bacteria allowing passage of plasmid DNA into the organisms. A high electric field is required for bacteria and so bacteria should be suspended in a solution of low ionic strength compatible with survival of the bacteria. Preparation of the bacteria entails extensive washes in distilled water to remove salt from the broth cultures:

1. A small overnight culture of bacteria is inoculated into a flask containing a liter of broth. The culture is grown until an OD of 0.45 is reached.

2. Bacteria are pelleted and washed in 100 ml of distilled water.

3. Bacteria are pelleted and washed in 50 ml of distilled water and this is repeated with decreasing amounts of distilled water, 25 ml, 10 ml and then the bacteria are resuspended in a volume of distilled water ($1–3 \times 10^{10}$ cells ml^{-1}) plus 10% glycerol and aliquoted in 50 µl amounts and snap frozen in a dry ice alcohol bath and stored at $-70°C$ until use. Each aliquot is sufficient for one electroporation or transformation.

4. For electroporation an aliquot is removed from the $-70°C$ and thawed on ice. 40 µl is removed and added to the electroporation cuvette and a small amount of the ligation reaction added. The ligation reaction should be diluted at least 1:5 and 1 µl used for electroporation. The dilution is necessary because of the salt content of the ligation mix.

5. The electroporation is carried out at 2.5 V at 96 µFad in a cuvette 0.2 cm wide for many of the commonly used *E. coli* bacteria. These conditions are for the Biorad Electroporator with a Pulse Controller and so the voltage may change slightly for other instruments.

6. Immediately after the voltage discharge 800 µl of SOC (Table 10.5) is added and the bacteria are incubated at 37°C for 1 h with shaking.

7. The bacterial suspension is diluted (usually 10^{-1} and 10^{-2}) and 200 µl of each is added to the LM plates containing appropriate antibiotics. It is usual to plate out 200 µl of the original culture along with dilutions.

This method will give efficiencies of 10^9 to 10^{10} transformants μg^{-1} of DNA, at least 10-fold higher than any other method.

Table 10.5. Bacterial media.

Compound	LM	SOB*	SOC*
Bactotryptone	1% (w/v)	2%	2%
Yeast extract	0.5%	0.5%	0.5%
KCl	–	2.5 mM	2.5 mM
NaCl	10 mM	10 mM	10 mM
$MgSO_4.7H_2O$†	10 mM	10 mM	10 mM
$MgCl_2$	–	10 mM	10 mM
Glucose	–	–	20 mM
Bacto agar	1.5%	–	–

* SOB and SOC are prepared without magnesium and autoclaved. Add Mg^{2+} salts from sterile solution adjusted to pH to 6.8–7.0 using KOH.
† For tetracycline plates omit Mg^{2+}.

Competent bacteria by the hexamine cobalt chloride method

This is the most efficient of the chemical methods and will give frequencies of 10^7 to 10^8 transformants μg^{-1} of DNA (Hanahan 1983).

The buffer for transformation is called TFB and is made as follows: MES (2-[4-morpholino]ethanesulfonic acid) is adjusted to pH 6.3 using KOH, sterilized by filtration and stored at −20°C.

10 mM MES
100 mM KCl
45 mM Mn_2 $Cl.2H_2O$
10 mM Ca $Cl_2.2H_2O$
3 mM $HACoCl_3$ [hexamine cobalt (III) chloride]

All salts are added as solids and the final solution is filtered through a pre-rinsed 220 nm Millipore filter and stored at 4°C. TFB is stable for at least one year at 4°C (final pH 6.15).

1. For preparation of bacteria, take a fresh overnight plate of bacteria and disperse one colony in 1 ml of SOB by moderate vortexing and then add to 10 ml of SOB in a 500 ml flask for good aeration.

2. Incubate at 37°C at 275 rpm in an orbital shaker until the cell density is between 4×10^7 ml^{-1} and 7×10^7 ml^{-1} ($OD_{550} = 0.45$–0.55 for DH-1). This usually takes 2–2.5 h.

3. Collect cells in a 50 ml polypropylene tube and place on ice for 10–15 min, then pellet at 1500 rpm for 10 min at 4°C.

4. Resuspend in 1/3 volume of ice-cold TFB by gentle vortexing and leave on ice for 10–15 min.

5. Pellet at 1500 rpm for 10 min at 4°C and resuspend in 1/12.5 volume of ice-cold TFB and add fresh DMSO (dimethylsulfoxide) or DMF (dimethylformamide) to 3.5% (7 μl/200 μl), swirl and leave on ice for 5 min.

6. Add DTT or β-mercaptoethanol to 75 mM (7 μl/200 μl), swirl and leave on ice.

7. Add a further 7 μl of DMSO as above and leave on ice for 5 min.

8. Place 221 μl samples into prechilled Eppendorf tubes, add DNA (add a maximum of 10 μl), swirl and leave on ice for 30 min.

9. Heat the tube at 42°C for **exactly** 90 s and immediately place on ice. This is for 1.5 ml Eppendorf tubes and the time may need to be adjusted for tubes of different thickness. Leave for 2–3 min and then add 800 μl of SOC

and incubate tubes at 37°C for 1 h at 225 rpm.

10. Plate 200 µl of the appropriate dilution on LM plates plus antibiotics.

If cells are to be stored rather than plating out immediately, they can be stored overnight in SOC. For longer storage periods dilute the cells with 40% glycerol/60% 1:1 SOB, chill on ice and snap-freeze in an ethanol dry ice bath. The bacteria are stored at −70°C. In each case the viability is ≥ 90%.

Note

A fresh bottle of DMSO should be opened and 100 µl aliquots placed in Eppendorf tubes and frozen at −20°C. Thaw an aliquot and use on that day and then discard. Oxidative products of DMSO are very inhibitory. The DMF alternative is not prone to oxidation and is stored at room temperature, although the efficiency of transformation is only 50% of that using fresh DMSO.

Competent bacteria for CaCl$_2$ method

This method is the least efficient, giving 10^6–10^7 transformants μg^{-1} of DNA. It is easy to carry out and can be used when efficiency is not critical.

1. A colony from a fresh culture plate is picked and transferred to 100 ml of SOB in a 1-liter flask and grown for 2–3 h at 37°C, shaking at 275 rpm. Harvest cells when the OD is 0.45–0.55 and transfer to two 50 ml polypropylene tubes and cool to 0°C on ice.
2. Centrifuge cells at 1500 rpm for 10 min at 4°C and resuspend the cells in 10 ml of ice-cold 0.1 M CaCl$_2$ and store on ice.

3. Pellet cells at 1500 rpm for 10 min at 4°C and decant supernatant and invert tube on a tissue to drain residual liquid. Resuspend cells in 2 ml of 0.1 M CaCl$_2$ for each 50 ml of original culture. The bacteria can at this stage be frozen in 200 µl aliquots at −70°C and stored, with a small decrease in the efficiency of transformation.
4. Add the DNA to the 200 µl aliquot, mix and store on ice for 30 min.
5. Transfer the tubes to a 42°C water bath for **exactly** 90 s, then rapidly cool on ice and add 200 µl of SOC and incubate for 1 h at 37°C with shaking.
6. Dilutions can then be plated on LM plates containing the appropriate antibiotic.

Mini-preps to test for successful cloning

If cloning has been successful, then a number of colonies should have grown on the plates. To confirm that the insert is in the vector, colonies are picked, grown overnight and the plasmid DNA extracted and analyzed by restriction enzyme digestion. If confirmation of cloning is the goal then the purity of the DNA is not so important, but if sequencing is the goal it is best to be more careful in the extraction process. Both methods are described below.

General purpose mini-prep

1. Take one colony and grow overnight at 37°C, with shaking, in 3 ml LB broth in a 15 ml tube.
2. Spin down bacteria and resuspend the pellet in 100 µl of lysis buffer.
   50 mM glucose
   25 mM Tris Cl, pH 7.0
   10 mM EDTA
   5 mg ml^{-1} lysozyme

Note

The solution can be made and stored at 4°C, but the lysozyme should always be added just before use.

3. Transfer to a 1.5 ml Eppendorf tube and incubate on ice for 5 min.
4. Add 20 µl of the following alkaline solution, which is made up **fresh**:
     250 µl of 4 N NaOH
     250 µl of 20% SDS
     add water to 5 ml
5. Mix gently by inverting the tube several times and then incubate for 5 min on ice.
6. Add 100 µl of a potassium acetate solution made up as follows:
     60 ml of 5 M potassium acetate
     11.5 ml of glacial acetic acid
     28.5 ml of distilled water
7. Vortex briefly and incubate on ice for 5 min.
8. Spin for 10 min in a microfuge and remove the supernatant to a fresh tube. Extract twice with phenol/chloroform.
9. Precipitate DNA with 0.1 vol of 3 M Na acetate and 2 vol of ethanol.
10. Wash pellet in 70% ethanol, dry and resuspend in 50 µl of distilled water. This method will give 20–30 µg of DNA, and is enough to carry out restriction analysis. The DNA can be used for further cloning.

Mini-prep for high quality plasmid DNA

This method is from Lee and Rasheed (1990).

1. Colonies are picked and grown overnight as above except that the broth is called 'terrific broth' and is made as follows:

     1.2% bacto-tryptone (w/v)
     2.4% bacto yeast extract (w/v)
     0.04% glycerol (v/v)
     0.17 M KH_2PO_4
     0.072 M K_2HPO_4

2. Of the overnight culture, 2 ml is taken, spun and the pellet resuspended in 200 µl lysis buffer as for general purpose (step 2) and vortexed for 5 s and then incubated at room temperature for 5 min.
3. Add 400 µl of the freshly prepared alkaline solution as for general purpose (step 4), invert the tube five times and incubate on ice for 5 min.
4. Add 300 µl of ice-cold 7.5 M ammonium acetate (pH 7.6), mix by inverting the tube and place on ice for another 5 min.
5. Spin in a microfuge for 5 min at room temperature, transfer the supernatant to a fresh tube and add 0.6 vol of isopropanol, incubate at room temperature for 10 min and spin in a microfuge for 10 min.
6. Add 100 µl of 2 M ammonium acetate, pH 7.4, to the pellet, vortex and incubate on ice for 5 min.
7. Centrifuge and save the supernatant, add 100 µl of isopropanol and incubate at room temperature for 10 min and spin as before.
8. Wash the pellet in 70% ethanol, remove the ethanol by centrifugation, dry the pellet and resuspend in 49 µl of TE and add 1 µl of RNAse (DNAse free), so that the final concentration of RNAse-A and RNAse-T1 is 100 µg ml^{-1} and 1000 U ml^{-1} respectively. Incubate at 37°C for 15 min, then add 25 µl of 7.5 M ammonium sulfate and 75 µl of isopropanol and leave at room temperature before pelleting DNA in a microfuge.
9. Wash the pellet in 70% ethanol, dry and resuspend in TE. Read the OD at 260 nm and 280 nm for concentration and purity. This method should yield 40–60 µg ml^{-1}.

DNA from either method can then be digested with restriction enzymes to determine the success of cloning. Sequencing of the fragment is only necessary if the sequence is unknown, or cloning was accomplished with an insert that was PCR amplified. If sequencing is necessary then it is best to use the second method described above and the DNA can be used directly.

DNA sequencing

It is sometimes necessary to sequence cloned genes, especially if the DNA fragment cloned is unique, or the fragment was produced by PCR, to ensure it has been faithfully copied. The most commonly used method is the Sanger Dideoxy-chain termination method (Sanger et al 1977). This method uses dideoxynucleotides (ddNTPs) which do not have the hydroxyl group at the 3-prime position in the deoxyribose and so while they can be added to a chain, nothing can be added to them so they act as chain terminators. If there are four reactions with the four different ddNTPs in each, then the result will be a series of chain terminations at A, T, C or G.

For the sequencing of a hitherto unsequenced piece of DNA, purified DNA is recommended, but if confirmation of a previously sequenced fragment is the goal, then miniprep DNA will suffice. Sequencing by the Sanger method can be carried out with single or double stranded DNA with only minor, but important differences in the protocol. Both will be described below.

Sequencing of single-stranded DNA templates

Preparation of M13mp single-stranded template

For single-stranded sequencing it is necessary to clone the fragment of interest into a vector which will give single-stranded DNA. Vectors such as Bluescript, or Genscribe-Z which contain the bacteriophage M13 origin of replication inserted in opposite orientations into the commonly used plasmid, pUC, are used for production of single-stranded DNA.

Cloning DNA fragments into M13 vectors

The actual procedure for cloning into the M13 vectors (Hu and Messing 1982; Messing 1983) is the same as described on page 213. With most of the M13 vectors the polylinker site is in the middle of the first 146 amino acids of the β-galactosidase gene (*lacZ*). The enzyme activity of this part of the β-galactosidase is complemented by a mutated *lacZ* gene on a F-factor plasmid carried by host cells of the M13 phage. This F-factor codes also for sex pili by which filamentous phage enter the host cell. Therefore for M13 cloning bacterial host cells with the F-factor present are used (e.g. JM101, JM109, TG-1 and DH-5αF′ are some of the commonly used bacteria). Cloning of a DNA fragment into M13 vector will disrupt the *lacZ* gene and successful experiments can be observed by the presence of white colonies on the petri dishes as opposed to blue colonies if no insert is present, when bacterial cells are plated on dishes containing IPTG (isopropylthio-β-D-galactoside) an inducer of β-galactosidase and X-gal (5-bromo-4-chloro-3-indolyl-β-D-galactoside).

To produce single-stranded DNA it is necessary to propagate the virus and this is accomplished as follows:

1. Grow an overnight culture of plating bacteria in SOB at 37°C.
2. Remove an aliquot of competent bacteria from the −70°C freezer, or produce some fresh as described above, and transfer 40 µl to each of three 5 ml culture tubes.
3. Add approximately 50–100 ng of the ligation mix to one tube, and to two control tubes add 5 pg of M13 double-stranded DNA to one and no

DNA to the other. Store the tubes on ice for 30 min.
4. Prepare a set of three tubes containing 3 ml of melted SOB agar and store at 47°C until later.
5. Heat-shock the three tubes containing the competent bacteria for 90 s at 42°C. Depending on the tubes used this time may need to be varied. The time for Falcon 2054 (5 ml) has been found to be 90 s, but glass tubes or thicker plastic ones will need more time.
6. Add aliquots of transformed bacteria to the SOB agar and add 4 μl of IPTG (200 mg ml^{-1}) and 40 μl of X-gal (20 μg ml^{-1}), then add 200 μl of the overnight culture from (1). Mix by vortexing, and pour the contents of the tube onto LB agar plate and label.

Plaques will appear at 12 h and recombinant white plaques should be picked and the virus amplified.

Analysis of recombinants

It is best to confirm the nature of the recombinant by isolation of the double-stranded replicative form (RF) of M13 bacteriophage and analyze with restriction endonucleases.

1. To isolate the double-stranded RF DNA, an isolated plaque is taken from the plate by touching the surface of the plaque with either a sterile tooth pick or micropipette tip and then vigorously shaking the tip into LB medium and incubating the small amount of agarose at room temperature for 1–2 h to allow the phage to diffuse out from the agarose.
2. Add 50 μl of a culture of plating bacteria to 3 ml of LB in a tube (use at least a 15 ml tube for good aeration). To this add a one-tenth volume of the phage suspension prepared above and incubate for 5–6 h at 37°C with shaking (225 rpm). Do not culture for longer periods or else deletion mutations will be selected.
3. Transfer 1.5 ml of the culture to a microfuge tube and centrifuge for 5 min at room temperature and transfer the supernatant to a fresh tube and store. The phage can be stored indefinitely at 4°C or −20°C without loss of infectivity. The remaining part of the culture can be used to isolate the double-stranded RF DNA.
4. The amount of RF DNA isolated from the rest of the bacterial culture is low (200–500 ng), but should be sufficient to analysis the recombinants.
5. The DNA is isolated essentially by the alkaline method described for plasmid DNA. One difference is that the lysozyme in solution I is unnecessary. In addition, it should be remembered that unlike plasmid isolation, there may be some contaminating single-stranded DNA in the RF DNA preparation. This may lead to confusing patterns upon restriction enzyme digestion. However, undigested controls should help interpretation.

Preparation of the single-stranded template

Once the recombinants have been confirmed it is then possible to culture sufficient single-stranded template for sequencing.

1. Add 0.5 ml of the phage stock to 2.5 ml of plating bacteria in LB broth and allow to sit at room temperature for 5 min to allow infection.

2. Add all of this culture to 250 ml of prewarmed LB and incubate at 37°C for 5 h.
3. Spin down the cells, transfer the supernatant to a 500 ml flask and add 10 g of polyethylene glycol (PEG 8000) plus 7.5 g of NaCl. Stir for 1 h at room temperature.
4. Pellet the phage particles by centrifugation for 10,000 g for 20 min, and drain the supernatant well before adding 10 ml of buffer (10 mM Tris Cl, pH 8.0; 10 mM NaCl and 100 mM EDTA) and resuspending the pellet.
5. Add an equal volume of phenol (tris-saturated) and mix the contents vigorously by vortexing and then centrifuge at 3000 g for 5 min. Transfer the upper aqueous layer to a fresh tube and extract with phenol/chloroform, spin and remove upper aqueous layer.
6. Add 1 ml of 3 M Na acetate and 20 ml of ethanol, mix and stand on ice for 1 h.
7. Recover the DNA by centrifugation at 10,000 g for 30 min at 4°C, discard the supernatant, wash the pellet with 70% ethanol and spin briefly.
8. Dry the pellet at room temperature and dissolve in 1 ml of TE. The DNA should be stored at −20°C for sequencing.

Sequencing reactions

There are a number of different DNA polymerase enzymes that can be used for sequencing and the template used will, to some extent, determine the type of enzyme. In addition there are a number of sequencing kits which supply all the reagents apart from the template and radiolabeled triphosphate. It is best to use one of these kits especially if your sequencing needs are limited. The DNA polymerase commonly used is the Sequenase version 2.0, which has high processivity (average number of nucleotides synthesized before the enzyme dissociates from the template), and a high rate of polymerization (number of nucleotides added per second). The *Taq* polymerase also has high processivity and polymerization and is used for determining the sequence of DNA templates that form secondary structures, since the reaction can be carried out at high temperatures (70–75°C).

1. The sequencing reactions need two sets of solutions, one for the initial short polymerization reaction to add approximately 25 bases to the primer using low concentrations of bases, and one set for the chain extension and termination.
2. Anneal primer (approx. 2 ng ml^{-1}) to single-stranded template (0.1–0.5 μg μl^{-1}) by placing both in a 0.5 ml microcentrifuge tube along with 2 μl of 5× Sequenase buffer (200 mM Tris HCl, pH 7.5; 100 mM MgCl$_2$; 250 mM NaCl) and distilled water to 10 μl. Warm to 65°C for 2 min and then place at room temperature and allow temperature to cool slowly. This will take 30–40 min.

Note

Using M13 means that there are primer sites at either end of the cloning site so different DNA fragments can be sequenced with the same primers and in both direction.

3. When cooled, add to the primer mix in the following order:
   Template primer reaction (10 μl)
   0.1 M DTT (1 μl)
   Diluted labeling mix (7.5 μM dGTP; 7.5 μM dCTP; 7.5 μM dTTP) (2.0 μl)
   [α-^{35}S] dATP (1000 Ci mmol^{-1}) (0.5 μl)
   Sequenase enzyme (diluted 1/8 in enzyme diluting buffer – 10 mM Tris Cl, pH 7.5 5 mM DTT; 0.5 mg ml^{-1} BSA) (2.0 μl)

4. Incubate at room temperature for 4 min.

5. While the primer is annealing in step 2 make up the termination reactions ready to add to it the reactions from step 3. The four termination reactions each contain one of the dideoxy bases, so in four different tubes labeled A, G, T, C add 2.5 μl of ddATP, ddGTP, ddTTP, and ddCTP termination mixes. The termination mixes can be made up as stock solutions and frozen at −20°C and should be aliquoted and warmed to 37°C before the next step.

Termination mixes

All the four different mixes contain:
50 mм NaCl
80 μм of each dNTP except for the termination base added at 8 μм.
For ddG termination:
50 mм NaCl
80 μм each of dTTP, dATP and dCTP and 8 μм ddGTP.
For ddA:
ddATP would substitute for dATP, and dGTP would be added at 80 μм etc. for the other two termination reactions.

6. To the termination mix add 3.5 μl of the reaction from step 3, and incubate at 37°C for up to 20 min.

7. Add 4 μl of the stop buffer to each reaction and store on ice until loaded onto the sequencing gel. It can be stored for up to a week at −20°C if it is ^{35}S-labeled, but must be run the same day if it is ^{32}P-labeled.

8. Heat the samples at 80°C for 2 min before loading onto the sequencing gel.

Stop buffer

95% formamide
20 mм EDTA
0.05% bromophenol blue
0.05% xylene cyanol blue

Note

The bromophenol runs at 26 base pairs and the xylene at 106 base pairs in a 6% acrylamide gel. This gives an indication of resolution.

Sequencing double-stranded DNA templates by the dideoxy-chain termination method

1. Place 4 μg of DNA in 500 μl microcentrifuge tube and add water up to 30 μl. It will help if more template is used compared to single-stranded DNA.

2. Add 3 μl of 2 N NaOH and incubate at room temperature for 5 min.

3. To neutralize the reaction add 5 μl of 3 м Na acetate and to precipitate add 120 μl of ethanol and leave at −20°C for 10 min.

4. Pellet DNA in a microfuge for 20 min, wash in 70% ethanol, dry and resuspend in 7 μl of distilled water, 2 μl of Sequenase reaction buffer and 1 μl of primer.

5. Add 2 μl of the sequencing reaction buffer and anneal for 45 min at 37°C.

Note

At this point the protocol is the same as for single-stranded DNA sequencing.

Table 10.6. Polyacrylamide gel.

	Stock solution	Final concentration	For 100 ml gel
Acrylamide (DNA sequencing grade)	40%	7%	17.5 ml
N′N′-methylbisacrylamide	2%	0.37%	18.5 ml
Urea	powder	7 M	42 g
TBE	5×	0.7×	14 ml
Ammonium persulfate (fresh)	0.1 g ml^{-1}	0.8 mg ml^{-1}	0.8 ml
TEMED*	100%	0.05%	50 µl
dH$_2$O	–	–	18.2 ml

* Before adding TEMED take 5–10 ml of the gel solution and add 20–30 µl of TEMED to this small volume and pour to the bottom of the gel to seal the spacers at the bottom. Wait 10 min and add 50 µl of TEMED to the remaining gel solution and pour carefully, placing the glass plates at an angle of 30° to the bench and avoid the creation of bubbles.

Preparaton of sequencing gel

Polyacrylamide gels are used to resolve the different band lengths and the standard method above will allow the sequencing of 200–300 base pairs. Below are the components of a 7% gel of 0.4 mm thickness. Thinner gels of 2 mm can be used and give better resolution, but are fragile.

Glass plates should be clean and one of them siliconized on one side to allow easy separation of the plates when the gel run is completed. This is done by placing several drops of Sigmacote (Sigma) onto the glass, spreading the drops over the plate's surface with a tissue, and then rinsing with distilled water. The plate is dried before use. The average size of sequencing plates is 30 cm × 40 cm and this size of plate can resolve 200–300 bases. Longer plates can be used to allow greater resolution. The glass plates are taped together with 3MM electrical tape, or any other brand of strong water resistant adhesive tape, and then large bulldog clips are placed over the tape as pressure to keep the plates tightly together during pouring. After pouring is complete, insert the comb in upside down and clip to make sure there is no gel between the glass plates and the comb. This can be achieved by placing bulldog clips at either side and along the top of the glass plates. Rest the gel at an angle to allow polymerization, which should take 30 min. The gel should be made at least 2 h before running, and should be pre-run for 30 min before loading. The gel can be left overnight, but to prevent drying Saran wrap should be placed around the top of the gel.

To load the gel the comb is removed and placed the right way up. It is best to use shark-toothed combs as the wells are then close to each other, allowing easy reading of

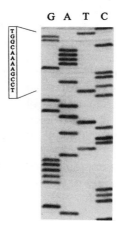

Figure 10.7. DNA sequence of the non-coding strand of part of the upstream regulatory region of HPV-11 showing one of the E2-binding sites (E2BS, ACCN$_6$GGT is the consensus sequence of the coding strand, i.e. complimentary to the sequence shown on the gel) at the origin of replication.

the gel. The comb should be placed so that the teeth touch the top of the acrylamide gel. The boiled samples are loaded and the gel is run at around 1800 V. The high voltage causes heat generation which helps to prevent renaturation of DNA strands or formation of secondary structures. However, heat may crack the glass plates, so most new gel rigs now come with a metal backplate, which helps to dissipate the heat evenly over the glass. After completion of the run the glass plates are separated, and the gel washed in a buffer containing 10% acetic acid and 12% methanol, to remove the urea and fix the gel for drying. The gel is transferred to 3MM Whatman filter paper, covered with Saran wrap, dried and exposed to X-ray film. If the radiolabel is ^{35}S then expose without Saran, but if it is ^{32}P-labeled then the Saran can remain over the gel during exposure. Figure 10.7 is an example of sequencing double-stranded DNA from the upstream regulatory region of HPV-11, showing one of the E2 binding sites (E2BS, ACCGAAAACGGT) at the origin of replication.

Transfection of mammalian cells

It is often desirable to transfect DNA into mammalian cells. This technique is used if you wish to

- transiently or stably express a viral gene in mammalian cells;
- investigate the activities of certain elements of a viral promoter;
- study the activities of a viral transactivation protein.

There are a number of methods used to transfect cells, three of which are described below.

Calcium chloride precipitation method

This method was first used by Graham and van der Eb (1973), and modified by a number of individuals to increase the efficiency. These changes can be during the calcium precipitation where temperature and CO_2 concentration are altered, or after calcium treatment, involving addition of glycerol, or chloroquine.

Cells

Cells are seeded the day before transfection at a density of no greater than 10^4 cells cm^{-2}. Typically 5×10^5 cells are seeded onto a 100 mm diameter petri dish. Next day, 3 h prior to transfection, the media is changed and the transfection mix prepared.

Preparation of precipitate

1. DNA is diluted to 40 µg ml^{-1} in distilled water, and calcium chloride (2 M $CaCl.6H_2O$ [10.8 g], made up to 20 ml, filtered through a 0.22 µm filter and stored at room temperature) is added to a final concentration of 250 mM. Typically 10 µg of DNA in 0.25 ml of distilled water is added to 62 µl of 2 M $CaCl_2$ in 0.25 ml of distilled water to make a final volume of 0.5 ml.

2. Add 0.5 ml of $2\times$ HBS (280 mM NaCl [1.6 g]; 10 mM KCl [0.074 g]; 1.5 mM $Na_2HPO_4.2H_2O$ [0.027 g]; 50 mM HEPES [1 g]; dH_2O [to 100 ml]; pH to 7.05 with 0.5 N NaOH, stored at room temperature) to a separate tube.

3. Now add dropwise the DNA/$CaCl_2$ mix to the $2\times$ HBS while the mixture is continually stirred by means of a jet of nitrogen directed onto the surface through a cotton plugged sterile Pasteur pipette, or mixed by gently tapping the tube after the addition of alternate drops. This procedure ensures adequate mixing and the formation of a fine precipitate. Precipitation should be carried out in plastic tubes, or siliconized glass tubes.

4. Precipitates are allowed to form undisturbed at room temperature for 15–20 minutes and then the mixture added to the 10 mm dish. If glycerol is going to be added (250 mM NaCl; 50 mM HEPES, pH 7.0; 15% glycerol) then the plates are incubated for 3–5 hours depending on the sensitivity of the cells to the $CaCl_2$ treatment. Where no glycerol shock is included the precipitate is left on the cells overnight.

5. If glycerol is used then the precipitate is removed and the cells washed twice

with serum-free medium and 2 ml of the glycerol solution is added for no more than 3 min. The time of glycerol treatment will depend on the cell type, and the optimum time will need to be assessed. After glycerol treatment the cells should be washed three times in serum-free medium, and then growth medium added for the remainder of the culture time.

6. Chloroquine can be added to the calcium precipitate during the incubation. This compound is a weak base and can neutralize endosomal pH and inhibit the activity of lysosomal hydrolases which may degrade the DNA during passage to the nucleus. Concentrations will vary with the cell type, but are commonly 100 µM.

7. Alteration of the temperature and CO_2 concentration during transfection can increase the efficiency nearly 100% in certain cell types as measured by stable transformants. Typically transfection is carried at 35°C in 2–4% CO_2, depending on the cells, and is carried out overnight with no glycerol shock included (Chen and Okayama 1987).

After calcium treatment, the cells are incubated in growth medium until harvested.

Electroporation

Electroporation uses an electric field passed through cells (as for bacterial cells described earlier) in suspension, to introduce DNA into the cells. The voltage used varies between cell types, so it is best to try different settings when using a cell type not previously tested. Cells are placed in small cuvettes somewhat similar to those used in a spectrophotometer except that there are metal strips down two sides to conduct the electrical current. Generally we have found that for transient transfections with cells which can be electroporated with great efficiency (30–40%) then circular as well as linear DNA can be used with little difference in the number of cells transfected. However, for stable cell lines it is more efficient to use linear DNA. Since this method tends to kill many of the cells in suspension (up to 50% of cells at particular settings) it is usual to use $1-2 \times 10^6$ per electroporation.

The following methods are for use with the Biorad Gene Pulser, or electroporator plus a Capacitance Extender when 960 microfarads (µF) is used and 0.4 cm wide cuvettes.

1. Cells are trypsinized and placed in 0.25 ml of either PBS or growth medium in small cuvettes ready for addition of the DNA. The cuvettes are placed on ice before DNA is added.

2. A wide range of DNA concentration can be used, from 250 ng up to 10 µg and DNA is added to the cells by mixing.

3. The cells are electroporated and then immediately placed on ice before being plated. The higher the voltage or the longer the time to deliver the electrical pulse then the more cell death is observed. The conditions are

Table 10.7. Electroporation conditions.

Cells or cell lines	µg of DNA	Voltage	Microfarads (µF)	% efficiency
NIH 3T3	0.5 µg	210	960	20–30
Chinese hamster ovary	0.5 µg	220	960	20–30
Human 293	0.5 µg	170	960	30–40
Primary human keratinocytes	10 µg	1000	96	0.1–2

always a compromise between efficiency of transfection and cell death. Table 10.7 gives the conditions for some of the cell types we have used.

The efficiency of transfection was measured using a β-galactosidase expressing plasmid, and staining for β-galactosidase activity. As a general rule the conditions for cell lines appear to be high microfarads (μF) and low voltage. So if testing a cell line for the first time then use 960 μF and vary the voltage between 150 and 270. Most commonly used cell lines will fall into this voltage range. The situation for primary cells and lymphocytes may be quite different and will need to be tested over a range for both voltage and μF.

The high efficiency of this method and the smaller amounts of DNA needed make it an attractive technique if an electroporator is available. However, it is not always the best method for certain cells and alternative methods have been developed as described below.

Lipofection

This method uses cationic lipids which, when mixed with DNA preparations, will form liposomes that will presumably transport the DNA into cells from fusion with the lipid-containing cytoplasmic membrane. There are a number of different lipid preparations commercially available but because high concentrations of the lipids need to be used for certain cell types the experiments can cost as much as $2 per plate. Fortunately liposomes can be made very cheaply and the following is one method we have used (Rose et al 1991). This method gives 20–30% transfection in a monkey kidney cell line (CV-1P), but only 2–5% with primary human keratinocytes.

Components

L-a-phosphatidylethanolamine dioleoyl (PtdEtn) and dimethyldioctadecylammonium bromide (DDAB) from Sigma. The concentration of DDAB is important with the normal range between 0.4–1.0 mg ml^{-1} and toxicity should be tested on each cell type used. PtdEtn is supplied as a 10 mg ml^{-1} solution in chloroform. For keratinocytes the normal concentration for each are 0.5 mg ml^{-1} for DDAB and 1 mg ml^{-1} for PtdEtn.

Preparation of a 10 ml batch of lipids

1. Add 5 mg DDAB to 1 ml of PtdEtn in a microfuge tube.
2. Evaporate to dryness in speed-vac.
3. Add 10 ml sterile distilled water to 15 ml sterile tube and using sterile technique resuspend the pellet with the water. The pellet will not dissolve at this stage and it is sufficient to get it resuspended.
4. Sonicate the lipid mix by placing the tube in a beaker of iced water. This sonication step is important and should be carried out until the solution is homogeneous and no large particles remain. This will take 1–2 hours.
   This lipid mixture is stable for several months at 4°C.

Transfection

The quantities used are for 60 mm dishes, but smaller or larger Petri dishes can be used as long as there is a proportional decrease or increase in the quantities of the components.

1. Add together 1.5 ml of serum free medium, 45 μl of the lipid mix and 10–20 μg of DNA.
2. Mix gently and stand at room temperature for 5–10 min.

3. Rinse cells twice with PBS and then add the DNA/lipid mixture.
4. Incubate cells at 37°C for 4 h, rocking every half hour to ensure an even distribution of the mix.
5. After 4 h add an equal volume (1.5 ml) of medium containing serum.
6. Incubate cells for a further 2 h, wash twice with PBS and then add the appropriate growth medium.

The cells are then usually harvested 48–72 hours later. Lipofection is probably the most versatile transfection method in that it is very effective with a wide variety of cell types with efficiencies of up to 30%.

Transfection using poly-l-ornithine

This method has been successfully adapted for use with primary human keratinocytes (Nead and McCance 1995), which are refractory to efficient transfection by most other methods (Table 10.7). This method was modified from a previously published report of Bond and Wold (1987). Human keratinocytes are difficult to transfect, with a maximum of 2% efficiency using electroporation (Table 10.7). In our hands higher frequencies have not been obtained using other methods. The poly-l-ornithine method gives frequencies of 15% to 20% and the method might be adapted to other cell types that are difficult to transfect by other methods.

1. Primary human keratinocytes are plated on 60 mm dishes in KGM medium (Clonetics, Utah, USA). This is a medium specifically for growth of human keratinocytes.
2. At 40% to 50% confluence the cells are washed twice with warm PBS and then warm Ham's F12 or KBM (Clonetics Inc. Utah, U.S.A.) containing 21 μg poly-l-ornithine and 10 μg of DNA are added. It is critical to keep the DNA/poly-l-ornithine ratio between 0.42 and 0.48. For example, we use 2.1 μl of 10 mg ml^{-1} poly-l-ornithine and 10 μg of plasmid DNA giving a ratio of 0.48. If the DNA amount is changed then the poly-l-ornithine concentration has to be altered to keep a ratio between 0.42 and 0.48. Transfection frequencies decrease if the ratio is outside this range and at some ratios we observed toxicity. The volume of the final mixture is not critical, but 1.8 ml is optimal for 60 mm plates.
3. The plates are placed at 37°C for 6 h with gentle rocking every hour.
4. After the incubation period the KGM is aspirated off and 3 ml of 27.5% DMSO in KGM is added for exactly 4 min. The percentage of DMSO is important and for keratinocytes 30% gives good results, but reduces significantly the viability of the cells. Therefore for other cell types the DMSO concentration may need to be altered to optimize transfection frequencies.
5. Immediately aspirate off the DMSO/KGM and wash three times with warm KGM and add fresh KGM and incubate cells until harvested.

This method is best with supercoiled DNA and can be used for both transient assays and stable transfectants. This is the first inexpensive method that, in our experience, results in high transfection frequencies of primary human keratinocytes.

Acknowledgements

All of the techniques described have been used in the laboratory over the years and the research has been funded by the Medical Research Council, U.K., Cancer Research Campaign, U.K. and the National Institutes of Health, U.S.A.

References

Angerer LM, Cox KH, Angerer RC (1987) Methods Enzymol 152: 649–661.

Bond VG, Wold B (1987) Mol Cell Biol 7: 2286–2293.

Chen C, Okayama H (1987) Mol Cell Biol 7: 2745–2752.

Collins JE, Jenkins D, McCance DJ (1988) J Clin Pathol 41: 289–295.

Dewhurst S, Chandran B, McIntyre K, Schnabel K, Hall CB (1992) Virology 190: 490–493.

Dower WJ, Miller JF, Ragsdale CW (1988) Nucl Acid Res 16: 6127–6145.

Feinberg AP, Vogelstein B (1983) Anal Biochem 132: 6–13.

Feinberg AP, Vogelstein B (1984) Anal Biochem 137: 266–267.

Graham FL, Van Der Eb AJ (1973) Virology 52: 456–467.

Gross-Bellard M, Oudet P, Chambon P (1973) Eur J Biochem 36: 32–38.

Hanahan D (1983) J Mol Biol 166: 557–580.

Hirt B (1967) J Mol Biol 26: 365–369.

Hu N, Messing J (1982) Gene 17: 271–277.

Innis MA, Gelfand DH (1990) In PCR Protocols: A guide to methods and applications. Innis MA, Gelfand DH, Sninsky JJ, White TJ Eds. Academic Press, San Diego, pp. 3–12.

Kopchik JJ, Cullen BR, Stacey DW (1981) Anal Biochem 115: 419–423.

Lee S-Y, Rasheed S (1990) Biotechniques 9: 676–679.

Messing J (1983) Meth Enzymol 101: 20–78.

Nead M, McCance DJ (1995) J Invest Dermatol 105: 668–671.

Rentrop M, Knapp B, Winter H, Schweizer J (1986) Histochem J 18: 271–276.

Rigby PWS, Dieckman M, Rhodes C, Berg P (1977) J Mol Biol 113: 237–251.

Rose JK, Buonocore L, Whitt MA (1991) Biotechniques 10: 520–525.

Sambrook J, Fritsch EF, Maniatis T (1989) In Molecular Cloning: A Laboratory Manual. 2nd Edition. Cold Spring Harbor Laboratory Press, New York, pp. 1.38–1.39.

Sanger F, Nicklen S, Coulson AR (1977) Proc Natl Acad Sci U.S.A. 74: 5463–5467.

Southern EM (1975) J Mol Biol 98: 503–517.

Studier FW, Rosenberg AH (1981) J Mol Biol 153: 503–525.

Taketo A (1988) Biochim Biophys Acta 949: 318–324.

Virus mutants

K. N. Leppard and C. R. Pringle

Virus mutants have been of crucial importance in the elucidation of the function of virus gene products. Classically, such mutants have been isolated by random mutagenesis and screening for phenotypic variants; only subsequently is the genetic defect characterized and the underlying basis for the phenotype determined. More recently, reverse genetics has offered the opportunity to make planned, directed mutations in virus genomes, the phenotypic effect of which can then be investigated. Whilst the latter is now the approach of choice, there remain situations in which it is necessary or desirable to follow the more classical route. The methodologies associated with these two approaches, together with further background information, are described in this chapter.

Isolation of mutants by classical genetic approaches

Mutation can be defined as a discontinuous event that results in a change in information content. Mutation and recombination are both the means of classical genetic analysis and the sources of variation upon which the evolutionary survival of viruses depends. However, in certain types of RNA viruses (mostly classified in the Order *Mononegavirales*), recombination and genome subunit reassortment do not occur, consequently mutation is the only process by which variation can arise. Perhaps as a consequence, the average rate of spontaneous mutation in viruses with RNA genomes tends to be high. High rates of mutation are achieved because RNA proofreading and RNA mismatch repair systems are absent in both prokaryotes and eukaryotes. The average error frequency at individual sites in viruses with negative stranded RNA genomes, which are recombination-deficient, has been estimated by direct sequence analysis to be in the range 10^{-4} to 10^{-5} (Parvin et al 1986; Steinhauer and Holland 1986; Steinhauer et al 1989). The error frequency measured by the same approach is about ten-fold lower in the recombination-competent positive-stranded poliovirus type 1 (Parvin et al 1986). Holland (1993) has argued from both theoretical considerations and observation that for most RNA viruses the mean replicase error rate is near maximal and approximately the reciprocal of genome length. Thus during replication of a rhabdovirus such as vesicular stomatitis virus (VSV), which has a genome size of approximately 1.1×10^{4} nucleotides, on average one mutation will be generated per replication event. Consequently in any VSV population in an infected animal or a culture vessel every possible base change may be represented at least once. Hence such viruses probably exist as an average (consensus) sequence maintained by positive selection. Another consequence is that the frequency of mutation at individual sites can only be increased slightly by mutagenesis. Several-fold increases were the maximum quantitative changes in mutation frequency observed at single sites in the VSV genome by direct nucleotide sequence analysis in response to treatment with a variety of chemical mutagens (Holland et al 1990). Nonetheless, high frequencies of mutants following chemical mutagenesis of VSV have been observed (Pringle 1970), presumably because the reduced virus yields accompanying mutagenic treatment favour the survival of minority components in the population. Similarly, although the inherent mutation frequency in DNA-containing viruses is low because of the existence of efficient proofreading and mismatch excision-repair systems, observed mutation frequencies in DNA viruses are often high (Smith and Inglis 1987). This could come about by the selection of anti-mutator genes (Hall et al 1984), by suppression of mismatch repair synthesis, by compartmentalization of virus genome replication, by synthesis of single-stranded DNA, etc.

The degeneracy of the genetic code means that not all nucleotide changes result in amino acid substitutions, and perhaps half of all nucleotide changes result in silent mutations. Missense, nonsense, frameshift, duplication and deletion mutants have been described for most types of animal viruses and these mutants can occur spontaneously or be induced by mutagenic treatment of either extracellular non-replicating virus or of replicating virus in infected cells. Spontaneous deletion mutants of viruses are common and are frequently present in the form of defective-interfering (DI) particles whenever viruses are propagated by undiluted passage.

Mutants of animal viruses may have specific phenotypes, such as resistance (to an inhibitor, an antiviral drug, or an enzyme), sensitivity (to heat, acidity), failure to be neutralized by particular monoclonal antibodies (escape mutants), host range or tissue specificity (receptor-binding mutants), or cytopathology (plaque size mutants). Historically, such mutants have been less useful than conditional lethal mutants where a common phenotype (e.g. temperature-sensitivity or suppressor-sensitivity) has been used to identify essential genes and analyze their functions. More recently the use of conditional lethal mutants has been superseded by the development of the more direct and definitive approaches of reverse genetics (see page 241). As a consequence conventional genetic analysis is now focussed predominantly on the use of mutants with specific phenotypes, e.g. drug resistance and monoclonal antibody escape mutants. A selection of representative methods applicable to both aspects of conventional genetic analysis follows, together with a description of methods of direct determination of mutation rates at specific sites in the viral genome.

The mutagenic agents which have been used widely in animal virology are listed in Table 11.1; ultra-violet light or ionizing radiation have been used less frequently to induce mutations in animal viruses, except in special circumstances (e.g. radiation leukaemia virus).

Direct measurement of mutation rate at specific sites in the viral genome

The methodology and its applications are described in detail by Steinhauer and Holland (1986) and Steinhauer et al (1989). The site-specific analysis of base substitution frequencies in RNA viruses depends on the high specificity of RNase T_1 for cleavage immediately following guanine residues. A brief outline of the method as it applies to VSV will be given here; the original papers should be referred to for a fuller description and alternative procedures.

Principle of the method

It is necessary initially to identify target guanine sites at the junction between two large T_1-resistant oligonucleotides (i.e. guanine residues with no guanine neighbours) in the region of the genome chosen for analysis. Complete digestion of such sequences will yield two large oligonucleotides representing the consensus sequence. Nucleotide substitution at the target guanine (junction) site will yield a larger T_1-resistant oligonucleotide product. Separation and quantitation of these oligonucleotides can provide an estimate of the ratio of the error oligonucleotide to the consensus oligonucleotides and an indication of the substitution frequency at that specific site. Synthetic cDNA is required which will anneal to and target the region of the genome chosen for analysis. The appropriate synthetic cDNA should be prepared and purified before proceeding further.

Procedure

1. Initially cells infected with wild type virus, which has been cloned by repeated cycles of reisolation from single plaques, are radiolabeled by incubation in the presence of ^{32}P orthophosphate. When cytopathic effect is extensive, released virus is purified and genomic RNA extracted by standard procedures.

2. The purified *in vivo* labeled RNA is then mixed with a large excess (100–500 µg) of unlabeled viral RNA and

Table 11.1. Mutagenic agents suitable for use with DNA viruses, RNA viruses and retroviruses.

Class	Mutagen	Action	Use	Conditions of exposure/ effective concentration	Representative references
Deaminating agents	Nitrous acid	Two-way transitions	Treatment of virions or nucleic acid	1–10 min. exposure to 1.0 M $NaNO_2$ in 0.25 M Na acetate (pH 4.8)	Williams et al 1971
	Hydroxylamine	One-way transitions; (CG → TA)	Treatment of virions or nucleic acid	1–30 min. exposure to 1.0 M H_3NO in 0.05 M Na phosphate buffer (pH 7.5)	Williams et al 1971
Base analogues	5-Bromodeoxyuridine	Misincorporation; two-way transitions	Replicating DNA viruses; retroviruses	5–30 µg ml^{-1}	Brown et al 1973; Bader and Brown 1971
	5-Fluorouracil (or 5-fluorouridine)	Misincorporation; two-way transitions	Replicating RNA viruses; retroviruses	10–200 µg ml^{-1}	Pringle 1975; Gharpure et al 1969
	5-Azacytidine	Misincorporation: two-way transitions	Replicating RNA viruses; retroviruses	1–100 µg ml^{-1}	Pringle 1975; Wyke 1973
	Ethyl methane sulphonate (or ethyl ethane sulphonate)	Alkylation (predominantly position N7 of purines) and depurination – one-way transitions/ transversions	Treatment of virions or nucleic acid	1–30 min. exposure to 0.05% EMS in 0.25 M Na acetate	Pringle 1975
	N-methyl-N-nitro-N-nitrosoguanidine	Alkylation (predominantly position N7 of purines) and depurination – one-way transitions/ transversions	Treatment of virions or nucleic acid	1–10 min. exposure to 1 mg ml^{-1} NTG in phosphate buffer (pH 7.6)*	Rettenmier et al 1975
Intercalating agents	Proflavine, ICR compounds and other acridines	Frameshifting in phage, but probably indirect in animal viruses	Replicating DNA and RNA viruses	1–10 µg per ml	Fields 1981; McKay et al 1988

*NTG is also an effective mutagen when incorporated into culture fluid at a ten-fold dilution.

annealed to the synthetic cDNA at a three-fold molar excess of DNA in 500 mM NaCl; 4 mM MgCl$_2$ buffered at pH 7.5 with 10 mM Tris HCl. The time and temperature of annealing can be determined by reference to page 7.63 of Sambrook et al (1989).

3. Unprotected single-stranded RNA is then digested with 25 μg of RNase T$_1$ per millilitre and 100 units of RNase T$_2$ per millilitre at 30°C for 2 h. (Digestion with RNase T$_1$ and RNase T$_2$ under these conditions will not digest single base mismatches in the hybrids).

4. Samples are then deproteinized by proteinase K digestion and phenol-chloroform extraction, concentrated by ethanol precipitation, and purified on a 20% polyacrylamide gel.

5. The purified hybrids are now treated with 100 μg per ml DNase 1 for 45 min at 37°C, followed by 5 min at 50°C. The samples are then proteinase K digested, phenol-chloroform extracted three times (avoiding transfer of gel fragments and debris), and ethanol precipitated two to three times followed by a final 70% ethanol wash.

6. After drying, the RNA should be suspended thoroughly in 20 μl of 1 mg ml^{-1} RNase T$_1$ buffered with 10 mM Tris HCl (pH 7.6). The samples should be transferred to new microcentrifuge tubes before digestion at 37°C for 30 min. Mid-way through digestion the samples should be heated to 100°C for 10 s and again transferred to a new microcentrifuge tube. (This procedure is intended to denature any remaining double-stranded molecules and to achieve complete digestion; RNase T$_1$ is resistant to 100°C for short periods.) The RNA is then loaded directly onto the first dimension of a large two-dimensional gel of the type described by de Wachter and Fiers (1972) and run in both dimensions as described by Holland et al (1979). The oligonucleotides are excised from the gel together with background gel slices and quantified by Cerenkov counting. (It should be noted that the error nucleotide will run as a laterally diffused broad band rather than single well-defined spot. This is a consequence of the presence of different base substitutions at the selected site and at adjacent sites.) The relative amount of ^{32}P in the error versus the consensus RNA gives an approximate value for the error frequency.

7. The error frequency has to be adjusted to take account of the proportion of guanine residues which escaped digestion. This can be achieved as follows. After quantitation, the error RNA is isolated from the gel slice and 3'-end labeled by ligation to 5'[^{32}P]Cp. The end-labeled error nucleotides are then gel-purified and sequenced by the direct chemical method of Peattie (1979). An aliquot should be redigested with RNase T$_1$ by the foregoing procedure to estimate the quantity of undigested guanine residues. The value obtained is used to correct the error frequency estimate.

Critical points

The initial virus inoculum should be rigorously plaque purified to obtain a homogeneous stock by repeated (at least three) cycles of re-isolation from single plaques.

All scintillation vials and microcentrifuge tubes used for sample counting should be precounted. Gel slices for counting should be of equal size and samples should be counted for a minimum of 50 min to ensure a random error of less than 10% for background samples and 5% for error RNA.

Isolation of conditional lethal mutants

Temperature-sensitive mutants

Temperature-sensitive (*ts*) mutants have proven their value in the analysis of gene function in virtually all groups of vertebrate viruses. The method described here is applicable to both DNA and RNA viruses and has been used successfully by one of us (C.R.P.) for isolation of temperature-sensitive mutants of pseudo-rabies virus, foot-and-mouth disease virus, VSV, Chandipura virus, respiratory syncytial (RS) virus, and several bunyaviruses. The advantage is that a single easily measured phenotype can be used for isolation of mutations in any essential gene function. This version of the method describes isolation of *ts* mutants of RS virus and is adapted from Pringle (1985).

Procedure

1. Choose appropriate permissive and restrictive temperatures. As a guide, the restrictive temperature should be the highest temperature at which plaque formation occurs without appreciable ($< 1 \log_{10}$ unit) diminution of plaque count relative to the permissive temperature. For most viruses restrictive temperatures are in the range 37–42°C and permissive temperatures in the range 31–33°C.

2. Produce a genetically homogeneous wild type stock of virus by repeated cycles of isolation and amplification of virus from monolayers with single plaques. (With certain paramyxoviruses up to ten cycles may be required, but for most viruses three cycles will suffice.) This should be carried out at the restrictive temperature; 39°C for RS virus. The next step depends on the type of mutagen employed. A list of the mutagens used successfully in animal virology is given in Table 11.1. In the case of deaminating and alkylating agents, proceed to (3a), (4a) and (5a). In the case of base analogue and intercalating mutagens proceed to (3b), (4b) and (5b).

3a. Expose aliquots of the cloned wild type virus to the mutagen as indicated in Table 11.1: i.e. 1.0 M $NaNO_2$ in 0.25 M Na acetate (pH 4.8); or 1.0 M H_3NO in 0.05 M Na phosphate buffer (pH 7.5); or 0.025% ethyl methane sulphonate (EMS) in 0.25 M Na acetate; or 1 mg ml^{-1} *N*-methyl-*N*-nitro-*N*-nitrosoguanidine (NTG) in phosphate buffered saline (pH 7.6). NTG is also an effective mutagen when incorporated into the culture fluid at 10-fold lower concentration; in this case steps (3b)–(5b) should be followed.

4a. Incubate at 4°C for varying periods and terminate reactions by dilution and rapid dialysis against the culture incubation medium.

5a. The virus yields at each time point should be determined by titration on monolayers of susceptible cells at the permissive temperature. Inactivation curves should then be plotted and samples from the linear portion of the curve should be used for mutant isolation.

3b. Inoculate monolayers of susceptible cells (BS-C-1 cells by preference for RS virus) in 50 mm Petri dishes or 30 ml screw-capped flasks with the cloned stock of wild type virus. Adsorb at the restrictive temperature for 1 h. The multiplicity of infection should be low; 0.01 pfu cell^{-1} for RS virus.

4b. Wash off the inoculum with three washes of serum-free culture medium and add 3 ml of medium containing 2% serum, antibiotics and an appropriate base analogue mutagen. (The medium for RS virus by preference would be the Glasgow version of Eagle's medium supplemented with 2% foetal calf serum, glutamine and antibiotics. Experience has shown that the composition of the culture medium and washing fluids is generally not a critical factor.) Base analogue and intercalating mutagens suitable for DNA viruses, RNA viruses and retroviruses are listed in Table 11.1. Choose 5-bromodeoxyuridine for DNA viruses and 5-fluorouracil for RNA viruses, or either of these for retroviruses, in the first instance, since they are known to be effective mutagens for most viruses at non-cytotoxic concentrations. A range of concentrations of mutagen should be chosen to determine the highest concentration of mutagen that can be tolerated by the host cell without loss of viability. (The optimal mutagen concentration within the ranges given in Table 11.1 has to be determined empirically because host cell sensitivity may vary).

5b. Incubate cultures at permissive temperature until viral cytopathic effect becomes visible in control unmutagenized cultures. Harvest the culture fluids, clarify by low speed centrifugation, and reduce the concentration of the mutagen by rapid dialysis for 2 h at 4°C. In the case of highly cell-associated viruses, the infected cells should be harvested into a small volume of culture fluid and lysed by two cycles of freezing to −70°C and rapid thawing, or by sonication.

6. Plate out dilutions of the mutagen-exposed samples on replicate monolayers of susceptible cells such that the majority of plates will contain one or a few plaques. Six-well cluster plates are best for this purpose. Incubate under agar or agarose-solidified nutrient medium with 2% foetal calf serum and antibiotics until well defined plaques are visible. The plaques can be visualized by staining with neutral red stain applied in a thin second agar- or agarose-containing overlay. Diffusion will require 2–4 h and the cultures should be kept in the dark to limit the photodynamic activity of neutral red.

7. Pick plaques using sterile Pasteur pipettes, removing an agar plug over the plaque and transferring it to an uninfected culture in a screw-capped flask. Plaques should only be taken from low-count or single-plaque plates as this will avoid the need to reclone plaque isolates before the next stage.

8. Screening for temperature sensitivity is carried out by inoculating duplicate series of wells in pairs of 96- or 24-well blocks, followed by incubation of one block at the permissive temperature and the other at the restrictive temperature. Alternatively, screening can be carried out by stabbing isolates onto corresponding sectors of agar-overlaid uninfected cells in 50 mm Petri dishes. After adsorption, a top layer of agar is applied to seal the plates and incubation at permissive or restrictive temperature is begun. Presumptive *ts* mutants are propagated by recovering virus from the wells or sectored plates incubated at the permissive temperature.

9. Stocks of presumptive *ts* mutants should only be established after at least two cycles of reisolation of virus from single plaques, followed by confirmation of the *ts* phenotype by differential plaque counting at permissive and restrictive temperatures. Generally a difference of $\geq 4 \log_{10}$ units in plaque count at the two temperatures is adequate. Differences of $2 \log_{10}$ units are useable, however, and indeed may be the maximum difference obtainable depending on the nature of the gene product (Pringle 1987).

Isolation of cold-sensitive mutants

Cold-sensitive (*cs*) mutants are the reciprocal of *ts* mutants. This phenotype tends to involve proteins that are incorporated into macromolecular structures in a temperature-dependent manner. Consequently the isolation of *cs* mutants can increase the spectrum of mutants obtainable. The procedure for isolation of *cs* mutants is the same as that for isolation of *ts* mutants, except that the restrictive temperature is the lower temperature and the permissive temperature is the higher temperature.

Isolation of temperature-dependent host range (tdCE) and non-temperature dependent host range (hrCE) mutants

Mutants with a conditionally temperature dependent phenotype (tdCE) have been described for both VSV and influenza virus. The VSV tdCE mutants multiplied at 31°C and 39°C in BHK-21 cells, but only at 31°C in secondary chick embryo cells. The tdCE mutants appeared to be present at higher frequency than *ts* mutants in stocks of 5-fluorouracil-mutagenized virus (Pringle 1978). The available evidence suggests that this phenotype is determined by the interaction of specific host factors with the viral polymerase (Szilyagi and Pringle 1975). Such mutants may have particular value in the study of virus–host interactions; e.g. the differentiation of pluripotent embryonal carcinoma cells to embryoid bodies was accompanied by a decrease in the restrictiveness of these cells for tdCE virus multiplication (Pringle 1978). Non-temperature dependent host range mutants (hrCE) were present at much lower frequency.

Procedure

(1) to (7) as for *ts* mutants.
8. tdCE mutants can be screened by plating mutagenized virus onto mixed culture monolayers seeded with BHK-21 and secondary CE cells in the proportions 3:1; 1:1 and 1:3 respectively. After adsorption and incubation at 31°C, hazy and small diameter plaques should be picked preferentially in order to enhance the recovery of host range mutants. Plaque isolates obtained in this way can be screened on replicate BHK-21 and CE monolayers at 31°C and 39°C to reveal simultaneously the presence of tdCE, hrCE and *ts* mutants. Presumptive mutants should be reisolated from plates with solitary plaques before further propagation.

Comments

This method depends on the existence of good facilities for cell culture since it requires the simultaneous availability of cell lines and secondary embryo cultures. However it is highly productive because mutants of different conditional phenotypes (*ts*, tdCE and hrCE) and non-conditional phenotypes (hr) can be isolated from a single mutagen treatment.

Monocultures of BHK-21 and CE cells can substitute for the mixed culture selection system described above. This option is more demanding in terms of space and effort, but the frequency of isolation of mutants of the different phenotypes is unlikely to be very different from that obtained by the mixed culture approach.

The spontaneous mutation frequency may be high enough in RNA-containing viruses to obviate the need for mutagenesis.

Isolation of suppressor-sensitive (amber) mutants

This approach has had little application in animal virology owing to the lack of cell lines expressing tRNA molecules able to suppress nonsense codons. However, in recent years a few cell lines have been engineered to express nonsense suppressor tRNA. Proven methods of isolating amber mutants will only be described in outline here as they depend on the use of non-standard cell lines. The L39 su⁺ cell line stably expresses a tyrosine-inserting tRNA giving a 4% suppression of nonsense (amber) mutations. These cells and the parental su⁻ LMTK⁻ cell line have been used successfully for isolation of amber mutants of VSV (White and McGeoch 1987). Sevidy et al (1987) have described an inducible suppressor system which has potentially greater discriminatory power. A human amber suppressor tRNA gene linked to the SV40 origin of replication and a second DNA with a *ts* SV40 large T antigen were cotransfected into monkey cells to obtain stably integrated cell lines (BSC-40*sup*D). In cell line BSC-40*sup*D12, transfer from restrictive to permissive temperature was accompanied by expression of a serine-expressing suppressor tRNA giving 50–70% suppression. A poliovirus amber mutant could be propagated efficiently in these cells at the permissive temperature.

Procedure

1. A mutagenized stock of virus is produced by growth in L39 su⁺ cells (or in induced su⁺ cells at their permissive temperature) in the presence of a base analogue or alkylating mutagen.
2. The mutagenized virus is then plated out at limiting dilution in monolayer cultures of L39 su⁺ cells (or induced su⁺ cells at their permissive temperature) under agar- or agarose-containing overlay, and incubated long enough to obtain large well defined plaques on control plates inoculated with unmutagenized virus.
3. Well isolated small or hazy plaques (or any plaques in the induced BSC40*sup*D12 cells) should then be picked and screened directly by inoculation into cultures of L39 su⁺ and LMTK⁻ su⁻ cells (or of cultures of BSC-40*sup*D at permissive and restrictive temperature). Screening of these plaques may reveal the presence of partially suppressible amber mutants.
4. Isolates which multiply in su⁺ cultures and fail to multiply in su⁻ cultures should be propagated in su⁺ cells for recloning and verification of phenotype by differential plaque counting on su⁺ and su⁻ cell monolayers. In practice, isolates showing 30-fold or greater differences in plaque count proved to be genuine amber mutants in the case of VSV mutagenized in L39 su⁺ cells.

Isolation of mutants with specific phenotypes

The procedure for mutagenesis and plaque isolation are similar to those described for *ts* mutants, on page 236, steps (1)–(5a) and (1)–(5b). The differences are in the screening, identification and verification of mutants. Some specific examples are listed below.

Monoclonal antibody escape mutants

Usually the mutagenesis steps (*ts* mutants, 1–5) are omitted and spontaneous mutants are selected.

6. Selection is carried out by incubating

a small volume of high titre virus with an equal volume of hybridoma fluid at 37°C for 60 min. Susceptible cells are infected and incubated until cytopathic effect is observed in control unneutralized cultures. If no cytopathic effect is observed in the neutralized virus cultures, consecutive cycles of infection in the presence of the selecting antibody are continued until resistant virus appears. Alternatively, if escape mutants are present at high frequency, virus can be isolated directly from surviving plaques on monolayers overlaid with an agar overlay containing the selecting monoclonal antibody.

7. Cloning by propagation of virus from individual plaques is carried out in the normal manner (page 237).

Isolation of drug resistant mutants

Mutants which are resistant (independent) or in some instances dependent on a particular anti-viral drug can be obtained by direct plating of mutagenized or untreated wild type virus under solid agar containing a range of non-cytotoxic, inhibitory concentrations of the drug in question. Resistant (or drug dependent) virus can be obtained by isolating and cloning virus from surviving plaques in susceptible cell cultures in the presence of the selecting drug. Resistant mutants can be distinguished from drug dependent mutants by differential plaque counting in the presence and absence of the anti-viral drug.

Alternatively, if the frequency of resistant mutants is low, the wild type virus should be propagated in the presence of progressively increasing sub-inhibitory concentrations of the drug until good growth is obtained. After cloning in the presence of the drug, resistant and dependent mutants can be discriminated by differential plaque counting. This second procedure is less desirable than the first as the resistant virus obtained may be genetically more complex than the resistant virus obtained by the first method.

Other specialized methods

More specialized methods which cannot be dealt with here include the isolation of the interference-resistant (Sdi⁻) mutants of VSV (Horodyski et al 1983); the specific protease-activation (pa) mutants of Sendai virus (Scheid and Choppin, 1976); the noncytopathic (nc) mutants of Newcastle disease virus (Madansky and Bratt, 1978); the thymidine kinase (Tk) mutants of vaccinia virus and the deoxypyrimidine kinase mutants of herpes simplex virus (Jamieson et al 1974); and many others.

General comments

The isolation and characterization of revertants should be an integral part of any experiment involving mutants obtained by the methods of random mutagenesis described here.

Dohmen et al (1994) have described a method of inducing *ts* mutations in specific genes of yeast, which may become applicable in animal virology. Their technique would overcome the limitations of the random mutagenesis approach of classical genetic analysis.

Construction of virus mutants by directed mutagenesis

The possibility of designing and constructing an animal virus mutant carrying a specific pre-determined genetic change is presently avail-able only for certain virus types. These viruses are, in general, those whose naked genetic material is infectious and they include viruses with either single- (parvovirus) or double-stranded (polyoma, adeno, herpes and pox viruses) DNA genomes and those with posi-tive sense single-stranded RNA genomes (picornaviruses and retroviruses). The lack of suitable tissue culture systems presently pre-vents the application of these techniques to the papilloma and hepadna viruses. Tech-niques for directed mutagenesis in negative sense RNA viruses are only just emerging and it is not yet possible to generalize them.

The methodology for the construction of virus mutants is similar for each of these virus systems. However, there is a distinction between those viruses where the genome is short enough to be cloned (as cDNA if neces-sary) and handled as a single entity (parvo, polyoma, picorna, retroviruses) and those where manipulations must be performed with a genome fragment which is then rebuilt into a complete genome (adeno, herpes, pox viruses), normally by homologous recombina-tion *in vivo*. A general method for the isolation of viral mutants by a directed approach is set out below. There are a number of alternatives at various points and these are described as fully as possible. This method should be read in conjunction with the relevant basic molecu-lar biology protocols (see e.g. Sambrook et al 1989), since these have not been reiterated here in full detail.

Isolation and cloning of viral genomic material

The approach to genome isolation and cloning for each of the virus families under considera-tion is listed in Table 11.2. Viral nucleic acid may be isolated either from infected cultured cells or from purified virions. A key point is the structure of the ends of the genome (if linear) since these will require special steps to permit their cloning. Large genomes must be frag-mented with an appropriate restriction enzyme and cloned as a library of fragments. RNA genomes must be converted to cDNA for cloning. This can be achieved for picorna-viruses by reverse transcription of infected cell RNA primed with oligo dT; for retro-viruses, it is more convenient to clone the appropriate fragment of infected cell genomic DNA containing the viral genome in its inte-grated proviral form.

Directed mutagenesis of cloned genetic material

Once cloned as DNA, viral genetic material is amenable to the full range of directed muta-genesis techniques that have been described. These can be divided into methods where existing restriction sites in the DNA are exploited to alter the sequence in a planned way and methods where a synthetic oligonu-cleotide, largely homologous to a segment of the clone but having one or more planned mismatches with the sequence, is used to direct the alteration of the DNA sequence

Table 11.2. Strategies for the directed mutagenesis of viruses.

Virus type	Genome type	Source material	Cloning
Parvovirus	Linear ssDNA (both strands present in particle populations).	Infected cell DNA.	GC tail vector and genome ends, hybridize and ligate; or use synthetic linkers.
Polyomavirus	Circular dsDNA.	Infected cell Hirt supernatant (Hirt 1967).	Linearize naked DNA by restriction and ligate to vector.
Adenovirus	Linear dsDNA.	Purified virions.	Restrict, and ligate fragments to vector; genome ends need deproteination before cloning (Rekosh 1981).
Herpes virus	Linear dsDNA (circular form in infected cells).	Purified virions or infected cell DNA.	Restrict, and ligate fragments to vector; ends can be cloned as a junction fragment from infected cell DNA.
Pox virus	Linear dsDNA.	Purified virions.	Restrict, and ligate fragments to vector; genome ends are covalently closed and must be opened with S1 nuclease and repaired before cloning.
Picornavirus	Linear (+) ssRNA.	Infected cell RNA.	Standard cDNA cloning.
Retrovirus	Linear (+) ssRNA.	Infected cell genomic DNA.	Identify fragment for cloning by Southern analysis and screen appropriate genomic library.

during *in vitro* DNA synthesis. Procedures of the latter type, being more general in their potential application, have largely displaced other methods. Methods utilizing a mismatched oligonucleotide can be further subdivided into procedures which exploit repair synthesis on a primed single-stranded DNA template and PCR-based procedures. The method described in detail here employs this latter approach.

There are many published PCR protocols for directed mutagenesis. The one detailed here was described by Ito et al (1991) and has been applied successfully by one of us in the mutagenesis of adenovirus (L. Miersman and K. Leppard, unpublished); it offers the advantage that a series of mutations across an amplifiable region can be constructed for an initial outlay of three primers plus one further primer for each mutation desired. The amplification scheme is represented in Fig. 11.1 and described in detail below.

Design of PCR primers

The hybridization sites for the PCR primers should be positioned on the target DNA according to Fig. 11.1. Primers A and B flank the target region for mutagenesis. Primer M is designed to eliminate an existing restriction site, **m**, at one end of the target region; the method also requires a second restriction site, **n**, at the other end of the target region. These sites define the sequence within which mutagenesis can be achieved. Primer X is designed specifically to generate the desired mutation in the target region. Primers A and B need only be 20–25 nucleotides in length; primers M and X should be approximately 30 nucleotides long and should have the mismatched nucleotide(s) at their centre. Ideally, all primers should be of 40–60%

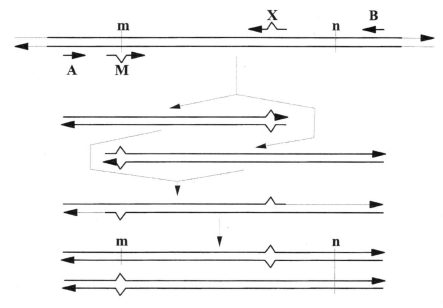

Figure 11.1. A flow diagram of the products of the two-step PCR protocol for DNA mutagenesis of Ito et al (1991) is shown below a diagram of the target DNA for mutagenesis. A, B, M and X are oligonucleotide primers with homology to the target DNA at the positions indicated. m and n are sites for restriction enzyme cleavage. All DNA strands are shown with arrow heads indicating their 3′ ends.

GC content and should have either G or C at their 3′ end. Selected primer sequences should be checked for chance alternative homologies to the target DNA prior to synthesis. Computer programs (e.g. Primer Design, Scientific and Educational Software, State Line, PA, U.S.A., for PC Windows, or OSP, free on anonymous ftp, for UNIX) are available which can aid PCR primer choice. A number of commercial organizations offer rapid delivery of synthetic oligonucleotides to order if 'in-house' synthesis facilities are not available.

First stage amplification

Two reactions are required. Each should be set up as follows:
  200 ng target DNA
  200 ng primer A (primer B)
  200 ng primer X (primer M)
  0.1 mM each dNTP
  1× Taq polymerase buffer (use the stock supplied by the enzyme supplier)

2.5 mM $MgCl_2$ (if not included in stock buffer)
  2–4 units Taq polymerase
  to 25 µl final volume with sterile distilled H_2O,
overlayed with paraffin oil and incubated through 20 cycles of denaturation, annealing and extension (94°, 1 min; 55°, 1 min; 74°, 3 min; extension time increased to 7 min for the final cycle). The quality of the reactions should then be assessed by analyzing 2.5 µl of the reaction mix on a flat-bed agarose gel alongside appropriate DNA markers.

Second stage amplification

The reaction should be set up as follows:
  2.5 µl first stage reaction 1 (primers A plus X)
  2.5 µl first stage reaction 2 (primers B plus M)
  200 ng primer A
  200 ng primer B
  to 12.5 µl with sterile distilled H_2O

and denatured at 85° for 2 min and allowed to cool to room temperature. The mix should then be further supplemented as follows:

0.1 mM each dNTP

1× *Taq* polymerase buffer

2.5 mM $MgCl_2$ (if not included in stock buffer)

2–4 units *Taq* polymerase

to 25 µl final volume with sterile distilled H_2O

overlayed with paraffin oil and incubated through 20 cycles of denaturation, annealing and extension (94°, 1 min; 55°, 1 min; 74°, 3 min; extension time increased to 7 min for the final cycle). The quality of the reactions should then be assessed by analyzing 1–2 µl of the reaction mix on a flat-bed agarose gel alongside appropriate DNA markers.

Selective cloning of mutated amplified product

Recover the amplified DNA from the reaction mix by extraction with phenol:chloroform and ethanol precipitation. Digest the product with restriction enzyme(s) cutting at sites **m** and **n** and purify DNA of length expected for cleavage at these sites by agarose gel electrophoresis. Only amplified product mutated at site X should retain restriction site **m**. Ligate the recovered fragment to an appropriately cut plasmid or M13 vector and recover clones. In theory, all of the clones should be mutated at the desired site; in practice, screening of 6 clones by DNA sequencing should permit the identification of the desired mutant.

Comment

If only a single, defined mutation in a sequence is required, it may be more convenient to use a variation of the above procedure in which primers M and X overlap in the region of the mutation, and each carries the desired mutant sequence (or its homologue). Cleavage of the second stage PCR product at sites **m** and **n** should produce a homogeneous, mutated DNA fragment. Note that this procedure is also generally applicable, but requires two specific oligonucleotides for each mutation to be generated.

Plasmid reconstruction

In order to permit mutant virus reconstruction, it is necessary to transfer the mutated fragment into the appropriate viral genomic clone or subclone. Careful choice of the sites **m** and **n** (page 242) will facilitate this process. Ideally, sites **m** and **n** will be unique in the viral genomic clone into which the mutation is to be moved. Failing this, the sites should be chosen to minimize the number of reconstruction steps required. In the simplest case, the genomic clone is digested with enzyme(s) **m** and **n** and the fragment produced is replaced with the mutated fragment produced above, to create the mutated cloned fragment for virus reconstruction. The sequence of the clone at the mutation site should be re-validated before proceeding further.

Rescue of virus from mutated cloned genetic material

If mutagenesis is being performed to define the function of a virus gene product, it is possible that the rescue will fail because of a lethal phenotype. The rescue of a mutation into virus particles demands either that the mutation is non-lethal or that the function affected can be provided *in trans*, either from a helper virus or from a helper cell line which expresses the relevant viral function(s) and in which both virus reconstruction and growth must be performed. Various helper cell lines that have been described are listed in Table 11.3.

Table 11.3. Cell lines which complement specific viral gene defects.

Cell line	Description	Reference
Cos1, Cos7	from monkey CV1 cells; express SV40 T antigens	Gluzman 1981
Cop5	from mouse C127 cells; express polyoma T antigens	Tyndall et al 1981
293	from human embryo kidney cells; express adenovirus 5 E1a and E1b functions	Graham et al 1977
KB8, 16, 18	from human KB cells; express adenovirus 2 E1a, E1a and E1b, or E1b functions respectively	Babiss et al 1983
gmDBP1, 2, 3, 4	from Hela cells; express adenovirus 5 E2a DNA binding protein	Klessig et al 1984
W162	from Vero cells; express adenovirus 5 E4 functions	Weinberg and Ketner 1983
ψ-2	from NIH3T3 cells; express Moloney MuLV structural proteins	Mann et al 1983
ψ-AM	as ψ-2 but expressing amphotropic envelope proteins	Cone and Mulligan 1984
D6	from Vero cells; express HSV 1 gB	Cai et al 1987
L3153$_{28}$	from Ltk$^-$ cells; express HSV 1 gC	Arsenakis et al 1986
L65, Z4, 2–6	from BHKtk$^-$, Ltk$^-$aprt$^-$, Vero cells respectively; express HSV 1 ICP4 (IE175)	Davidson and Stow; Persson et al 1985; DeLuca et al 1985
C34	from 293 cells (above); express adenovirus capsid protein IX	Caravokyri & Leppard, 1995

Direct rescue (parvo, polyoma, picorna, retroviruses)

For each of these viruses, infectious progeny can be generated by transfecting cloned genomic material into appropriate cells. The transfected material must either have the same overall form as true viral genomic material or be capable of giving rise to that form *in vivo*. For the parvovirus, AAV, and for retroviruses, infectious progeny will result from transfection of complete genome plasmid clones without further manipulation (Hager et al 1979; Samulski et al 1982); for retroviruses, continuously producing cell lines can be isolated. Picornaviruses can be rescued by transfection of cloned plasmid DNA (Racaniello and Baltimore, 1981) but the process is much more efficient if RNA is expressed *in vitro* from the clone and this material is then introduced into cells by electroporation (van der Werf et al 1986). For polyomaviruses, the cloned genome must be excised from the plasmid and recircularized by ligation before transfection.

Any of the established protocols for DNA transfection may be used in these procedures. The most widely used method is calcium phosphate-mediated transfection (Graham and van der Eb 1973).

1. Prepare the following transfection mixes:
   (a) 10 µg cloned viral DNA
       10 µg salmon sperm DNA
       250 mM CaCl$_2$
       in 0.5 ml
   (b) 275 mM NaCl
       10 mM KCl
       10 mM glucose
       50 mM hepes, pH 7.08
       1.4 mM Na$_2$HPO$_4$
       in 0.5 ml

   Add mix (a) slowly to (b) over approx. 1 min, then mix by gently blowing air bubbles through the solution for a further 60 s. Leave at room temperature for 30 min. (Note that the components of these mixes must be sterile; DNA for transfection should be purified by phenol:chloroform extraction and ethanol precipitation under aseptic conditions and redissolved in sterile H_2O before use.)

2. Re-feed a monolayer culture of approx. 5×10^6 cells at 50% confluence (for direct plaque isolation, 90–100% confluence) with fresh growth medium 3 h prior to transfection. (Transfection efficiency is maximized if the cells are growing rapidly.)

3. Add the DNA precipitate to the culture and incubate under the appropriate growth conditions for the cells for 4 h. (The transfection efficiency may sometimes be enhanced if the volume of growth medium is reduced prior to adding the DNA precipitate. In this case, care must be taken to ensure that the monolayer remains moist throughout the incubation by rocking the culture dish at intervals.)

4. Remove the medium and precipitate, and shock the cells with a solution of 20% glycerol in isotonic buffer (prewarmed to normal growth temperature) for 1 min. Remove the glycerol solution and wash the monolayer twice with isotonic buffer; it is important that the glycerol is rapidly and completely removed from the cells. Return the cells to normal growth medium (for viruses which are able to give plaques on the chosen cell line, this growth medium may be substituted by a suitable nutrient semi-solid overlay under which discrete plaques can form).

5. Incubate the culture until either cytopathic effect or plaques are seen (for continuously producing retroviral lines, harvest the culture medium at intervals) and then harvest the culture, or discrete plaques.

Rescue by recombination (adeno, herpes, pox viruses)

For viruses with larger genomes, the general principle for reconstruction is to achieve recombination *in vivo* between the cloned mutated sequence and viral genomic material. This can be done by providing a sufficient length of viral sequence in the cloned fragment, flanking the mutated site on both sides, and introducing this DNA into permissive cells, either with viral genomic DNA or fragments thereof (adeno, herpes), or in the presence of wild-type virus (pox). Unless some selection against the wild-type is available (e.g. select against tk^+ in construction of mutants in the *tk* gene of vaccinia), only a small proportion of the virus from such cultures is likely to be recombinant and so carry the mutation.

For adenovirus, the genome is of a manageable size such that its infectivity can be destroyed by digestion with a single-cutting restriction enzyme. This means that the problem of high non-recombinant background mentioned above can be largely eliminated in this system. Enzyme(s) is/are chosen so that the fragment(s) resulting overlap(s) with the cloned mutated fragment. Only by homologous recombination between these fragments can intact, potentially infectious, genomes result. When such a DNA mixture is transfected, a high proportion of the resulting plaques contain mutated virus. An example of this strategy, suitable for isolating viral mutants in the left 10% of the adenovirus genome is shown in Fig. 11.2.

Alternatively, fragments are chosen so that a complete genome can be precisely reconstituted by 3-fragment ligation *in vitro*. Unless the wild-type genome fragment equivalent to the cloned mutated fragment is removed by appropriate size-based purification techniques, it is crucial to treat the mixture of genomic fragments with alkaline phosphatase prior to adding the cloned mutated fragment to the ligation mixture.

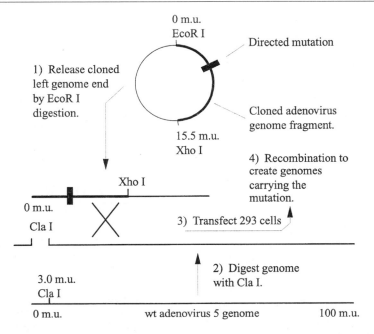

Figure 11.2. Representation of the reconstruction strategy for adenovirus type 5 mutations within the left 10–15% of the genome. Related strategies are available to introduce mutations into other parts of the genome. The cloned adenovirus fragment is shown as a heavy line and the position of the targeted mutation introduced into this DNA by *in vitro* manipulation is indicated by a filled box. The sequence of steps required to reconstruct virus from this DNA is indicated by numbers 1–4.

1. Select an appropriate reconstruction strategy and prepare the necessary adenovirus genomic DNA fragment(s). (For herpes use intact wt viral DNA for co-transfection; for pox virus, superinfect with wt virus.)
2. Perform transfection procedure as described for direct rescue, p 245, using a mixture of DNA fragments (or ligated DNA) to a total mass of 10–20 μg. The ratio of fragments is important to the final outcome; the cloned, mutated fragment should generally be in a 2–3× molar excess over the wt DNA or DNA fragment(s) in the mix (or in the ligation).
3. Incubate the culture until either cytopathic effect or plaques are seen and then harvest the culture, or discrete plaques. If a bulk lysate is obtained, this must next be used to generate an array of discrete plaques for further analysis.

Comment

Customarily, 293 cells (Table 11.3) are used for transfections in the reconstruction of adenovirus 2 or 5 mutants and for plaque assays, unless the specific complementing ability of another cell type is required, since they have a high plaquing efficiency. 293 cell monolayers are fragile, especially during glycerol shock and subsequent application of the agar overlay. Great care is needed during these procedures to avoid major disruption of the monolayer. For direct isolation of recombinant adenovirus plaques on monolayers of 293 cells, transfection efficiency is increased by maintaining cultures in medium containing 10% newborn calf serum and transferring to medium containing 10% fetal calf serum at the re-feeding which precedes transfection.

Validation and purification of isolated mutant virus

Viruses reconstructed from infectious cloned mutated genetic material

The principal origin of contaminants in such mutant virus stocks is recombination between the input nucleic acid or, subsequently, virus and endogenous sequences in the helper cells. Either individual plaques should be screened and selected mutant plaques grown on (see below) or, if this is not possible, the genomic nucleic acid of the mutant virus stock must be monitored on an ongoing basis to ensure retention of the desired mutation and absence of unexpected features that might indicate the evolution of variants in the culture.

Viruses reconstructed by ligation or recombination

The above procedures (page 247) will generally produce a background of non-recombinant virus against which the desired mutant must be identified. Either directly, or following ampli-fication of the virus stock, the viral genome content of individual plaques must be analyzed for the presence of the desired mutation.

1a. If the frequency of mutants is expected to be high, this can be done either by applying traditional molecular techniques (restriction analysis, sequencing) to purified viral genomic material or to the products of PCR amplification, or by PCR-based assays wherein the production of an amplified band of a defined size is diagnostic of the presence of the expected mutation.

1b. If the frequency is likely to be low, other techniques more suited to the throughput of large numbers of isolates may be appropriate (hybridization screening of infected cell nucleic acid; phenotypic screening – growth on non-complementing vs. complementing cells).

2. Once a mutant plaque has been isolated, the virus must be further plaque-purified twice more to ensure homogeneity.

Chapter 11

References

Arsenakis M, Tomasi LF, Speziali V, Roizman B, Campadelli-Fiume G (1986) J Virol 58: 367–376.

Babiss LE, Young CSH, Fisher PB, Ginsberg HS (1983) J Virol 46: 454–465.

Bader JP, Brown NR (1971) Nature New Biol 234: 11–12.

Brown SM, Ritchie DA, Subak-Sharpe JH (1973) J Gen Virol 18: 329–346.

Cai W, Person S, Warner SC, Zhou J, DeLuca N (1987) J Virol 61: 714–721.

Caravokyri C, Leppard KN (1995) J Virol 69: 6627–6633.

Cone RD, Mulligan RC (1984) Proc Natl Acad Sci USA 81: 6349–6353.

Davidson I, Stow ND (1985) Virology 141: 77–88.

DeLuca NA, McCarthy AM, Schaffer PA (1985) J Virol 56: 558–570.

DeWachter R, Fiers W (1972) Anal Biochem 49: 184–197.

Dohmen RJ, Wu P, Varshavsky A (1994) Science 263: 1273–1276.

Fields BN (1981) Curr Top Microbiol Immunol 91: 1–24.

Gharpure MA, Wright PF, Chanock RM (1969) J Virol 3: 414–421.

Gluzman Y (1981) Cell 23: 175–182.

Graham FL, Smiley J, Russell WC, Nairn R (1977) J Gen Virol 36: 59–72.

Graham FL, Van der Eb AJ (1973) Virology 52: 456–467.

Hager GL, Chang EH, Chan HW, Garon CF, Israel MA, Martin MA, Scolnick EM, Lowy DR (1979) J Virol 31: 795–809.

Hall JD, Coen DM, Fisher BL, Weisslitz M, Randall S, Almy RE, Gelep PT, Schaffer PA (1984) Virology 132: 26–37.

Hirt B (1967) J Mol Biol 26: 365–369.

Holland JJ (1993) In Emerging viruses SS Morse (Ed.) Oxford University Press, New York and Oxford, pp. 203–218.

Holland JJ, Grabau EA, Jones CL, Semler BL (1979) Cell 16: 494–504.

Holland JJ, Domingo E, de la Torre JC, Steinhauer DA (1990) J Virol 64: 3960–3962.

Horodyski FM, Nichol ST, Spindler KR, Holland JJ (1983) Cell 33: 801–810.

Ito W, Ishiguro H, Kurosawa Y (1991) Gene 102: 67–70.

Jamieson AT, Gentry GA, Subak-Sharpe (1974) J Gen Virol 24: 465–480.

Klessig DF, Brough DE, Cleghon V (1984) Mol Cell Biol 4: 1354–1362

McKay E, Higgins P, Tyrrell D, Pringle CR (1988) J Med Virol 25: 411–421.

Madansky CH, Bratt M (1978) J Virol 26: 724–729.

Mann R, Mulligan RC, Baltimore RD (1983) Cell 33: 153–159.

Parvin JD, Moscona A, Pan WT, Leider JM, Palese P (1986) J Virol 59: 377–383.

Peattie DA (1979) Proc Natl Acad Sci USA 76: 1760–1764.

Persson RH, Bacchetti S, Smiley JR (1985) J Virol 54: 414–421.

Pringle CR (1970) J Virol 5: 559–567.

Pringle CR (1975) Curr Top Microbiol Immunol 69: 85–116.

Pringle CR (1978) Cell 15: 597–606.

Pringle CR (1985) In Virology: a practical approach BWJ Mahy (Ed.) IRL Press, Oxford, pp. 95–118.

Pringle CR (1987) In The Rhabdoviruses RR Wagner (Ed.) Plenum Press, New York and London, pp. 167–244.

Racaniello VR, Baltimore D (1981) Science 214: 916–919.

Rekosh D (1981) J Virol 40: 329–333.

Rettenmier CW, Dumont R, Baltimore D (1975) J Virol 15: 41–49.

Sambrook J, Fritsch EF, Maniatis T (1989) Molecular Cloning: A Laboratory Manual, 2nd ed. CSH Laboratory, Cold Spring Harbor.

Samulski RJ, Berns KI, Tan M, Muzyczka N (1982) Proc Natl Acad Sci USA 79: 2077–2081.

Scheid A, Choppin PW (1976) Virology 69: 265–277.

Sevidy JM, Capone JP, RajBhandary UL, Sharp PA (1987) Cell 50: 379–389.

Smith DB, Inglis SC (1987) J Gen Virol 68: 2729–2740.

Steinhauer DA, Holland JJ (1986) J Virol 57: 219–228.

Steinhauer DA, de la Torre JC, Holland JJ (1989) J Virol 63: 2063–2071.

Szilagyi JF, Pringle CR (1975) J Virol 16: 927–936.

Tyndall C, LaMantia G, Thacker CM, Favaloro J, Kamen R (1981) Nucl Acids Res 9: 6231–6250.

van der Werf S, Bradley J, Wimmer E, Studier FW, Dunn JJ (1986) Proc Natl Acad Sci USA 83: 2330–2334.

Weinberg DH, Ketner G (1983) Proc Natl Acad Sci USA 80: 5383–5386.

White BT, McGeoch DJ (1987) J Gen Virol 68: 3033–3044.

Williams JF, Gharpure M, Ustacelebi S, Armstrong JA (1971) J Gen Virol 11: 95–102.

Wyke JA (1973) Virology 52: 587–590. .

References

Polypeptides

12

D. R. Harper
B. F. Coles

Proteins are the structural and effector components of a virus, and the characterization of viral proteins is a necessary step in studying viruses. It is often necessary to remove contaminating proteins prior to such study. This chapter presents information on methods used to purify and characterize viral proteins.

It should be noted that many of the chemicals used are hazardous, for example monomeric acrylamide which is a potent neurotoxin. All chemicals should be used in accordance with approved safety procedures at all times.

Virology Methods Manual
ISBN 0–12–465330–8

Purification and characterization of viral proteins

Numerous methods exist to remove contaminating proteins and to enrich the protein of choice. These are summarized below.

Chromatography

Analytical and preparative chromatography use a range of matrices and solvent systems to separate proteins by different properties. The large number of separation criteria that can be used (size, charge, hydrophobicity, binding properties) make chromatography a very flexible approach to the separation of biomolecules. In a typical application, beads of a solid matrix (sepharose, agarose, etc.) are swollen in a solvent and poured into a columnar container. After equilibration with the solvent to be used, the sample is applied and solvent flows through the column either by gravity flow or under pressure. Pressurized solvent flow apparatus (HPLC) can give higher resolution with smaller sample volumes, and is better suited to analytical systems. For large scale purifications or crude samples, low pressure systems are more useful. Low pressure systems are also far less costly and complex, and allow columns to be prepared by the user to their specific requirements.

As with most analytical systems, there is an increasing tendency for columns to be obtained in ready-to-use form, even for low pressure applications.

Gel filtration (size exclusion) chromatography

This uses beads with pores of a specific size. The solid phase does not actually immobilize any components of the sample. However, large proteins do not enter the pores, and pass through the column rapidly. Smaller proteins enter the pores and are delayed in their passage through the column. Elution order is by size and shape, with the range resolved determined by the structure of the solid phase.

Application
Any system where separation by size is required (and the target protein may be resolved from others present on the basis of size).

Hydroxylapatite chromatography

Hydroxylapatite is a crystalline form of calcium phosphate which binds biological macromolecules (including proteins) by interaction with its surface calcium groups. Low molecular weight biomolecules are not adsorbed and are eluted. Bound macromolecules are eluted by gradually increasing the ionic strength of the solvent.

Application
The ability of this system to resolve different proteins is poor, and it is typically used for initial or final purification of proteins (or other biological macromolecules) from solutions containing high levels of low molecular weight material, with other methods used to resolve the target protein from other proteins.

Ion exchange chromatography

The matrix of the solid phase is charged (the strength and polarity of the charge can be selected from a broad range), and binds (immobilizes) charged material in the sample. Uncharged material or material with the same charge as the matrix is eluted. The solvent used is then changed, by gradually altering the pH (which will alter the charge on a protein and release it from the matrix) or by increasing the concentration of salt (the ions of which compete out the charged protein and release it from the matrix). Individual proteins will elute at specific pH or salt levels.

Application

Separation of proteins in a mixture where the target protein may be resolved from others present on the basis of its charge. The pH of the loading buffer determines the charges of the different proteins in the mixture.

Affinity chromatography

The matrix of the solid phase is covalently linked to a group or molecule (often an antibody) which specifically binds to the target protein, immobilizing it. Unbound proteins are eluted in the solvent flow. The solvent is then changed by altering the pH, using salt solutions or organic solvents or by addition of a competing molecule, all of which interfere with binding of the target molecule to the solid phase and result in its elution. Multiple bound molecules may be differentially eluted by the use of a gradually changing solvent.

Application

Where the protein to be separated has specific binding properties such as DNA binding proteins, receptor binding proteins, etc., the appropriate ligand will be bound to the solid phase. Where specific adsorbents are available such as monoclonal or monospecific antibodies, lectins (for glycoproteins) etc., these may be bound to the solid phase. This does not require the target protein to have specific binding activity. It should be noted that linkage to a solid phase may inactivate some monoclonal antibodies.

Hydrophobic chromatography

A hydrophobic solid phase adsorbs and immobilizes proteins with hydrophobic properties from a polar solvent. These are then eluted by gradually reducing the polarity of the solvent, either by reducing salt concentration (hydrophobic interaction chromatography, HIC) or by increasing the amount of organic components in the solvent (reverse phase chromatography). It should be noted that organic solvents may denature the target protein. The bound proteins will elute in order of increasing hydrophobicity (the most hydrophobic proteins eluting last).

Application

Separation of hydrophobic proteins, particularly from proteins which are less hydrophobic (or are hydrophilic). Used to purify large amounts of proteins.

Electrophoresis

Electrophoresis separates macromolecules by filtering them through a gel matrix (except in CZE, see p 254). The macromolecules are moved by the application of an electrical field. For protein separations, the gel matrix is almost always polyacrylamide (crosslinked polymers of acrylamide).

SDS-polyacrylamide gel electrophoresis (SDS-PAGE)

A development of electrophoresis where the presence of the negatively-charged detergent sodium dodecyl (or lauryl) sulfate linearizes polypeptides and coats them in a uniform charge dependent almost solely on size. Other denaturing agents are usually present (sulfhydryl reagents), ensuring excellent protein solubility. It is important to note that proteins are highly denatured and may not retain epitopes or other properties of the native form. Also, proteins composed of subunits are usually resolved as individual polypeptides.

Application

Probably the most widely used system of protein separation, often regarded as the definitive system. Post-electrophoresis processing may involve staining of polypeptides, detection of radioisotopes, or transfer of proteins from the gel to an adjacent membrane ('Western blotting').

Native electrophoresis

Non-denaturing, relies on the native charge to mass ratio of proteins. The charge is determined by pH, and may not be sufficiently variable to allow good resolution. Many proteins will not resolve due to poor solubility.

Application

Rarely used for protein purification. May be used to resolve proteins with relatively intact epitopes, but resolution is poor. For very large protein aggregates, the gel matrix may be agarose.

Isoelectric focusing (IEF)

Relies on the formation of a pH gradient within a gel matrix when current is applied due to the presence of *ampholytes* (which define the pH gradient formed, and may be altered across a wide range). Proteins migrate to the pH at which they do not carry a charge. The migration may be allowed to proceed to completion (isoelectric focusing) or be halted part way through the run (non-equilibrium pH gel electrophoresis, NEPHGE).

Application

Where proteins are to be separated on the basis of their isoelectric properties (that is, the pH at which they do not have an electrical charge). Large protein aggregates (up to the size of intact viruses) may be separated in an agarose matrix.

Two-dimensional electrophoresis (2-D PAGE)

A combination of an IEF separation followed by SDS-PAGE of the resolved proteins in a second dimension from the intact IEF gel. One separation will resolve thousands of individual proteins.

Application

This is the highest resolution electrophoretic system, but is complex and difficult to perform. Automation and standardization of reagents are reducing variability, although this is still a major problem.

Capillary zone electrophoresis (CZE)

This is a purely analytical system where molecules are separated by their native electrical properties in a liquid phase contained in a capillary tube. Due to the small size of the tube, separation is very rapid, and sample quantity can be extremely small (picograms). Apparatus for this application can be expensive. Capillary IEF is also possible using coated tubes.

Application

Usually used for smaller molecules such as oligopeptides, but can be used for some proteins. Very small structural changes can be detected (slight structural variation in hemoglobin or monoclonal antibodies can be detected easily). Proteins are usually detected by UV absorption.

Summary

Any of the above methods may be used to allow the preparation of purified proteins. This may involve removal of proteins from the gel matrix by digestion, elution, or protein blotting. Alternatively, scaled up systems may be used (except for 2-D PAGE and CZE) which allow collection of buffer fractions as proteins exit from the end of the gel.

Precipitation, centrifugation, filtration

Radioimmune precipitation

Specific antibodies are mixed with the target antigen and allowed to bind. The antigen–antibody complexes are then precipitated either by high-speed centrifugation (direct immunoprecipitation) or, more frequently, by binding to an antibody-specific particulate material followed by low-speed centrifugation (indirect immunoprecipitation).

Application
Radioimmune precipitation to identify viral proteins present in radiolabeled cells. The particulate phase is usually fixed bacterial cells with specific antibody binding proteins on the cell surface, or such proteins bound to agarose beads.

Salt or solvent precipitation

Proteins will precipitate from solution when the nature of the solvent is altered by increasing the amount of a salt or organic constituent in the solvent. The point at which an individual protein will precipitate varies according to their particular properties.

Application
The addition of specific concentrations of ammonium sulfate to concentrate antibodies from protein-rich solutions. The ability of this system to resolve individual proteins is poor, and it is most frequently used to concentrate the target protein rather than to purify it.

Density gradient centrifugation

This relies on differing densities in the material to be separated. A tube containing a range of solute concentrations (densest at the bottom, least dense at the top) is loaded with the sample and centrifuged at high speed. The sample is resolved into bands of different density which may be extracted individually. The solute may be sucrose (separation by the rate of sedimentation), caesium chloride (equilibrium density centrifugation) or another solute which allows the formation of a density gradient.

Application
Normally used for material of larger than molecular size, such as viruses or viral capsids. However, sucrose gradients may be used to separate IgG and IgM antibodies for serological testing. If correctly used, can give high resolution. Simple centrifugation (at different speeds to precipitate material of different sizes, such as cell nuclei and intact viruses) may be used for initial separations.

Filtration

Membranes are available which have relatively precise properties, and can be used to separate proteins by molecular weight.

Application
While useful, this method is not precise, and is normally used as an initial step to remove impurities of very different molecular weight. Membranes are often used in cartridge form where centrifugation is used to assist filtration. Examples of molecular weight cutoffs are M_r of 10,000, 30,000 or 100,000. Membranes with a low molecular weight cutoff may be combined with absorbent materials to remove excess solvents ('concentrators').

Other methods exist, but the material presented above covers the systems most commonly used for protein purification. Most of these applications are also used for other biological and chemical separations.

Chromatography

The range of chromatographic techniques is so vast that this chapter can make no attempt to do more than summarize the methods used. In all cases the manufacturer's instructions should be followed for the preparation and use of solid phases. Typical protocols are shown in Table 12.1.

Table 12.1. Examples of chromatographic protocols.

Technique	Column	Starting buffer	Eluting buffer	Notes
Affinity	Agarose beads with reactive surface groups (e.g. Bio-Rad Affi-Gels) to which specific adsorbents (such as monoclonal antibodies or enzyme ligands) are coupled by the user.	Phosphate-buffered saline (PBS) or other physiological buffer.	0.1–2.0 M NaCl in linear 0.1 M steps; specific chaotropic or ligand-competing agents such as 2-mercaptoethanol or NADP (all in starting buffer as solvent).	Wide range of possible adsorbents makes generalized protocols difficult to specify.
Anion exchange	Quaternary amine e.g. MonoQ, 5 × 50 mm; flow of 0.35 ml min^{-1}, 20 ml total volume	Variable according to protein. e.g. 20 mM tris/HCl pH 7.5–8.0; 20 mM piperazine/HCl pH 9.5–9.8.	0–0.3 M NaCl in starting buffer.	Equilibration essential; sample is concentrated onto column during loading.
Cation exchange	Carboxylic acids e.g. Mono S as above	Variable e.g. 50 mM morpholinoethane sulfonic acid pH 5.5–6.5.	0–0.3 M NaCl in starting buffer.	Prolonged equilibration essential.
Hydroxylapatite	e.g. 25 × 160 mm, flow of 0.6 ml min^{-1}, 450 ml total	10 mM sodium phosphate, pH 6.8.	10–400 mM sodium phosphate, pH 6.8.	Equilibration is easy but sample must be concentrated.
HIC	E.g. phenyl, hexyl and butyl columns: 4.7 × 100 mm column run at 0.3 ml min^{-1}	1.5 M ammonium sulfate (enzyme grade) 0.1 M sodium phosphate pH 6.8.	20 mM sodium phosphate.	As samples elute in low salt, this is a desalting step.
Size exclusion	Many size ranges e.g. M_r 2000–80,000	50 mM sodium chloride or phosphate, pH 7.0.	As starting buffer.	Desalting is possible using small columns.

Gel electrophoresis

Gel electrophoresis relies on the sieving properties of a gel matrix, retarding the migration of proteins in an applied electrical field in direct proportion to their size. There is a wide range of electrophoretic techniques, summarized in page 253, but owing to limitations of space, methods are given only for the most popular system, that of sodium dodecyl sulfate polyacrylamide gel electrophoresis (SDS-PAGE). As described in page 253, this resolves SDS coated proteins in a matrix of crosslinked acrylamide. The SDS prevents protein folding from affecting mobility and provides a uniform charge-to-mass ratio, ensuring that protein mobility is inversely proportional to protein size. While some groups on the protein (such as phosphate) may interfere with SDS binding and increase the apparent size of a protein, the relationship between mobility and size is generally reliable when compared to 'marker' proteins of known size resolved on the same gel.

Many manufacturers will supply 'pre-cast' gels, which simplify the procedures involved but increase the cost. The range available may also be limited. It is possible to run polyacrylamide gels where the concentration of acrylamide increases down the gel, allowing the resolution of high and low molecular weight proteins on the same gel. However, these gradient gels are very awkward to prepare, and pre-cast gels provide a sensible alternative where such gels are required. Linear gels (with a constant concentration of acrylamide) are relatively easy to prepare.

Where small proteins are being resolved, the concentration of acrylamide required (method below) may make the gel brittle. In such circumstances, alternative systems may be used. Two examples are the use of tricine (N-tris[hydroxymethyl]methyl-glycine) instead of glycine in the reservoir buffer (Schagger and von Jagow 1987) or of a 10% acrylamide gel containing 50% (w/v) sucrose (Chambers and Samson 1982). Both of these methods allow resolution of proteins down to M_r 1000.

General method for SDS-PAGE

Stock solutions

All water used should be of high purity. The level of ionic contaminants is particularly important, since high levels will result in rapid running and diffuse bands.

Resolving gel buffer ×2

90.6 g Tris base, 2.0 g sodium dodecyl sulfate, adjust pH to 8.8 with hydrochloric acid, make volume up to 1 litre with water.

Stacking gel buffer ×2

30.24 g Tris base, 2.0 g sodium dodecyl sulfate, adjust pH to 6.8 with hydrochloric acid, make volume up to 1 litre with water.

Acrylamide/bisacrylamide

200 g acrylamide, 4.4 g NN'-methylene bisacrylamide, make volume up to 500 ml with water.

Ammonium persulphate

0.4 g ammonium persulphate, make volume up to 20 ml with water. Store at 4°C and use within two weeks.
NNN'N'-Tetramethylethylenediamine (TEMED): Used as supplied.

Buffer-saturated n-butanol

Shake 200 ml of n-butanol with 100 ml of resolving gel buffer ×2 and 100 ml of water. Allow phases to separate (approximately one hour minimum). Store at room temperature, use upper phase as gel overlay.

Reservoir buffer

6.05 g Tris base, 2.0 g sodium dodecyl sulfate, 28.8 g glycine, make volume up to 2 litres with water.

Sample buffer

2 g sodium dodecyl sulphate, 10 g glycerol, 2.5 ml 2-mercaptoethanol, 1 ml 0.1% bromophenol blue in water, 25 ml Bx2, make volume up to 100 ml with water. Omission of 2-mercaptoethanol will leave sulfhydryl bonds intact but may result in poor resolution of proteins; samples with and without 2-mercaptoethanol should never be mixed on the same gel since the sulfydryl reagent will diffuse between lanes. Sample buffer may be made up as a 2x concentrate where the protein sample is already in solution, and mixed 1:1 to achieve the correct final concentration.

Gel mixtures

The amount of acrylamide/bisacrylamide used will vary with the final desired concentration of acrylamide in the gel. Resolving gels can range from 6% to 20% acrylamide: a 10% gel will resolve proteins from M_r 12,000 to 200,000. A gel containing less than 6% acrylamide will be very difficult to handle, while with acrylamide concentrations above 15% the gel may become brittle, and alternative approaches may be used as described previously.

Stacking gels are usually made with final concentrations of 4% acrylamide.

Resolving gel (for 50 ml): 25 ml Ax2, 1 ml ammonium persulfate, acrylamide/bisacrylamide as desired (25 ml for 10% acrylamide), water to 50 ml.

Stacking gel (for 15 ml): 7.5 ml Bx2, 0.4 ml ammonium persulphate, 1.5 ml acrylamide/bisacrylamide, 5.6 ml water. Polymerization and resolution will be improved if gel mixtures are degassed under vacuum for 5–10 min, prior to the addition of TEMED. The mixture should be swirled at intervals to help with degassing.

Pouring the gel

SDS-PAGE gels are normally 1–2 mm thick and are run vertically, using commercially supplied slab gel equipment such as the Bio-Rad Protean IIxi or the Hoefer SE600.

1. Set up the slab gel apparatus in accordance with the manufacturer's instructions, and test for leaks by filling with water. After leak testing, empty out water and remove residue with absorbent paper.
2. Immediately before pouring the gel, add 40 µl 100 ml^{-1} (resolving gel) or 150 µl 100 ml^{-1} (stacking gel) TEMED to initiate polymerization.
3. Gently swirl the mixture, and pour the gel using a large-volume pipette.
4. After pouring, the resolving gel should be overlaid (gently) with 1-butanol saturated with Ax1 to prevent uneven polymerization.
5. When the gel is set (approximately 30 min), a double meniscus will be visible under the butanol layer. Gel setting can be checked by gently tilting the apparatus.
6. Remove the butanol and wash thoroughly with water before placing the well-forming comb in position and pouring the stacking gel around it.
7. Setting requires approximately 30 min, after which the comb is gently removed and the wells washed with water and drained with a hypodermic needle.

Sample loading

1. Samples are heated to 100°C for 1–3 min immediately before loading to ensure thorough denaturation.
2. Samples are loaded into the wells using an air displacement micropipette, changing the tip for each sample.
3. After loading, gently fill each well with reservoir buffer, then fill the upper and lower chambers.

Running the gel

If the apparatus is water cooled, this will prevent heat-induced distortion of the band pattern and allow higher currents (and shorter run times) to be used.

1. SDS-PAGE gels are normally run at constant currents, in the range of 15–35 mA per gel, giving run times from 7 to 3 h in a typical apparatus. When the blue band of the dye front enters the resolving gel it can be seen to sharpen, and this also occurs with protein bands.
2. When the dye front is approximately 5 mm from the end of the gel, the current is switched off and the apparatus dismantled. The gel should be handled only while wearing wet gloves to avoid tearing (gels with a lower concentration of acrylamide tear more easily, below 7.5% handling is difficult).

Gel staining

There are a large number of protein stains available. If maximum sensitivity is desired, a high-resolution silver stain may be used, in accordance with the manufacturer's instructions. However, for routine and economical staining, the following system is suitable, giving blue bands on a clear background.
Stain: 0.5 g Coomassie brilliant blue R-250, 250 ml 2-propanol, 100 ml acetic acid, 650 ml water, mix to dissolve stain.
Destain: 250 ml 2-propanol, 100 ml acetic acid, 650 ml water.
The gel is stained for 3–18 h, and destained until the background blue staining is removed (at least four hours). If using short staining or destaining times, the gel should be gently shaken.

Autoradiography and fluorography

If a gel is not stained prior to autoradiography or fluorography, the proteins should be fixed within the gel matrix. This can be achieved by incubation of the gel for 30 min in 25% 2-propanol/10% acetic acid.

Radiolabeled proteins may be detected by drying the gel under vacuum (gel dryers should be used in accordance with the manufacturers instructions) and placing the gel next to an X-ray film (autoradiography). The exposure time typically ranges from 2 to 21 days, and is dictated by the level of radioactivity present.

If the radioisotope is of low emission energy (such as ^{3}H), or present in very low amounts, impregnation of the gel with a radiation-sensitive fluor prior to exposure to the X-ray film will greatly increase detection. However, if the isotope is of moderate energy and not present in very low amounts, fluorography will result in blurring of bands, so autoradiography is used. For high-energy isotopes, most emissions will pass through the film, and a solid fluor placed behind the film will enhance detection. These 'intensifying screens' work in a similar way to direct fluorography. Suggested detection systems are shown in Table 12.2.

Several convenient proprietary water based fluors are available (such as 'Amplify' from Amersham International) and should be used in accordance with the manufacturer's instructions. An alternative system is as follows:

Table 12.2. Sensitivities of autoradiography and fluorography with different radionuclides.

Radioisotope	Method	Temperature (°C)	Preflashed film	Sensitivity (d.p.m.)*	Enhancement factor†	
					Dried gel	Filter or TLC
^{3}H	Autoradiography,	RT	No	$> 2 \times 10^6$		
	fluorography	−70	Yes	5000	1000	100
^{14}C/^{35}S	Autoradiography,	RT	No	4000		
	flurography	−70	Yes	250	15	10
^{33}P	Autoradiography	RT	No	1000		
^{32}P	Autoradiography,	RT	No	350		
	intensifying screen	−70	Yes	30	10	14
^{125}I	Autoradiography,	RT	No	1000		
	intensifying screen	−70	Yes	60	16	17

* Results obtained by loading samples into 5 mm gel slots, followed by electrophoresis and drying. Units are d.p.m. of acid-precipitable material needed to produce a detectable image (0.02 A_{450}) after 24 h exposure under the conditions shown.

† Enhancement factor = increase in sensitivity by use of fluorography or intensifying screen. RT, room temperature.

This table is reproduced from *Virology Labfax* with permission from BIOS Scientific Publishers Ltd.

1. The gel is dehydrated with three 30 min incubations in dimethyl sulfoxide (a powerful hygroscopic).
2. This is followed by incubation for 2 h in 20% (w/v) 2,5-diphenyl oxazole (PPO) in dimethyl sulfoxide. PPO is the radiation-sensitive fluor.
3. PPO is precipitated by incubation for 1 h in water.
4. The gel is dried and exposed as for autoradiography. This method may cause cracking on drying with gels above 12% acrylamide.

Western (immuno) blotting and radioimmune precipitation

Most immunoassays will indicate the presence of reactive antibodies, but both immunoblotting and radioimmune precipitation will also provide evidence of the specificity of those antibodies. Using either technique one test can identify thirty or more reactive antigens in a single assay. However, each technique has significant advantages and disadvantages.

Proteins detected by immunoblotting are highly denatured, and configuration-sensitive epitopes will be destroyed. In practice this means that many antibodies will not bind, and some proteins may not be detected even with polyclonal sera. While blotting techniques do exist that are described as 'non-denaturing', this is not the case. Simply pulling the proteins through a gel and adsorbing them to a solid matrix will destroy many epitopes. As a result, it is important to remember that a negative result by immunoblotting does not indicate that no specific antibodies are present. Due to the highly denaturing sample preparation, resolution of proteins is very high. Most viral and cellular structures are disrupted, and even poorly soluble proteins are solubilized. Antibody binding occurs to individual proteins, so larger structures will not be detected.

In contrast, radioimmune precipitation uses very mild solubilization conditions which preserve proteins in their native configuration and will retain most epitopes, even those which depend on protein folding or (some) protein–protein interactions. These gentle conditions mean that large structures such as whole viral nucleocapsids may not be disrupted and will be removed when the antigen is clarified, which may prevent the detection of proteins contained in such structures. Other poorly soluble proteins will also be removed on clarification. In addition, non-reactive proteins associated with antigenic proteins may remain associated throughout the procedure until resolved by SDS-PAGE and show up as separate bands, even though no specific antibodies are present.

The relative advantages and disadvantages of each technique must be considered when using them. Using both methods in the same investigation can bypass these limitations and provide valuable comparative data.

General method for immunoblotting

Stock solutions

Blotting buffer

3.03 g Tris base, 14.4 g glycine, 200 ml methanol, make up to 1 litre with water. The addition of 0.15 g of sodium dodecyl sulfate per litre has been found in this laboratory to enhance the transfer of high molecular weight proteins. Variations in the concentration of methanol used may also enhance transfer, although this varies with the protein under study.

Blocking solution

1% (w/v) casein in phosphate buffered saline (Dulbecco 'A') (PBS).

Reaction buffer

1% (w/v) casein, 2% (v/v) normal rabbit serum, in PBS.

Method	TANK	SEMI-DRY
Electrodes	Platinum wire	Conductive plates
Transfer time	16 hours	1 to 3 hours
Buffer required	2 to 3 litres	1 litre
Maximum capacity	2 gels	6 gels
External cooling	Required	Not required

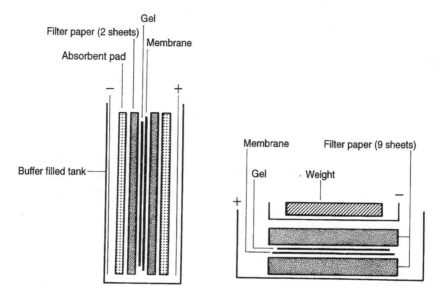

Figure 12.1 Comparison of tank and semi-dry electroblotting systems.

Wash buffer

0.1% Tween-20 in PBS.

Transfer

After electrophoresis, the gel is equilibrated in transfer buffer for 30 min.

Transfer membrane is cut to the size required and soaked in transfer buffer for 30 min. Most commonly, nitrocellulose is used, but polyvinylidene difluoride (Immobilon-P, Millipore) or nylon-supported nitrocellulose (Hybond C-super, Amersham International) may also be used. If polyvinylidene difluoride is used, the membrane must be pre-wetted in methanol, in accordance with the manufacturers instructions. Electroblotting may use either tank or semi-dry apparatus (Fig 12.1).

Tank system

Gel and membrane are inserted, between sheets of filter paper and absorbent pads, into clamping cassettes, then immersed in a tank of buffer between two platinum wire electrodes. Transfer is usually overnight at 30 V (constant voltage), with the option of an additional short, high intensity transfer (200 V, which requires extra cooling) to enhance protein recovery. Up to two gels may be transferred at the same time.

Chapter 12

Semi-dry system

Gel and membrane are placed in a buffer saturated filter paper stack, with sheets of dialysis membrane between the paper/gel/membrane transfer units sandwiched between plate electrodes. Since reactive metal anodes will oxidize, the electrodes may be graphite, conductive plastic, or an oxide or platinum coated anode with a metal cathode. Transfer is usually at 0.8 mA cm^{-2} cross-section for 1–2.5 h. Alternatively, transfer may be performed at 0.12 mA cm^{-2} overnight. Semi-dry transfers may be performed on up to six gels simultaneously, and use far less buffer than tank transfers.

All gel equipment should be assembled and used in accordance with the manufacturer's instructions.

Electroblotting for protein sequencing

In addition to the normal considerations for electroblotting of proteins, when using electroblotting to prepare proteins for sequencing it is necessary to ensure that:

- The resolving gel is allowed to set for at least 12 h to ensure complete polymerization.
- The membrane used is compatible with the sequencing protocol. Nitrocellulose membranes will dissolve and should not be used. Polyvinylidene difluoride (PVDF) membranes are generally suitable.
- Tris buffers are removed during washing of the membrane, since the amino groups of Tris will interfere with sequencing.
- There is enough protein present on the membrane to allow sequencing. As a general guide, a band which is clearly visible when stained as described with amido black will contain sufficient protein. Colloidal metal stains will interfere with sequencing and should not be used.
- The membrane binding sites must not be blocked with additional protein (see below).

Staining

If staining is required, a number of methods are available. One system for nitrocellulose membranes is as follows:

1. Stain for 5 min in 40% methanol/10% acetic acid/0.5% amido black, with gentle agitation.
2. Destain for 2–5 min in 40% methanol/10% acetic acid, with gentle agitation.

For PVDF membranes, use the above solutions, staining for not more than one minute.

Blocking

Unused protein binding sites on the membrane must be blocked prior to immunodetection to prevent non-specific binding of antibodies. Blocking is performed by rocking for 1–2 h in a suitable blocking solution at room temperature. Alternatively, the membrane may be incubated overnight (without rocking) in blocking solution at 4°C. Limited renaturation of proteins may occur during blocking. After blocking, antigen-bearing strips are cut using a fresh scalpel blade. These may be folded into foil and stored at −20°C for several months prior to immunoreaction, if desired. Blocking solutions normally contain high levels of non-reactive protein in a physiological buffer (e.g. the solution of 1% casein in PBS described on page 261), but 0.05% Tween 20 (a non-ionic detergent) in PBS may also be used (Baetteiger et al 1982).

Immunoreaction

Immunoreaction can take place in rolling drums, plastic boxes, or dedicated reaction trays. This last option is particularly suited to multiple immunoreactions. Volumes of reaction and wash solutions should be sufficient to thoroughly irrigate the strips, typically filling a flat-bottomed reaction container to a depth of 1–3 mm when stationary. All incubations require agitation, either on a rocking table or (for drums) by rolling of the reaction vessel. An effective procedure for immunoreaction is as follows:

1. Antigen-bearing strips are incubated at 37°C for 2–3 h in reaction buffer containing a 1:150 dilution of the test serum.
2. The strips are washed four times, for fifteen minutes each time.
3. Labeled probe antibody, diluted to working concentration in reaction buffer, is added to the strips and these are then incubated at 37°C for 1.5–2 h.
4. The strips are again washed four times.

Detection of bound probe

If the probe is directly stained, bands will be visible on the membrane.

If a radiolabeled probe has been used, the strips are then dried, covered with clingfilm, and exposed to X-ray film, using fluorographic intensifying screens if the radiolabel is the gamma-emitting ^{125}I. Exposure to film may require days or weeks.

If an enzyme-labeled probe has been used, reaction with substrate must be allowed to occur. For the production of coloured bands [chromogenic detection, many substrates are available (Cunningham and Simmons 1993)]. A commonly used substrate is 4-chloro-1-naphthol, which gives purple bands and

is used with probes conjugated to horseradish peroxidase. For this reaction, the procedure is:

1. Strips are washed in 0.05 M Tris/HCl pH 7.4 + 0.2 M NaCl (TBS).
2. The strip is incubated for 5 min in fresh TBS containing 0.6 mg ml^{-1} 4-chloro-1-napthol and 2μl ml^{-1} 30% H_2O_2 solution.
3. The reaction is stopped by rinsing in TBS.
4. If required, the bands may be further developed by overnight incubation of the strip in the TBS rinse at 4°C.
5. With any chromogenic system, bands are visible only on the nitrocellulose strip itself, which is fragile when dry and becomes extremely fragile with age. The band pattern should be recorded by photography and/or photocopying.

Luminescent immunodetection may use alkaline phosphatase or horseradish peroxidase, with a substrate such as AMPPD or luminol (respectively), which emit light during reaction (Cunningham and Simmons 1993; Stanley and Kricka 1991). Commercial systems such as the ECL system from Amersham International use chemical enhancers of the reaction to give more intense and stable luminescence. The strip is exposed to X-ray film for a few seconds or minutes. However, light is a product of the ongoing reaction, and depletion of available substrate can cause bands to become less intense, which can give a relatively short 'window' for successful exposure. Luminescent systems give a durable film image, with the potential for multiple exposures, combining a major advantage of radiometric detection with the speed of chromogenic systems.

Band quantitation

Unlike most immunoassays, immunoblotting does not give results which are easily reduced to numerical data. The varying background observed on membrane strips makes densitometry unreliable, and visual inspection is usually the method of choice. This contrasts with direct protein staining of gels, where variable background intensity is not usually a problem, and densitometry may be a useful method of quantitation. Where immunoblotting is used diagnostically, it has been found that detection of a single band should not be regarded as indicative of a positive result. If multiple bands are required, the incidence of false positives is greatly reduced.

General procedure for radioimmune precipitation

Stock solutions

TD buffer

100 ml phosphate buffered saline (Dulbecco 'A') (PBS) plus 1 g Triton X-100, 0.5 g sodium deoxycholate, 17.4 mg phenyl-methyl sulphonyl fluoride (PMSF), 36.1 mg hydroxymercuribenzoate sodium salt (HMB), 0.1 g sodium azide.

PBS-CR

10 ml PBS, 0.1 g casein, 0.2 ml normal rabbit serum

PBS-T

100 ml PBS, 0.1 g Tween-20

Antigen preparation

1. Virus-infected cells must be radiolabeled (see page 267)
2. Wash the cells with PBS.

3. Put TD buffer onto cell sheet (adherent cells) or resuspend cells in TD buffer (non-adherent cells). Use 1 ml of TD buffer for 25 cm^2 of confluent cell sheet or 2×10^6 to 4×10^6 cells.
4. Freeze at $-70°C$ overnight.
5. Thaw at 37°C.
6. Scrape off cell sheet (adherent cells) and sonicate at 20 kHz for 15 s.
7. Pellet debris at 40,000 g for 1 h.
8. Assay radioactivity present in 5 μl aliquot of antigen.
9. Store antigens at $-20°C$.

Radioimmune precipitation

1. In a 1.5 ml centrifuge tube, mix 1 ml 'Omnisorb' protein G (for IgG detection) (Calbiochem) and 0.5 ml PBS. Mix, spin for 1 min at 'slow' speed setting (3100 g) in an MSE Micro-Centaur centrifuge. Resuspend in 1 ml PBS, repeat spin. Repeat wash at least three times, until the supernatant is clear. Take up the final pellet in 1 ml PBS-CR . Each vial will provide enough washed protein G for assaying five sera for IgG.
2. Mix antigen containing 50,000–100,000 CPM with 100 μl washed protein G, make volume up to 200 μl with PBS-CR if required.
3. Incubate for 1 h at 37°C, with mixing at least once by inversion.
4. Spin for 1 min at slow speed setting, and mix 170 μl of the supernatant with 15 μl of test serum. As a general guide, when using monoclonal antibodies use 10–20 μl of ascitic fluid or 100–200 μl of unconcentrated tissue culture supernatant.
5. Incubate for 2 h at 37°C, with at least three mixings
6. Add 100 μl of washed protein G, and mix.
7. Incubate for 1 h at 37°C, with at least one mixing.
8. Add 1 ml PBS-T.
9. Spin for 1 min at slow speed setting, resuspend pellet in 1 ml PBS-T by

pumping with a pipette tip. Repeat spin and wash three times, and resuspend pellet in 80 µl reducing sample buffer for SDS-PAGE (see page 258). Place in a 100°C water bath for 2 min, cool in a room temperature water bath.

Spin for 2 min at 'fast' speed setting (13,000 g) and take 60 µl of supernatant.

Store at −20°C prior to analysis by SDS-PAGE. Owing to the low recovery of antigen by this technique, it is often necessary to use fluorography even for isotopes such as ^{14}C and ^{35}S which are usually detected by autoradiography (Table 12.2).

Radiolabeling of cells

Radiolabeling is a versatile and simple method of identifying biological macromolecules produced by cells. For viral proteins, the use of specific radiolabels makes possible:

- Detection of particular classes of proteins (for example, use of sugars which are incorporated only into glycosylated proteins).
- Structural studies of proteins (for example, use of different radiolabeled amino acids (e.g. cysteine for studies of disulfide bonds) or of chemical groups which may be attached by post-translational modification (e.g. radiolabeled orthophosphate) to determine which are present in a particular protein).
- Detection of proteins produced at specific times (for example, enhanced detection of viral proteins by adding radiolabel after cellular synthesis has been inhibited by the virus infection, use of short 'pulse' radiolabeling at different times after infection to obtain a 'snapshot' of viral and cellular synthesis at these times).
- Studies of protein processing (for example, 'Pulse-chase' analysis (see below) where proteins are labeled as they are produced and then analyzed at increasing intervals after their production, identifying processing or degradative events).
- 'Tagging' of proteins (for example, surface iodination, where the ^{125}I is chemically linked to the surface structures of a virus or cell, demonstrating their location).

General procedure for radiolabeling of viral proteins

Details of isotopes and commonly used radiolabels are given in Tables 12.3 and 12.4, respectively. Owing to the highly variable nature of viral infections of cells, it is only possible to give the most general of guidelines for radiolabeling of viral proteins:

- With those viruses that produce cytopathic effect, antigen production is likely to be maximal when cytopathic effect is relatively advanced, although not to the point where cells have stopped synthesizing proteins.
- In order to maximize the labeling of viral proteins relative to those of the cell, labeling should be for a relatively short period, late in infection. The period of radiolabeling with a particular molecule will be affected by the amount of the unlabeled equivalent in the cell. For example, amino acids and sugars are generally turned over rapidly and short labeling periods may be used, while fatty acids (which are present in large amounts in cellular lipids) require longer labeling periods. For amino acids labeling periods will generally vary from 0.5–6 h, although shorter or longer periods may be used if required, with appropriate alterations in the amount of label present: short labeling times require high levels of radiolabel, longer labeling times can use reduced levels.
- As a general guideline, for radiolabels where there is not a large cellular pool of the equivalent unlabeled molecule, a labeling period of one twelfth of the time since infection (e.g. for harvest at 24 h post-infection, label from 22–24 h post-infection) is a good starting point from which to investigate the optimum labeling time.
- Incorporation of a radiolabeled molecule may be increased by starving the cell of the unlabeled form. This will usually involve the formulation of the label itself in depleted medium, and (where the labeling period is short, e.g. of 2 h or less) may also involve pre-incubation in depleted medium to decrease cellular reserves. Media lacking individual amino acids are available, and are used with dialyzed serum (from which

Table 12.3. Isotopes used for biological radiolabelling.

Isotope	Half life	Emission energy	Detection on gel
Beta emitters:			
^{3}H	12.4 years	Very low	Fluorography
^{14}C	5740 years	Moderate	Autoradiography
^{35}S	87.4 days	Moderate	Autoradiography
^{33}P	25 days	Moderate	Autoradiography
^{32}P	14.3 days	High	Intensifying screen
Gamma emitters:			
^{125}I	60 days	High	Intensifying screen

Table 12.4. Details of commonly used radiolabels.

Radiolabel	Advantages	Disadvantages
Total protein:		
^{35}S methionine	Inexpensive, available at high specific activities.	Methionine is not a common amino acid, some proteins will label poorly while others will appear very intense, short half life.
^{3}H leucine	Inexpensive, available at high specific activities, leucine is present almost all proteins, long half life.	Low emission energy requires fluorographic detection.
^{14}C amino acid mixture	Will label all proteins, long half life.	Very expensive, only available at low specific activities.
Glycoproteins:		
^{3}H glucosamine hydrochloride	Long half life, inexpensive.	Low emission energy requires fluorographic detection.
^{14}C glucosamine hydrochloride	Long half life.	Expensive, low specific activity.
Phosphoproteins:		
^{32}P orthophosphate	Cheap, high specific activities available.	High emission energy requires stringent safeguards, short half life.
^{33}P orthophosphate	High specific activities available, moderate emission energy.	Expensive, short half life.

Many other radiolabels are used for specific applications, notably ^{125}I for 'tagging' of biomolecules all low molecular weight compounds have been removed). Depletion of sugars, phosphates or many other molecules is less simple since depleted media are not practical, although dialyzed or lipid-stripped serum may still be used. Depleted media are often toxic to cells during prolonged exposure, and should not be used for more than 6–12 h in total. Methods should be optimized for individual systems.

A radiolabeling protocol of this type has the general plan:

Infect – Incubate under complete media until cytopathic effect is advanced – (starve) – Radiolabel – Harvest

This is 'pulse labeling', where a short 'pulse' or radiolabel gives a snapshot of synthesis in the cell at a particular time. With 'pulse-chase' radiolabeling, the radiolabel is then removed and replaced with complete medium highly enriched for the equivalent unlabeled molecule (typically at least five times normal levels unless this would be toxic). This has the effect of swamping any residual label present, so that all proteins synthesized in the 'chase' period are unlabeled. As a result, any changes to proteins produced during the pulse can be observed. Pulse-chase radiolabeling is often used to determine precursor-product relationships, but can also be used to determine the half-life of a particular protein or proteins.

Expression of viral proteins in heterologous systems

While many viruses grow well in cell culture and produce very high levels of proteins, this is not always the case. For those viruses which do not grow in culture, purification of viral proteins from natural sources may be possible. However, it is often simpler to clone the viral gene of interest into an expression system designed to produce high levels of the cloned protein. Many such systems exist (Kinchington 1993), and the procedures used for cloning and expression lie outside the concerns of this chapter. However, a brief summary of the major points of commonly used expression systems may be of value.

In general, viral genes are usually cloned into gene libraries maintained in prokaryotic plasmids, and then sub-cloned into expression systems. The range and number of cloning systems available is huge, and many excellent systems are available in complete form from biotechnology companies such as Pharmacia, Invitrogen, or Promega. Unless the investigator has good contacts with another laboratory able to supply such systems it is usually easier to purchase them.

Despite the ease of use of such systems, prokaryotic expression systems will produce proteins very different from those made by a virus infecting a eukaryotic cell. As a result, it may be better to use a eukaryotic expression system such as yeast, baculovirus or mammalian cell/plasmid systems. Unfortunately, the general principle that the more 'realistic' products are produced by systems that are more difficult to use applies, and the importance of 'authentic' post-translational processing must be balanced against the difficulties of expression. The advantages and disadvantages of producing viral proteins in different expression systems are summarized in Table 12.5.

Table 12.5. Features of eukaryotic and viral proteins expressed in heterologous systems.

	Bacteria	Yeast	Insect cells	Mammalian cells
Correct protein folding	− to +; may precipate	± to +	Usually, may precipitate	Yes
Proteolytic cleavage	No	± to +	Usually	Yes
Glycosylation	No	Usually, but different (unbranched, O-linked)	Usually, but different (branched)	
Acylation	No or different	Usually	Usually	Yes
Phosphorylation	No	Usually, may be different	Usually, may be different	Yes
Secretion	No, but may be engineered	Usually	Usually	Yes
Compartmentalization	n/a	± to +	Usually	Yes
Functional activity	Occasionally	Often	Often	Usually
Major systems for high-level expression	(i) Fusion proteins (ii) Strong/inducible promoters	Yeast shuttle and expression vectors	Baculovirus expression systems	(i) Viral expression systems (ii) Amplifiable cell lines*
Effort required	Easy; easy to scale-up	Considerable; easy to scale-up	Considerable; possible for scale-up	Considerable; possible for scale-up (CHO-DHFR)
Possible levels of expression (% wt)	Up to 30%	Up to 1%	Up to 30%; usually less than 10%	Up to 10%; usually much less than 1%

Features in this table are to act as a general guide and should not be considered comprehensive.

* Amplifiable cell lines are not detailed in this chapter, but are used for expression, particularly if large scale-up is required. The two most commonly used systems are chinese hamster ovary cells with dihydrofolate reductase amplification (CHO-DHFR) and plasmids bearing the SV40 replicon amplified in T-antigen-expressing cells, such as COS cells (SV40-COS). (This table is taken from 'Expression of Virus Genes in Heterologous Systems' by P. R. Kinchington, in *Virology Labfax*, D. R. Harper (Ed.), 1993, BIOS Scientific Publishers Ltd, and is presented here with the permission of the publishers).

Amino acid sequencing of polypeptides

Amino acid sequence analysis is, at present, performed by highly sensitive, automated Edman degradation. In this technique the polypeptide N-terminus is reacted with an aromatic isothiocyanate and the product then cleaved under acid conditions to yield a characteristic amino acid derivative with the concomitant generation of a polypeptide one amino acid shorter than the original. Sequential degradation and HPLC analysis of the amino acid derivatives establishes the sequence. Methods for C-terminal analysis are not yet sufficiently developed to be of practical use.

In practice, virologists will submit their samples to a protein sequencing service for analysis.

The amount and reliability of amino acid sequence information is highly dependent upon the quantity of material, its purity and the sequence of the polypeptide chain itself. A prerequisite for sequencing is a free N-terminus and in many cases the N-terminus is covalently modified (Aitken, 1990). There is no easy way to 'free' the N-terminus of a polypeptide and in these cases peptides must be generated with free N-termini (see below). A second requirement is that the polypeptide must be immobilized on an inert support; either glass fibre or a polyvinylidene difluoride (PVDF) membrane.

Quantitation

Modern protein sequencers can detect as little as 0.2 pmol of amino acid. However, there is a threshold of approx. 0.5 μg below which no reliable sequence information is obtained.

Any protein assay method may be used but none are reliable for dilute solutions and workers frequently greatly overestimate the amount of protein present. In practice, therefore, it is as good to use the UV absorption of a sample at 214 and/or 280 nm. A protein solution of 1 mg/ml has an approximate A214 of 10 and A280 of 1 at 1 cm path length. Note that almost all impurities and buffers will affect this quantitation. For quantitation of bands blotted from gels use a dye stain (e.g. Coomassie blue or amido black) and judge the amount using a set of standards. The rule is – if you can't see it clearly with a dye stain there isn't enough material.

Guidelines for preparation of samples for sequencing

- Use the most highly purified reagents and water possible.
- Avoid amine or ammonium salt buffers. Ammonium salts, primary and secondary amines will produce derivatives during sequencing. These will be in vast excess over peptide and may prevent successful analysis. *Note that tris is a primary amine.* (To some extent this problem can be overcome by concentration of samples onto a membrane.)
- Avoid high salt concentrations e.g. > 0.5 M. Salt may precipitate during handling and cause problems.
- Thiols and detergents are less of a problem than amines but use them judiciously. Consult the protein sequencer staff.
- Avoid excessive dilution of samples (e.g. < 1 μg ml^{-1}).
- Use concentrating conditions during purification if possible, e.g. desalting via a size exclusion column can lead to loss of polypeptide due to dilution – an HPLC technique may be suitable (see below).

- Use appropriately small columns and vessels; do not transfer samples from one vessel to another frequently; keep vessels in which polypeptides have been stored in case material remains bound to the vessel.
- Do not store dilute samples, but work on them immediately.
- Do not repeatedly freeze and thaw dilute samples.
- Do not concentrate samples to dryness as recovery may be difficult (e.g. freeze drying and 'gyrovap' concentrators).
- Be aware that concentration through a membrane may lead to sample losses. The use of a stream of nitrogen (with heating to no more than approximately 37°C) is convenient as volume reduction is always visible. Small amounts of detergent may be added if essential, e.g. SDS to a *final* concentration of less than 0.1%.

Digestion of polypeptides

It is frequently necessary to digest polypeptides in order to gain sequence information away from the N-terminus.

General procedure for enzymic digestion in solution

1. Ensure that the polypeptide is in an appropriate buffer and check pH (see Table 12.6).
2. Use the protease at at least 0.1 μg ml^{-1}. This may require a small volume to keep the protease/substrate ratio reasonable, i.e. < 1:10.
3. Perform a protease blank.
4. Isolate peptides by RP-HPLC (see below).

Digestion with cyanogen bromide

1. Work in an efficient fume hood, Hydrogen cyanide is a by-product of the reaction.
2. Dissolve the polypeptide in 50–200 μl of approx 60% formic acid in a small (5 ml) pear shaped flask with a ground glass joint.
3. Add a small crystal of CNBr (approx. 2 mg) and leave overnight at 4°C.
4. Remove formic acid and by-products with a rotary evaporator. Do not heat above 40°C, and remove from the heat when solvent has been removed.
5. Add 10 μl of 100% trifluoroacetic acid and allow this to run around the flask to dissolve the peptides.
6a. Add approx 200 μl of water (i.e. an appropriate volume for the HPLC setup) and purify by reverse phase (RP)-HPLC.
6b. Add buffer for SDS-PAGE. Adjust the pH with bicarbonate buffer until correct and run on SDS-PAGE using the method for low MW peptides (Schagger and von Jagow 1987), followed by blotting onto PVDF membrane.

Table 12.6. Protease digestion of samples for amino acid sequencing.

Protease	Sites of cut	Buffer
Trypsin	K, R	50–100 mM ammonium bicarbonate, pH 8.4
Chymotrypsin	F, Y and hydrophobic regions	50–100 mM ammonium bicarbonate, pH 7–9
S. aureus V8 protease	E	50–100 mM ammonium bicarbonate, pH 7.8
Lysylendopeptidase*	K (+ 0.1% SDS)	100 mM tris, pH 9.0

* From *Endobacter*. This protease retains complete activity in 0.1% SDS. It is obtainable from the WAKO chemical company.

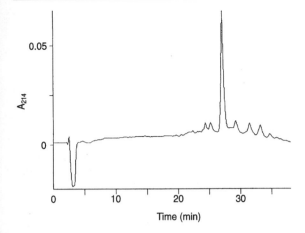

Figure 12.2. HPLC separation of a sample of azo-reductase by HPLC.

Approximately 8 μg of protein was applied to an Aquapore RP 300 column (a 30 nm pore C-8 reverse-phase column from Applied Biosystems) 2.1 mm internal diameter and 100 mm long and eluted with a 70 min linear gradient of 2–70% acetonitrile in water, both solvents containing 0.1% trifluoroacetic acid. The flow rate is 130 μl min⁻¹ and the eluant was monitored at 214 nm.

The negative peak at approx 7 min is the buffer which flows straight through the column. Sequence analysis of the sample prior to HPLC caused ambiguity of sequence due to the protein and buffer contaminants. These ambiguities were resolved by using the HPLC purified material. Note that from the peak height, flow rate and the cell path of 5 mm it can be estimated that the major peak contains approximately 6 μg of protein.

Sequencing polypeptides bound to membranes

Normal transfer methods should be used taking note of the precautions given above.

Digestion of polypeptides on PVDF membranes

(Method taken from Pappin, personal communication.)

1. Cut out the band of interest and soak it for 5 min in the minimum volume of 1% octylglucoside containing the appropriate pH buffer for the protease of choice (e.g. 20–100 μl). Check pH.
2. Prepare a control lacking polypeptide.
3. Add protease to each sample so that protease concentration is at least 0.1 μg ml⁻¹ and protease is at no more than one tenth the amount of polypeptide.
4. Leave to digest at 20–25°C overnight.
5. Remove supernatant and purify peptides by RP-HPLC.

Note

Octylglucoside acts as a detergent to wet the membrane and at the same time blocks protein binding sites on the membrane which would otherwise bind the protease. Peptides are released into solution.

HPLC purification of polypeptides

Polypeptides may be purified by means of RP-HPLC provided that wide-pore packings are used. The technique is also useful for desalting samples using a short column and rapid gradient. It is not appropriate to go into detail here and a single example is given here (Fig. 12.2).

Amino acid analysis

The same criteria of purity and contaminants that apply to amino acid sequencing apply to amino acid analysis. However, the background of amino acid contaminants and amine buffers is even more critical since while sequencing the levels of contaminants will drop during cycles, this is not possible in amino acid analysis. The guidelines on page 271 should be followed but for accurate analyses several samples of a single polypeptide should be analyzed and these samples should include at least a solvent/buffer blank treated in an identical way to the sample.

Suppliers quoted in text

Amersham International

USA: 2636 South Clearbrook Drive, Arlington Heights, IL 60005.

UK: Amersham Place, Little Chalfont, Bucks. HP7 9NA.

Applied Biosystems

USA: 850 Lincoln Center Drive, Foster City, CA 94404.

UK: Kelvin Close, Birchwood Science Park North, Warrington WA3 7PB.

Bio-Rad Laboratories

USA: 3300 Regatta Blvd., Richmond, CA 94804.

UK: Bio-Rad House, Maylands Avenue, Hemel Hempstead, Herts. HP2 7TD.

Hoefer Scientific Instruments

USA: 654 Minnesota Street, PO Box 77387, San Francisco, CA 94107.

UK: Unit 12, Croft Road Workshops, Croft Road, Newcastle-under-Lyme, ST5 0TH.

Invitrogen

USA: 3985B Sorrento Valley Blvd., San Diego, CA 92121.

UK: R&D Systems Europe Ltd., 4-10 The Quadrant, Barton Lane, Abingdon, Oxford OX14 3YS.

Millipore

USA: 80 Ashby Road, Bedford, MA 01730.

UK: The Boulevard, Blackmoor Lane, Watford, Herts. WD1 8YW.

Pharmacia Biotech

USA: 800 Centennial Avenue, P.O.Box 1327, Piscataway, NJ 08855.

UK: 23 Grosvenor Road, St. Albans, Herts. AL1 3AW.

Promega

USA: 2800 Woods Hollow Road, Madison, WI 53711

UK: Epsilon House, Chilworth Research Centre, Southampton SO1 7NS.

WAKO Chemical Company

USA: 1600 Wellwood Road, Richmond, VA 23237.

Europe: Nissanstrasse 2, D-41468 Neuss, Germany.

References

Aitken A (1990) Identification of Protein Consensus Sequences. Ellis Horwood, New York.

Baetteiger B, Newhall VWJ, Jones RB (1982) The use of Tween 20 as a blocking agent in the immunological detection of proteins transferred to nitrocellulose membranes. J Immun Meth 55: 297–307.

Chambers P, Samson ACR (1982) Non-structural proteins in Newcastle-disease virus-infected cells. J Gen Virol 58: 1–12.

Cunningham MW, Simmonds AC (1993) In Virology Labfax, Harper DR (Ed.) Bios Scientific Publishers, Oxford, pp. 123–149.

Kinchington PR (1993) In Virology Labfax, Harper DR (Ed.), Bios Scientific Publishers, Oxford, pp. 265–287.

Schagger H, von Jagow G (1987) Tricine-sodium dodecyl sulphate-polyacrylamide gel electrophoresis for the separation of proteins in the range from 1 to 100 kDa. Anal Biochem 166, 368–379.

Stanley PE, Kricka LJ (Eds) (1991) Bioluminescence and Chemiluminescence: Current Status. John Wiley & Sons Ltd., Chichester.

Bibliography

General

Deutscher MP (1990) Guide to Protein Purification. Methods in Enzymology 182, Academic Press, New York.

Harper DR (1993) Virology LabFax. Bios Scientific Publishers, Oxford.

Harris ELV, Angal S (1989) Protein Purification Applications: A Practical Approach. IRL Press, Oxford.

Harris ELV, Angal S (1989) Protein Purification Methods: A Practical Approach. IRL Press, Oxford.

1 Purification and characterization of viral proteins

Ford TC, Graham JM (1992) An Introduction to Centrifugation. Bios Scientific Publishers, Oxford.

Horvath C, Nikelly JG (1990) Analytical Biotechnology: Capillary Electrophoresis and Chromatography. American Chemical Society, Washington DC.

2 Chromatography

Dean PDG, Johnson WS, Middle FA (1985). Affinity Chromatography: A Practical Approach. IRL Press, Oxford.

Bidlingmeyer BA (1992) Practical HPLC Methodology and Applications. Wiley, New York.

Braithwaite A (1985) Chromatographic methods (4th edn). Chapman and Hall, London.

Horvath C, Ettre LS (1993) Chromatography in biotechnology. American Chemical Society, Washington DC.

Oliver RWA (1989). HPLC of macromolecules: A Practical Approach. IRL Press, Oxford.

Ravindranath B, (1989) Principles and Practice of Chromatography. Ellis Horwood, Chichester.

Yamamoto S, Nakanishi K, Matsuno Y (1988). Ion-exchange chromatography of proteins. Marcel Dekker, New York.

3 Gel electrophoresis

Dunn MJ (1994) Gel electrophoresis: proteins. Bios Scientific Publishers, Oxford.

Hames BD, Rickwood D (1990) Gel Electrophoresis of Proteins: A Practical Approach (2nd edition). IRL Press, Oxford.

4 Western (immuno) blotting and radioimmune precipitation

Dunbar BS (1994) Protein Blotting: A Practical Approach. IRL Press, Oxford.

Harper DR, Liu KM, Kangro HO (1990) Protein blotting—ten years on. J Virol Meth 30, 25–40.

Slater RJ (1990) Radioisotopes in biology: A practical approach. IRL Press, Oxford.

5 Radiolabeling of cells

Billington D, Jayson GG, Maltby PJ (1992) Radioisotopes. Bios Scientific Publishers, Oxford.

Morgan SJ, Darling DC (1993). Animal Cell Culture. Bios Scientific Publishers, Oxford.

Slater RJ (1990) Radioisotopes in biology: A practical approach. IRL Press, Oxford.

6 Expression of viral proteins in heterologous systems

Kinchington PR (1993) 'Expression of Virus Genes in Heterologous Systems' in Virology Labfax, Harper DR (Ed.) Bios Scientific Publishers, Oxford, pp. 265–287.

Sambrook J, Fritsch EF, Maniatis T (1989) Molecular Cloning: A laboratory manual. Cold Spring Harbor Laboratory Press, New York.

7 Amino acid sequencing of polypeptides

Manton CT, Hodges RS (1991) High performance liquid chromatography of peptides and proteins: separation, analysis and conformation. CRC Press, Boca Raton.

Shively JE (1986). Methods of protein microcharacterization. Humana Press, Clifton NJ.

The assay of viral enzymes

M. McCrae

Although the replication cycles of viruses are in all cases closely interwoven with the metabolism of the cells that they infect there are virus specific steps which require the virus to encode enzymes capable of catalyzing the process in question. These enzymatic activities can be subdivided into two broad categories; first those required to ensure that the nucleic acid of the virus is both transcribed and replicated accurately and efficiently and second those needed to ensure that virus encoded proteins are either processed and/or modified appropriately. The absence of RNA-dependent RNA polymerase activities in eukaryotic cells dictates that all RNA-containing viruses must encode the transcriptase/polymerase activity needed to transcribe and replicate their genomes. These activities are either a component of the infectious virion (Baltimore class III, V and VI) or synthesized in infected cells from the input virion RNA (Baltimore class IV). In the case of DNA viruses the extent to which the virus relies on the transcription and replication machinery of the cell is governed largely by the size of the viral genome and the sub-cellular localization of the transcription/replication process. Thus the small DNA viruses such as SV40 which replicate in the nucleus rely entirely on cellular enzymatic activities whereas the poxviruses such as vaccinia virus which have a large genome and replicate in the cytoplasm of the cell encode virtually all of the activities needed for transcription/replication of their genomes. With the exception of the poxviruses which carry a DNA-dependent RNA polymerase activity and several other enzyme activities in the infectious virion, the enzymatic activities encoded by DNA viruses are confined to the virus-infected cell. Thus the enzymes encoded by viruses can be broadly subdivided into those associated with nucleic acid metabolism and those involved in processing/modifying proteins and each of these subdivisions can be further divided into activities found in both the purified virion and virus infected cell and those restricted to the infected cell. These subdivisions form a convenient basis on which to categorize the various virus-encoded enzyme activities and will be used in this chapter to try and simplify the description of the enzyme assays.

Virology Methods Manual
ISBN 0–12–465330–8

Enzymes concerned with nucleic acid metabolism

Viruses encode a variety of enzyme activities associated with nucleic acid metabolism ranging from synthetic polymerases through RNA-modifying activities to enzymes such as thymidine kinase which are concerned with synthesis of the nucleotide triphosphate substrates for DNA and RNA synthesis. These different categories of enzyme will be dealt with in turn using a number of specific examples to illustrate the assay protocols used.

Virion-associated polymerases

These activities are normally quiescent in the intact virus particle and hence the assay procedure consists of two steps. First the infectious virus particle must be treated either chemically or enzymatically to unmask the polymerase activity. Normally this involves the 'loosening' or removal of the outer layer(s) of the virus particle to allow the substrates for the enzymatic reaction to gain access to the catalytic centre of the polymerase and the synthetic products to be released into the supernatant of the reaction. The second step is the reaction itself which normally involves measuring the synthesis of nucleic acid on the endogenous template contained within the virus particle although in some cases, e.g. reverse transcriptase an exogenous template is often employed. To illustrate the assay protocols four specific examples will be used, the RNA-dependent RNA polymerase of reovirus (Skehel and Joklik 1969; McCrae 1985), the RNA-dependent RNA polymerase of vesicular stomatitis virus (VSV) (Baltimore et al 1970; Szilágyi and Pringle 1972), the DNA-dependent RNA polymerase of vaccinia virus (Kates and McAuslan 1967; Munyon et al

1967) and the RNA-dependent DNA polymerase (reverse transcriptase) of HIV (Popovic et al 1984; Spira et al 1987).

Reovirus RNA-dependent RNA polymerase

In the case of this activity, unmasking requires the removal of the outer virion shell which is achieved by proteolytic digestion with chymotrypsin. Digestion is carried out in 20 mM Tris-HCl buffer pH 8.0–0.12 M KCl at 37°C for 60–65 min using freshly diluted chymotrypsin at a final concentration of 50 μg ml^{-1} and purified virus at a final concentration of 1mg ml^{-1}. The virus cores produced in this digestion are a great deal more resistant to protease digestion than the intact virus particle but it is important to adhere to the conditions given to ensure that there is no loss of RNA transcriptase activity as a result of over digestion. Enzymatically active cores are collected by centrifugation (30,000 g 4°C, 20 min) and resuspended directly in the synthesis reaction mix at a final concentration equivalent to 1 mg ml^{-1} of purified virus. The reaction mixture for simple assay of enzymatic activity which is carried out at 37°C has the following constitution: 100 mM Tris-HCl buffer pH 8.0, 5 mM ATP, 5 mM CTP, 5 mM GTP, 0.5 mM UTP, 0.5 mM S-adenosyl methionine, 500 units ml^{-1} Pancreatic RNAase Inhibitor, 100 μCi ml^{-1} [^{3}H] UTP. The reaction is started by adding MgCl$_2$ to a final concentration of 10 mM and activity monitored by taking small samples (10 μl) every 15 min from the reaction onto 2.5 cm Whatman filter paper disks (labeled using a pencil) which are dropped into cold 5% trichloroacetic acid (TCA). These are then washed in cold 5% TCA (twice), ethanol (twice) and ether (twice) and the incorporation of radioactivity into acid insoluble material measured by liquid scintillation counting.

The high activity and stable nature of the reovirus RNA-dependent RNA polymerase means that it can be used to synthesize large amounts of viral m-RNA *in vitro*. For such large scale synthesis of viral mRNA the synthesis reaction mix should contain the following per 10 ml:

1. 30 mg ATP
2. 20 mg CTP
3. 20 mg GTP
4. 10 mg UTP
5. 37.5 mg Phospho-enol-pyruvate
6. 50 µl Inorganic Pyrophosphatase (100 units ml^{-1})
7. 1 mg Rabbit skeletal pyruvate kinase
8. 1 ml 1 M Tris-HCl buffer pH 8.0
9. 0.5 ml 10 mM S-adenosyl methionine (fresh)
10. 5000 units Placental RNA-ase Inhibitor
11. 200–500 µCi[^{3}H] UTP

After warming the reaction mixture to 37°C, synthesis can be initiated by adding 1 M MgCl$_2$ to a final concentration of 10 mM. Synthesis is allowed to proceed with gentle stirring and its progress monitored by the removal of small aliquots (10 µl) at 1 h intervals and measuring the incorporation of [^{3}H] UTP into acid-insoluble material. After 4–6 h the synthesis reaction will stop but this is due to the exhaustion of enzyme substrates rather than inactivation of the virion transcriptase. Therefore after 5 h incubation viral cores can be collected by centrifugation (30,000 g, 4°C, 20 min), the mRNA containing supernatant removed and retained and the cores resuspended in fresh reaction mixture and a second cycle of synthesis allowed

to proceed for a further 5 h. This process can be continued for five or six cycles giving a very significant (several mg) yield of viral mRNA.

RNA-dependent RNA polymerase of VSV

The unmasking of this activity is achieved by disrupting the lipid containing envelope of the virus by treatment with neutral detergent in the presence of a reducing agent (Szilágyi and Pringle 1972).

Purified virus particles ($2 \times 10^{10} - 8 \times 10^{10}$) in 20 mM Tris-HCl buffer pH 8.0 are treated with 0.08% Triton N101 (Sigma Chemical Co.) and 7 mM B-ME in a final volume of 200 µl for 10 min at 0°C. Then 200 µl of polymerase reaction mix are added. This mix has the following constitution: 200 mM Tris-HCl buffer pH 8.0, 200 mM NaCl, 1.25 mM ATP, CTP and GTP, 0.125 mM UTP, 5 mCi [^{3}H] UTP and 32 mg ml^{-1} actinomycin D. After removing a 20 µl time 0 sample onto a Whatman 2.5 cm filter paper that is transferred immediately into cold 5% TCA containing 40 mM sodium pyrophosphate, the reaction is started by warming the mix to 37°C and adding 1 M MgCl$_2$ to a final concentration of 5 mM. Further 20 µl samples are then removed as before at 10 min intervals for 90 min. The collected samples are washed in cold 5% TCA containing 40 mM sodium pyrophosphate (twice), ethanol (twice) and ether (twice) and the incorporation of radioactivity into acid insoluble material measured by liquid scintillation counting.

Vaccinia virus DNA-dependent RNA polymerase

The activation step in this case involves treating purified virions (100 μg–1 mg) in 50 mM Tris-HCl buffer pH 8.5 with a neutral detergent (0.1% Triton-X-100) in the presence of a reducing agent (32 mM β-mercaptoethanol) at 20°C for 20 min in a reaction volume of 3 ml. The neutral detergent is removed by centrifuging the virus through a 20% sucrose cushion (1.75 ml) containing 50 mM Tris-HCl buffer pH 8.5, 5 mM dithiothreitol (DTT) at 25,000 rpm and 4°C in the Beckman SW 50.1 rotor for 30 min. The treated virus pellet (viral cores) obtained is resuspended in 0.3 ml of 50 mM Tris-HCl buffer pH 8.5, 5 mM DTT, 5% glycerol and 0.1 ml of polymerase reaction mixture added. The polymerase reaction mixture contains Tris-HCl buffer (200 mM), ATP (8 mM), GTP (4 mM), CTP (4 mM), UTP (0.4 mM), $[^3H]UTP$ (20 μCi ml^{-1}), Phospho-enol-pyruvate (30 mM) and rabbit skeletal pyruvate kinase (80 μg ml^{-1}). After removal of a time 0 sample (20 μl) the assay mixture is warmed to 37°C and the assay started by the addition of 1 M $MgCl_2$ to a final concentration of 7mM. Enzyme activity is followed by removing samples (20 μl) at 10 or 15 min intervals onto 2.5 cm Whatman filter disks which are transferred immediately to cold 5% TCA. At the end of the reaction the collected samples are washed in cold 5% TCA (twice), ethanol (twice) and ether (twice) before the incorporation of radioactivity into acid insoluble material is measured by liquid scintillation counting.

RNA-dependent DNA polymerase (reverse transcriptase) of HIV

The assay of reverse transcriptase (RT) normally makes use of an artifical exogenous template such as Poly rA:oligo dT_{12-18} rather than measuring activity on the endogenous virion template. Virus particles carrying the enzyme to be assayed are first concentrated from clarified tissue culture supernatants (centrifuged at 2000 rpm for 10 min to remove cells and large cellular debris) either by ultracentrifugation (100,000 g for 2 h) or if safety considerations do not allow this then by precipitation by polyethylene glycol (PEG).

PEG precipitation is carried out on 3 ml of culture supernatant by adding 1.5 ml of 30% PEG 8000 – 0.4 M NaCl, mixing well and leaving overnight at 4°C. The precipitated virus is collected by centrifugation at 800 g for 45 min. The virus pellet is resuspended in 150 μl of 25 mM Tris-HCl buffer pH 7.8, 0.25 mM EDTA, 0.025% Triton-X-100, 50% glycerol, 10 mM DTT, 100 mM KCl plus 75 μl of 0.9% Triton-X-100, 45 mM KCl. This buffer combination will disrupt the virus leading to both the unmasking of the RT activity and the inactivation of virus infectivity. Therefore all steps up to and including this resuspension should be carried out using a biohazard hood.

The assay involves setting up two parallel assays, one employing PolyrA:oligodT$_{12-18}$ and a second in which the exogenous template is PolydA:oligodT$_{12-18}$. The activity on the dA template represents nonspecific cellular polymerase activity and it is subtracted from the rA template value (which reflects the HIV specific RT activity) to obtain an accurate estimate of RT activity.

To carry out the assay 10 μl of the resuspended virus pellet is added to 90 μl of reaction mixture containing 40 mM Tris-HCl buffer pH 7.8, 8 mM DTT, 10 mM MgCl$_2$, 2.5 μCi[^{3}H] TTP, 5 mM NaCl and 0.05 units of either PolyrA:oligodT$_{12-18}$ or PolydA:oligo dT$_{12-18}$ template. Reactions are incubated at 37°C for 60 min after which time the reaction is placed on ice and 10 μl of t-RNA (10 mg ml^{-1}) followed by 1 ml of cold 10% TCA added to each tube to precipitate the reaction products. The precipitates are collected after 20–30 min of incubation on ice onto glass fibre filters. These are washed with cold 5% TCA and then 70% ethanol before being dried under a heat lamp and the acid insoluble radioactivity measured by liquid scintillation counting. After subtracting the dA template value from that obtained with the rA template the recommended cutoff value for clarified supernatants from primary cocultivation of HIV positive PBMC with HIV negative PBMC is 10,000 cpm ml^{-1}. If the clarified supernatant originates from an acute infection of continuous T cell lines or PBMC then a less stringent cut off value of 1000 cpm ml^{-1} can be taken to indicate a positive result. Obviously in dealing with HIV infected material care must be taken to adhere strictly to relevant safety regulations.

Viral polymerases found in infected cells

A major consideration in assaying this type of activity is that of ensuring that it is differentiated from contaminating cellular polymerases that will be present in the crude cellular extract often assayed. To illustrate the type of assay procedure that is followed for viral polymerases only found in infected cells two virus polymerases will be used, one from an RNA virus and one from a virus with a DNA genome.

Poliovirus RNA-dependent RNA polymerase

This activity is only expressed in virus-infected cells following translation of the + sense viral genome and is often termed the viral replicase. The realization that in copying the + sense genome the replicase must begin by synthesizing a poly U tract complementary to the poly A tract at the 3′ end of the genome led to the first assay protocol for poliovirus replicase, in which a poly U polymerase activity is assayed using exogenously added poly A template and an oligo U primer (Flanegan and Baltimore 1977a).

The first step in the assay procedure involves the preparation of a polymerase containing fraction from virus infected cells. For this 4×10^7 virus infected cells are collected by centrifugation at 3–6 h post infection, washed once in Earle's saline and resuspended in 2 ml of 10 mM Tris-HCl buffer pH 8.0–10 mM NaCl (TN buffer). A cytoplasmic extract is prepared from these cells by Dounce homogenization (40 strokes) and removal of nuclei and unlysed cells by centrifugation (5000 g, 4°C, 5 min). The viral polymerase is associated with membranes and can be concentrated by collecting the membrane fraction of the cytoplasmic extract by centrifugation (20,000 g, 4°C, 30 min). The polymerase activity is solubilized and endogenous RNA removed in a single step in which the membrane pellet is resuspended in 0.8 ml of TN buffer containing 1% Nonidet P-40, 0.5% sodium deoxycholate and 2 M LiCl. After 15 h at −20°C the precipitate containing both single stranded and replicative intermediate RNA is removed by centrifugation (17,000 g, 4°C, 15 min).

The supernatant obtained is dialysed for 20 h against TN buffer (2 changes) at 4°C. A final volume of approximately 1 ml of polymerase containing supernatant should be obtained from the 4 x 10^7 infected cells. The assay for poly U polymerase activity is set up in a final volume of 125 μl using 50 μl of dialysed polymerase fraction. The final reaction mixture contains the following: 50 mM Hepes buffer pH 8.0, 8 mM magnesium acetate, 10 μCi [^{3}H] UTP, 2.5 μg polyA, 1.25 μg oligo U$_{11-19}$, 4 mM phospho-enol-pyruvate, 0.3 units pyruvate kinase, and 1.25 μg actinomycin D. A 10 μl time 0 sample is removed onto a Whatman 2.5 cm filter disk which is transferred immediately to cold 5% TCA, the reaction is then warmed to 37°C and further samples taken at 10 min intervals for 1 h. The collected samples are then washed in cold 5% TCA (twice), ethanol (twice) and ether (twice) before measuring the incorporation of radioactivity into acid insoluble material by scintillation counting.

This polymerase activity can also be assayed using its natural template, i.e. poliovirus RNA (Flanegan and Baltimore 1977b). In this case the procedure is the same as for the poly U polymerase assay but the reaction conditions are somewhat modified such that the final reaction mixture has the following constitution:

42 mM hepes buffer pH 8.0, 7 mM magnesium acetate, 3 mM phosphoenol pyruvate, 0.3 units pyruvate kinase, 7 μM [^{3}H] UTP (5 × 10^4 cpm pmol^{-1}), 1 mM each of ATP, CTP, GTP, 8 mM DTT, 8 μg ml^{-1} actinomycin D, 150 μg ml^{-1} purified poliovirion RNA, and 6 μg ml^{-1} Oligo U$_{20}$. This assay is also normally carried out at 30°C as the enzyme gives a linear rate of UMP incorporation for a longer time at this temperature.

Herpes simplex virus (HSV) DNA-dependent DNA polymerase

The direct assay of viral DNA polymerase activities in infected cells is made difficult by the presence of cellular DNA polymerase activities. In the case of the HSV enzyme this problem can be circumvented to some degree by the use of high (150 mM) salt concentrations which inhibit most DNA polymerases but stimulate the HSV enzyme (Keir et al 1966). However in recent years the alternative approach that has been used for this and numerous other viral enzymes found in infected cells has been to exploit recombinant DNA technology to over-express the viral activity. Thus in the case of HSV-1 DNA polymerase it has been expressed in insect cells using a baculovirus recombinant (Marcy et al 1990). The enzyme can be assayed in a nuclear extract prepared from recombinant infected cells (24–36 hours p.i.).

The extract is prepared by first releasing nuclei from infected cells by Dounce homogenization (20–30 strokes). The nuclei are collected by centrifugation and resuspended in Buffer A (20 mM Hepes buffer pH 7.6, 0.5 mM DTT, 10 mM NaHSO$_3$, 0.5 mM PMSF, 2 μg ml^{-1} Leupeptin) and lysed by adding an equal volume of buffer A + 3.4 M NaCl. The lysed nuclei were then centrifuged at 100,000 g for 1 h and the resulting supernatant dialysed against Buffer A containing 10% glycerol and 0.5 mM EDTA. This dialysed extract is then used in enzyme assays. The assay measures the ability of the enzyme to carry out DNA synthesis on an 'activated' (i.e. high primer to template ratio) DNA template at high salt concentrations. The total reaction volume of 25 μl contains the following: 10 μl dialysed nuclear extract, 20 mM Tris-HCl buffer pH 7.5, 150 mM ammonium sulphate pH 7.5, 5% glycerol,

5 mM $MgCl_2$, 5 mM DTT, 2.5 µg activated calf thymus DNA (Sigma), 50 µM dATP, dGTP, dTTP, 5 µM dCTP, and 0.5 µCi[α-^{32}P] dCTP. The synthesis reaction is carried by incubation at 37°C for 30 min and stopped by the addition of 10 µl 0.25 M EDTA. 10 µl (twice) samples are spotted onto 2.5 cm Whatman DE81 filters which are washed in 0.5 M sodium phospate pH 7.0 four times, 80% ethanol and then 100% ethanol, allowed to dry and then radioactive incorporation measured by scintillation counting.

RNA modifying activities

These are concerned with making post transcriptional modifications to viral mRNA, i.e. 5′ RNA capping and 3′ polyadenylation.

5′ RNA capping activities

Two enzymatic activities are involved in the addition of the 5′ cap to mRNA. These are: a guanylyl transferase activity which actually adds the GTP residue to the 5′ end of the RNA through an unusual 5′–5′ phosphodiester linkage; and a methylase activity that adds methyl groups to the cap structure (Furuichi et al 1975; Cleveland et al 1986). In those viruses such as reovirus and vaccinia virus which replicate exclusively in the cytoplasm of the cell and hence cannot make use of cellular capping activities present in the nucleus, these activities are virion associated. Practically the simplest activity to assay for in connection with 5′ RNA capping is the methylase. The donor of methyl groups in the methylation reaction is S-adenosyl methionine and therefore methylase activity can be assayed simply by using [^{3}H] S-adenosyl methionine (100 µCi ml^{-1}) instead of labeled UTP in the transcriptase assays described above.

Vaccinia virus Poly A polymerase activity

This activity which is present in the virus particle (Kates and Beeson 1970) must be activated before being assayed and this is done by treating purified virions exactly as for assaying the virion associated DNA-dependent RNA polymerase.

The assay is then set up in a final volume of 100 µl in a reaction mixture that contains: vaccinia virus cores (50 µl), 50 mM Tris-HCl buffer pH 8.5, 10 mM β-ME, 5 mM $MgCl_2$, 20 µCi[^{3}H] ATP. After removing a 10 µl time 0 sample onto a Whatman 2.5 cm filter paper that is transferred immediately into cold 5% TCA, the reaction is started by transferring the reaction mixture from ice to 37°C and further samples are taken at 10 min intervals over 1 h of incubation. The collected samples are processed by washing in 5% TCA (twice), ethanol (twice) and ether (twice) before measuring the incorporation of ATP into acid insoluble material using scintillation counting.

Enzymes involved in nucleotide triphosphate biosynthesis

Several large DNA viruses, most notably herpes simplex virus and vaccinia virus, encode a thymidine kinase activity which is involved in the phosphorylation of thymidine to thymidine triphosphate. This activity is dispensible for virus growth in tissue culture but has been implicated in virus pathogenesis *in vivo*.

Herpes simplex virus thymidine kinase

As with all viral enzymes found only in infected cells, the major consideration in assaying this enzyme is establishing conditions that allow its activity to be differentiated from that of its cellular counterpart. In the case of the herpes simplex virus (HSV) enzyme this can be done because the viral enzyme is not subject to allosteric regulation and so its activity can be readily detected at high concentrations of TTP which inhibit the host enzyme (Preston 1977).

The assay can be carried out on an infected cell lysate. This can be prepared from a 90 mm plate of infected BHK cells (MOI = 20) at 7 h post infection by first scraping the cells into 1.5 ml of phosphate buffered saline and pelleting for 15 s in a microfuge. All subsequent steps are carried out on ice. The cell pellet is resuspended in 250 µl of extraction buffer (50 mM Tris-HCl buffer pH 7.5, 5 mM β-ME, 5 µM thymidine, 0.5% Nonidet P40) and incubated for 10 min. The extract is then microfuged for 1 min and the supernatant either used directly for enzyme assay or stored at −70°C for assay at a later time. The enzyme assay is set up in a final volume of 50 µl by mixing 25 µl of infected cell extract with 25 µl of a freshly made 2× reaction mix having the following constitution: 200 mM NaPO$_4$ buffer pH 6.0, 10 mM ATP, 20 mM MgCl$_2$, 200 µCi ml^{-1} [^{3}H] thymidine, 100 µM TTP. After 1 h of incubation at 31°C the reaction is terminated by adding 10 µl of 2 mM thymidine, heating to 100°C for 2 min and then microfuging for 1 min. 45 µl of the supernatant of this spin is spotted onto Whatman 2.5 cm DE81 filters and after drying these are washed for 5 min in 4 M ammonium formate pH 4.0 containing 10 µM thymidine (three times) at 37°C and then with ethanol (twice). After drying, the radioactivity incorporated into phosphorylated thymidine is measured by scintillation counting.

Enzymes concerned with viral protein processing/ modification

The extent to which any particular virus type needs to encode enzyme activities for post-translational processing/modification of its proteins is to some degree dependent on the replication strategy that its type of genome dictates. In a wide variety of viruses some or all of the protein information is initially translated into a polyprotein which must be co- or post translationally cleaved to give the final functional viral proteins. These cleavage events are in some cases carried out by cellular proteases but in many cases the virus encodes a protease or proteases to perform some of the required cleavages and such proteases represent the first of two major types of activity in this enzyme category. The initial type of viral protease assay relied on the ability of the enzyme specifically to cleave the appropriate viral precursor protein. These assays were in general laborious and not particularly quantitative since they normally involved the incubation of infected cell extracts with radioactive viral precursor (usually prepared by *in vitro* translation of the relevent viral information) and monitoring of precursor cleavage by polyacrylamide gel electrophoresis (PAGE) and autoradiography. This type of assay has now been largely replaced following the realization that viral proteases can usually be expressed from the relevant viral genetic information in active form in bacteria. Thus most viral proteases are now studied by first expressing the relevant viral gene at high level in *E. coli* and assaying the activity of the over expressed gene by its ability to cleave a short peptide carrying its specific cleavage site. An example

of this type of assay carried out on the HIV protease follows.

HIV protease

This enzyme is a member of the aspartic protease family and consequently has similarities to other members of the family such as pepsin. It has been expressed in an active form in *E. coli* using a variety of plasmid expression systems (Darke et al 1989; Ido et al 1991), all of which have in common an inducible promoter since high level expression of the enzyme is cytotoxic for the bacterium.

The over-expressed protein accumulates as inclusion bodies in the *E. coli*, therefore following induction of protease expression cells are lysed using a French press and the inclusion bodies collected by centrifugation (10,000 g, 10 min), resuspended in a buffer A (10 mM Tris-HCl buffer pH 8.0, 2 mM EDTA, 1 mM PMSF) containing 1% Triton-X-100 and pelleted as before. The inclusion bodies are dissolved by resuspending the pellet in 10 mM Tris-HCl buffer pH 7.5, 8 M urea, 10 mM DTT and filtered through a DEAE membrane. The denatured protease present in the filtrate is then acidified by the addition of 0.02 vol. of 10% TCA giving a final pH of 3.5 and then refolded either by dialysis overnight against 1 mM DTT, 10 mM sodium acetate buffer pH 3.5

or by rapid 10-fold dilution in the same buffer. This refolded material can be assayed for virus specific protease activity using a synthetic peptide whose sequence, SQNYPIVR, is based on the p17/p24 cleavage site found in the HIV Pr55^{gag} (Hanson et al 1988). The reaction is carried out by incubation for 30 min at 30°C in a final volume of 25 μl and contains 0.2 M NaCl, 1 mM DTT, 0.1% Triton-X-100 and 100 mM sodium acetate pH 5.5. Two approaches can be taken to measure cleavage of this short peptide at the correct site (Y-P). If non-radioactive peptide is used in the assay then fractionation and identification of the cleavage products can be done using HPLC on a C18 reverse phase column (SynChropak 4.6 × 250 mm, 5 μm) using gradient elution with 0–20% (v/v) in 0.1% trifluoroacetic acid and detecting the products by absorbance at 215 nm (Ido et al 1991). Alternatively the peptide can be acetylated at its amino terminus using [^{3}H] acetic anhydride and then cleaved in an enzyme assay (Kaplan et al 1994). If this second method is used then the reaction is terminated by the addition of Dowex X-50W-X4 (5% w/v) in 0.1M acetic acid, when the acetylated cleavage product is found in the supernatant and can be quantitated by liquid scintillation counting.

The second major class of viral enzymes concerned with protein processing/modification are protein kinases. A wide variety of viruses encode protein kinase activities which in some cases are associated with the virus particle and in others are only found in infected cells. Assays covering the two types of viral protein kinases will be described to illustrate the general principles of the assay protocols.

v-src tyrosine kinase activity of Rous sarcoma virus

The underlying strategy of this assay which is common to many aimed at measuring virus-specific tyrosine kinases is to use a viral kinase specific antibody to immunoprecipitate the protein from infected cell lysates and then carry out the actual kinase assay using the immunoprecipitate (Liebl et al 1992).

Therefore in this case, infected chick embryo fibroblasts from a 35 mm dish are lysed in 0.5 ml RIPA buffer (150 mM NaCl, 10 mM Tris-HCl buffer pH 7.5, 1 mM EDTA, 1% Nonidet P-40, 1% sodium deoxycholate, 0.5% SDS, 1 mM sodium orthovanadate, 100 μg ml^{-1} leupeptin, 20 μg ml^{-1} aprotinin) and clarified by centrifugation for 2 min at 14,000 g. 1 μl of ascitic fluid of anti-src monoclonal antibody (Mab 2-17 from Microbiological Associates, Bethesda, MD) is added to the supernatant and after 2 h of incubation at 4°C, the immune complexes are collected by adsorption for 45 min at 4°C to 20 μl of a 10% suspension of fixed *Staphylococcus aureus*. The adsorbed complexes are collected by centrifuging at 14,000 g for 2 min and washed (twice) in detergent wash buffer (150 mM NaCl, 10 mM Tris-HCl buffer pH 7.5, 1 mM EDTA, 0.5% Nonidet P-40, 1% sodium deoxycholate, 10 μg ml^{-1} leupeptin) before being resuspended in 60 μl of Buffer A (20 mM HEPES buffer pH 7.4, 5 mM MgCl$_2$, 5 mM MnCl$_2$). To quantitate the amount of pp60^{v-src} in the immunoprecipitate half of the material is run on an 7% SDS polyacrylamide gel (Laemmli discontinuous buffer system) and immunoblotted with Mab 2-17. The remaining half is re-pelleted and resuspended in 30 μl of Buffer A containing 1 μM [γ-^{32}P] ATP and 0.33 mg ml^{-1} acid-denatured enolase as kinase substrate. After 5 min of incubation at 30°C the reaction is terminated by the addition of 6 μl of 6× SDS gel sample buffer (1× = 2% SDS, 5% β-ME, 10% glycerol, 62.5 mM Tris-HCl buffer pH 6.8) containing 5 mM EDTA to prevent non-enzymatic tyrosine phosphorylation. The reactions are then boiled and fractionated on a 7% SDS polyacrylamide gel, the radiolabeled enolase band localized by autoradiography, excised, and digested overnight at 70°C in 0.75 ml of 30% hydrogen peroxide. The radioactivity incorporated and hence kinase activity are then measured by scintillation counting.

Herpesvirus seryl/threonyl protein kinase

Lytic infection of BHK cells with both pseudo-rabies virus and herpes simplex type 1 (HSV-1) have been shown to induce a new virus encoded seryl/threonyl protein kinase activity (Katan et al 1985; Purves et al 1986). As with other virus coded enzymes which have cellular homologues the major problem in specifically assaying the viral enzyme lies in differentiating it from the cellular activities. This can be most easily achieved in the case of these protein kinase activities by ion exchange chromatography of infected cell extracts. Therefore preparation of samples for specific assay of viral protein kinase activity involves the following:

Infected BHK cells (MOI 10–20) are harvested by scraping at 8 h post-infection in the case of pseudorabies virus or 18 h post-infection for HSV-1,

collected by centrifugation and resuspended in 50 mM Tris-HCl buffer pH 7.5, 10 mM KCl, 1.5 mM magnesium acetate, 1 mM PMSF, 10 μg ml^{-1} leupeptin. After incubation on ice for 10 min the cells are lysed by dounce homogenization (30–40 strokes) and then the ionic composition of the homogenate adjusted to 125 mM KCl, 5 mM magnesium acetate, 5 mM β-ME, 25 mM Tris-HCl buffer pH 7.5 and centrifuged at 30,000 g for 30 min. The post mitochondrial supernatant is then centrifuged at 165,000 g for 150 min to produce a post ribosomal supernatant. After overnight dialysis against 20 mM Tris-HCl buffer pH 7.5, 1 mM EDTA, 10 mM β-ME, 10% glycerol, this supernatant is loaded onto a DEAE-cellulose column equilibrated in the same buffer. For reasonable purification of the enzyme this column can be eluted with a 0–0.4 M gradient of KCl, but if only crude fractionation of the viral enzyme is required then cellular kinase contaminants can be removed by batch elution of the column with 0.2 M KCl and then the viral enzyme eluted with 0.4 M KCl. The viral enzyme is assayed using protamine sulphate as a substrate in a reaction mixture containing 20 mM Tris-HCl pH 7.4, 50 mM KCl, 10 mM MgCl$_2$, 10 mM β-ME, 0.1 mM ATP, 1 μCi [γ-^{32}P] ATP, 0.8 mg ml^{-1} protamine sulphate and 40 μl of column eluate in a final volume of 120 μl. After 30 min of incubation at 30°C, a 100 ml sample is taken onto Whatman 2.5 cm filter papers which are washed in 20% TCA (twice), 10% TCA (four times), ethanol (twice) and ether (twice) before being dried and radioactive incorporation into acid insoluble protein is measured by liquid scintillation counting.

Miscellaneous viral enzymes

The major enzyme activity in this category is the neuraminidase activity found as a component of ortho and paramyxoviruses which cleaves $\alpha(2–6)$- or $\alpha(2–3)$-ketosidic linkages between terminal sialic acid and adjacent galactose on glycoconjugates (Potier et al 1979; Woods et al 1993). It has been studied in greatest detail in influenza virus and the assay protocol that will be given is that for measuring the neuraminidase of influenza virus. It is a fluorimetric assay in which the fluoresence of the 4-methylumbelliferone liberated by cleavage of 2-{4-methylumbelliferyl}-a-D-N-acetylneuraminic acid is measured in a luminescence spectrometer.

The assay is carried out in microtitre plates (Dynatech MicroFLUOR). Virus is diluted in assay buffer (32.5 mM MES buffer pH 6.5, 4 mM $CaCl_2$) to 100 µl and serial 2× dilutions are made in the same buffer. The reaction is initiated by the addition of an equal volume of assay buffer containing 100 µM 2-{4-methylumbelliferyl}-α-D-N-acetylneuraminic acid and incubated at 37°C for 15 min with shaking. The reaction is terminated by the addition of 150 µl of 14 mM NaOH in 83% ethanol and the released 4-methylumbelliferone quantitated by fluorimetry in a luminescence spectrometer using an excitation wavelength of 365 nm and emission wavelength of 450 nm.

References

Baltimore D, Huang AS, Stampfer M (1970) Proc Natl Acad Sci USA 66: 522–526.

Cleveland DR, Zarbl H, Millward S (1986) J Virol 60 307–311.

Darke PL, Leu CT, Davis LJ, Heimbach JC, Diehl RE, Hill WS, Dixon RAF, Sigal IS (1989) J Biol Chem 264: 2307–2312.

Flanegan JB, Baltimore D (1977a) Proc Natl Acad Sci USA 74: 3677–36

Flanegan JB, Baltimore D (1977b) J Virol 29: 352–360.

Furuichi Y, Morgan M, Muthukrishnan S, Shatkin AJ (1975) Proc Natl Acad Sci USA 72: 362–366.

Hanson J, Billoh S, Schulze T, Suckrow S, Moelling K (1988) EMBO J 7: 1785–1791.

Ido E, Han HP, Kezdy FJ, Tang J (1991) J Biol Chem 266: 24359–24366.

Katan M, Stevely WS, Leader DP (1985) Eur J Biochem 152: 57–65.

Kates J, Beeson J (1970) J Mol Biol 50: 19–33.

Kates JR, McAuslan B (1967) Proc Natl Acad Sci USA 58: 134–141.

Keir HM, Subak-Sharpe J, Sheddon WIH, Watson DH, Wildy P (1966) Virology 30: 154–157.

Kaplan AH, Michael SF, Webbie RS, Knigge MF, Paula DA, Everitt L, Kempf DJ, Erickson JW, Swanstrom R (1994) Proc Natl Acad Sci USA 91: 5597–5601.

Liebl EC, England LJ, Dedue JE, Martin GS (1992) J Virol 66: 4315–4324.

Marcy AI, Olivo PD, Challberg MD (1990) Nucl Acids Res 18: 1207–1215.

McCrae MA (1985) Virology: A practical approach B.W.J. Mahy (Ed.) 151–169 IRL Press, Oxford.

Munyon WE, Paoletti E, Grace JT (1967) Proc Natl Acad Sci USA 58: 2280–2288.

Popovic M, Sarngadharan MG, Read E, Gallo RC (1984) Science 224: 497–500.

Potier ML, Mameli L, Belisle M, Dallaire L, Melancon SB (1979) Anal Biochem 94: 287–296.

Preston C (1977) J Virol 23: 455–460.

Purves FC, Katan M, Stevely WS, Leader DP (1986) J Gen Virol 67: 1049–1057.

Skehel JJ, Joklik WK (1969) Virology 39; 822–831.

Spira TJ, Bozeman LA, Holman RC, Warfield DT, Phillips SK, Feorino DM (1987) J Clin Microbiol 25: 97-99.

Szilágyi JF, Pringle CR (1972) J Mol Biol 71: 281–291.

Woods JM, Bethell RC, Coates JAV, Healy N, Hiscox SA, Pearson BA, Ryan DM, Ticehurst J, Tillings J, Walcott SM, Penn CR (1993) Antimicrob Ag Chemo 37: 1473–1479.

Section 3

Medical Virology

Initial *in vitro* screening of drug candidates for their potential antiviral activities

14

A. A. Al-Jabri
M. D. Wigg
J. S. Oxford

Recently chemotherapy of viral diseases has become a reality in clinical medicine. Remarkable progress has been made during the past decade in the development of new antiviral agents for the treatment of some common viral diseases. Preclinical evaluation of candidate agents for their antiviral activity *in vitro* with respect to both antiviral efficacy and cellular toxicity is the initial aim for antiviral drug development. Because of the existence of different viruses that grow in different cell lines, it is almost impossible to find a single specific antiviral test that can be applied for all viruses. For example, antiviral screening tests for inhibition of viruses that grow in cell suspension will differ from those growing in monolayer cell lines. As is the case in all biological assays, the exact concentration of an antiviral required to inhibit the replication of a virus will depend on the infectivity input of the virus, the cell type used, the duration of the experiment, the kinetic of infection in that particular cell type, and the sensitivity of the assay being used (Johnson 1991). As a practical illustration of these problems we note that studies on the assessment of antiviral agents vary greatly from one laboratory to another and it is often difficult to compare results reported by different laboratories (Holmes et al 1990).

In this chapter, we will describe the *in vitro* methods used in our own laboratories, for screening antiviral agents against HIV using cell suspension, and herpes simplex (HSV) and influenza viruses cultivated in monolayer cell lines. In addition we outline an assay for virucidal activity. These methods are not designed to identify the mechanisms of action of any compound. But the viruses chosen are the most commonly used in antiviral screening assays. The vast variety of other antiviral assays described in the literature are beyond the scope of this chapter and will not be reviewed here. Nor have we made any attempt to summarize tests which employ virus induced enzymes as specific targets (see Chapter 13). Such tests have the obvious advantage of specificity and ease of operation, but the inhibition will still have to be tested in the biological assays described herein. Fortunately the development of the MTT method

Virology Methods Manual
ISBN 0–12–465330–8

has provided a technique which can, with slighter modifications, be used for many virus cell combinations. The main prerequisite is that the virus should cause cell destruction. Finally it must be appreciated that antiviral chemotherapy is a very practical science and extremely commercial in its application. Thus candidate drugs have to be synthesized easily and cheaply, should have long storage lives and must be active at micromolar levels. No patient will swallow a 10 g tablet.

Evaluating the antiviral activity of a low number of candidate drugs with potential anti HIV-1 activity using cell suspension techniques

Note that specific national guidelines are enforced for category III laboratories which is a basic laboratory for safe cultivation of HIV-1. However, the most important factor is experience of the scientific staff who have been trained to handle life threatening pathogens in safety. The simplest category III laboratory would be equipped with class I (with hepair filter) and class II safety cabinets (with partially recirculating air flow) for culturing infected and uninfected cells respectively. A low speed centrifuge, an inverted microscope, a small autoclave, a CO_2 incubator and storage for frozen samples at 4°C, −20°C and −180°C (liquid nitrogen in gaseous phase) are other essential items. The virus is normally contained in plastic culture flasks which are themselves placed in sealed plastic boxes and these containers are opened only in the class I cabinet. The laboratory must have a clear protocol to explain procedures including waste disposal.

To illustrate our methodology we will use a compound X with potential anti HIV-1 activity. The weight of X, its solubility, chemical composition, and storage conditions should be recorded.

Materials and reagents

HIV-1 with known $TCID_{50}$, determined by prior titration in the cells to be used in the experiment protocol. Typically used laboratory strains of HIV-1 are RF, IIIB, and MN. Some of these viruses may have restrictions which only allow the virus to be used for non-commercial studies. In addition we often utilize a recent clinical isolate from an AIDS patient, since certain antivirals inhibit laboratory isolates but not clinical isolates.

H9 T-lymphoblastoid cell line, mycoplasma-free.
Azidothymidine (AZT) as a control antiviral compound.
Trypan blue (0.4%) (Sigma).
Haemocytometer.
96-well tissue culture plates (Falcon).
48-well tissue culture plates (Falcon).
CO_2 incubator.
Pipettes.
20 ml universal containers.
Cell culture medium, RPMI 1640 (Sigma).
RPMI 1640 complete growth medium (containing 10% heat, inactivated Fetal Bovine Serum, 50 IU ml^{-1} Penicillin, 50 µg ml^{-1} Streptomycin, 25 mm HEPES, and 2 mm L-Glutamine).
HIV-1 core p24 antigen assay (Coulter Corporation).
Empigen (Calbiochem-Novabiochem)
MTT (Sigma) 5 mg ml^{-1} in PBS.
0.04 N HCl in isopropanol.
Ordinary and inverted microscopes.
Centrifuge.
Gilson pipettes and tips.
Eppendorf pipetter.
ELISA plate reader.

Evaluation of cellular toxicity

1. Prepare H9 cells at a density of 2×10^5 cells ml^{-1} in complete growth

medium. Note that the viability of the H9 cells should be not less than 95% at the start.

2. Dispense 180 µl of cell suspension into wells of a flat bottomed 96-well tissue culture plate.

3. Prepare compound X (under sterile conditions) at 10× the desired final concentrations. For example, prepare the compound X at 10 mM then make 10-fold dilutions to 0.01 µM to give final concentrations of 1 mM to 0.001 µM in the test. It is always advisable to include higher concentrations when checking the cytotoxicity of the compound. AZT at 10× the desired final concentration should also be included as a positive control compound (concentration range of 1000 µM to 0.001 µM).

4. Add 20 µl of compound X in at least quadruplicate to give the final concentrations desired. Also utilize AZT as a control.

5. Incubate the plates at 37°C with 5% CO_2.

6. Check cell viability after 3, 5, 7, and 11 days, using the trypan blue exclusion method. Trypan blue stains only dead cells, while viable cells remain colourless. The test is robust, cheap and reliable.

7. Calculate the percentage of viable cells in each well, the mean and the time point for each individual concentration.

8. Plot the results as the percentage of viable cells versus the compound concentration at each time point and determine the toxicity of the compound X. A toxic compound will reduce the viable cell counts in a dose dependent fashion compared to a drug free control. An important point to remember is that certain drugs may have selective toxicity for certain other cells such as bone marrow cells and in this case the simple screen described above could give misleading results

when translated into a 'therapeutic index' in a patient.

Viral syncytium assay

This assay is cheap to perform and relatively rapid. It can be used to screen a compound library of 10–1000 compounds. However, some clinical virus isolates may not induce syncytia. The test is dependent upon viral replication and the consequence production of viral gp120 spike which mediates cell to cell fusion (syncytia formation). The syncytia are recognized using an inverted microscope and counted.

1. Compound X and AZT as a positive control are dispensed in the correct volume to give the desired final non-toxic concentrations of each compound. The dilutions of the drugs to be used will depend on the results of the toxicity testing above. Commonly the highest concentration of drug tested needs to be ten-fold less than the concentration which shows toxic effects.

2. Prepare H9 cells at a density of 2×10^5 cells ml^{-1} in complete growth medium. Dispense the cells at 180 µl per well into 96-well flat bottomed plates. Obviously, the number of plates used depends on the number of drugs under test and the desired different dilutions of the virus to be used. For example use HIV virus at 10, 100, and 1000 TCID$_{50}$ (tissue culture infectious dose 50%).

3. Add 20 µl of the appropriate virus dilution to each well of the plates leaving the last wells as controls free of compound X.

4. Observe and record syncytia formation and cytopathic effects (CPE) on days 3, 5, and 11 post-infection. Syncytia are multinucleated giant cells that can be seen as big ballooned cells directly in the wells of the plate (Fig. 14.1).

Initial *in vitro* screening of drug candidates

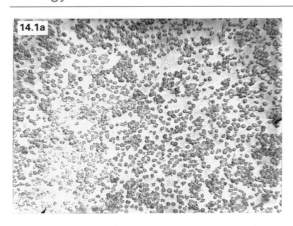
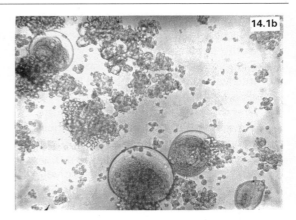

Figure 14.1. Cytopathic effects of HIV-1. (a) C8166 uninfected cells (day 5 in culture). (b) C8166 cells infected with HIV-1, MN isolate, at 1000 $TCID_{50}$ (day 6 post-infection), syncytia are shown as big multinucleated giant cells.

Evaluation of viral p24 core antigen levels

This assay is ELISA based and often scientists purchase commercial kits. The assay measures the release of HIV core p24 antigen from infected cells. It is exceedingly sensitive and also expensive. It can be used to detect replication of non-syncytium inducing viruses and can be automated for screening of 10–1000 compounds.

1. Prepare cells (H9) at a density of 1×10^6 ml^{-1} and add 450 µl of cells to 20 ml universal tubes labeled with the final desired concentration of the compound being tested.
2. Add 50 µl of 10× stock of the drug at the desired final concentration then incubate at 37°C for 30 min to allow for drug/cell equilibrium to be achieved.
3. Add 50 µl of the HIV isolate at 10, 100, 1000 $TCID_{50}$ to each of the universals at the different drug dilutions required including the controls.
4. Incubate for 3 h at 37°C.
5. Wash cells twice using 20 ml of RPMI 1640 by centrifuging at 1800 rpm (350 g). This step is important to remove any input virus which could be mistaken, subsequently, for newly replicated p24.
6. Resuspend the cells in each universal using 1.8 ml of complete growth medium.
7. Plate out cells in 48-well plates at 900 µl well^{-1} in duplicate, and add 100 µl of the 10× drug concentration to the appropriate wells.
8. Incubate plates at 37°C with daily inspection for CPE and syncytia formation.
9. Take samples of supernatants at days 3, 5, 7, and 11 after infection. Inactivate samples using 0.1% Empigen.
10. Determine the viral p24 antigen levels using a commercial, or 'in house', ELISA test (see below).
11. Plot the results as mean p24 production versus the compound concentration including the control drug used (e.g. AZT). A compound with anti HIV-1 activity will reduce or totally eliminate the subsequent production of the viral core p24 antigen (Fig. 14.2). By comparing the control drug AZT with X for the ability to inhibit p24 production and the levels of p24 in the presence or absence of X, a clear indication of the potential activity of X can be

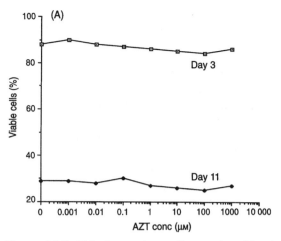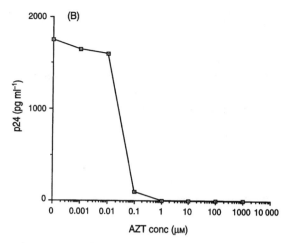

Figure 14.2. This figure shows the results of *in vitro* experiments on cellular toxicity and antiviral activity of Azidothymidine (AZT), as a positive control, in PBMCs using a clinical isolate of HIV-1. Toxicity of AZT after 3 and 11 days post-infection (A) and AZT versus HIV-1, 5 days post-infection (B).

established. A single word of caution here, however, is that exceeding low concentrations of AZT cause an apparent total inhibition of viral p24 antigen in the test, giving a therapeutic index in excess of 10,000. However, when this *in vitro* result is translated into the practical clinical use of AZT as a drug in HIV infected patients the therapeutic index drops to approximately 10.

'In House' ELISA for HIV-1 p24

Materials

Purified sheep anti p24 (D7320, Aalto Bioreagents)
96 well ELISA plates (Greiner, 655001)
Plate covers (ICN Flow 77–400–05)
TBS (25 mM tris-(hydroxymethyl) aminomethane, 144 mM sodium chloride, pH 7.4)
PBS (10 mM phosphate, 137 mM sodium chloride, 2.7 mM potassium chloride, pH 7.4)
Tween-20
Empigen (Calbiochem-Novabiochem)
Azide
Bovine serum albumin (BSA) (Sigma)
Baculovirus derived recombinant p24 antigen (MRC-ADP 620)

Biotinylated monoclonal antibody to p24 (MRC-ADP 454) [EH12]
Streptavadin-POD conjugate (Boehringer 500 U/ml)
Substrate [o-Phenylenediamine Dihydrochloride (OPD) tablets, Sigma P7288]
Substrate buffer [Phosphate Citrate buffer (50 mM sodium phosphate, 20 mM citric acid, pH 5.0)]
H_2O_2
3 M sulphuric acid
ELISA plate reader

Method

1. Coat ELISA plates with 100 µl of D7320 antibody (10 µg/ml) diluted in PBS. Leave plates overnight at room temperature in a moist chamber.
2. Wash plates 3 times with TBS and block with 2% BSA in TBS for 1 h at room temperature (200 µl/well). Aspirate solution from wells of plates and leave to dry at room temperature.
3. Prepare a standard curve (100 to 0.1 ng) using viral p24 antigen (MRC-ADP 620) in GM containing 0.1% Empigen, 0.02% azide. Add samples in triplicate (100 µl/well) as well as standard curve

in duplicate. Seal plates using plate covers.

5. Incubate plates at room temperature overnight in a moist chamber.

6. Wash plates 6 times with 300 µl/well TBS and tap plate on dry paper to remove excess fluid.

7. Add 100 µl/well EH12 diluted 1/1000 in TBS containing 2% BSA, 0.05% tween 20 and incubate at room temperature for 2 h.

8. Repeat step 6.

9. Add Streptavadin-POD conjugate at 100 µl/well (5 µl of streptavadin-POD conjugate at 250 U/ml in 10 ml TBS containing 2% BSA, 0.05% tween 20). Incubate for 1 h at room temperature.

10. Repeat step 6 and add substrate in substrate buffer containing 0.01% H_2O_2 (100 µl/well) and incubate for 15–30 min at room temperature.

11. Stop reaction with 3 M sulphuric acid (50 µl/well) and using an 'ELISA plate reader' read plates at OD 492.

Evaluating the anti-HIV activity of high numbers of candidate drugs

Colorimetric MTT (tetrazolium salt) assay

(Schwartz et al 1988; Pauwels et al 1988)

This simple colorimetric test was first widely used in HIV studies but variations have been applied to herpes and influenza. It has the potential advantage of automation, allowing a high throughput of antiviral drugs to be screened in excess of 10,000 drugs. Tetrazolium salt MTT {3-(4,5-dimethylthiazol-2-yl)-2,5-diphenyltetrazolium bromide} assay, described here, is a variation of the procedure of Mossman (1983).

1. Add 100 µl of cells at a concentration of 3×10^4 cells ml^{-1} to a 96-well plate.
2. Add 50 µl of complete growth medium with or without drug to be tested at the appropriate concentration.
3. Incubate for 2 h at 37°C in a 5% CO_2 incubator to allow drug-cell equilibration to be achieved.
4. Add 100 µl of virus at 2.5×10^3 infectious particles per ml.
5. After 7 and 10 days, resuspend the cells and remove 100 µl of cell suspension for the MTT assay.
6. Replace the wells with fresh medium, plus and minus drug, to obtain a final volume of 250 µl per well.
7. All assays should be carried out in triplicate. Add 10 µl of 5 mg ml^{-1} MTT in PBS to all microwells containing 100 µl of sample.
8. Incubate for 4 h at 37°C in a 5% CO_2 incubator.
9. Remove the supernatant and add 150 µl of acid-isopropanol (0.04 N HCl in isopropanol).
10. Mix thoroughly to dissolve the dark blue crystals.
11. Incubate for a few minutes at room temperature ensuring that all blue crystals are dissolved.
12. Read the plate in an ELISA reader using a wavelength of 540 nm.
13. Cells treated with drug but not infected with HIV are used to determine drug toxicity.
14. The anti-HIV activity of the drug is determined at nontoxic concentrations by calculating the infected–uninfected cell absorbency rates.
15. AZT should be included as a positive control.

Comments (high and low numbers of drugs)

1. Cell lines such as C8166, CEM and JM can be used instead of or as well as H9 cells. PBMCs in log phase growth can also be used in screening for potential anti HIV-1 activity, but usually only for special screening with restricted numbers of drugs.
2. The above procedures can be applied also when screening for anti HIV-2 candidates.
3. Active compounds should have the following characteristics: high potency with at least 50% inhibition of viral p24 antigen in the culture supernatants, at low drug

concentrations, as compared to a drug free control. The drug should obviously have low toxicity and the results should be reproducible.

4. H9, CEM, MT4, U937 cells as well as others can be used in the MTT assay.

5. Reverse transcriptase (RT) activity in the supernatant fluids can also be used as another method for the evaluation of antiviral replication.

6. *The Therapeutic Index* (TI) for each compound is calculated as follows: TI = Maximum nontoxic concentration/Minimum antiviral concentration. The higher the TI, the higher the compounds antiviral activity (AZT has a TI of >1000).

7. We recommend the use of the more economic 'in house' ELISA for large scale screening of samples when using cell lines with laboratory adapted strains. The more sensitive and expensive commercial ELISA (Coulter) should be used to confirm results expecially when using clinical isolates and PBMC, since clinical isolates may not replicate as highly as laboratory adapted strains.

8. If compounds show antiviral activity when tested as single compound (as above), it might be of interest to test more than one compound in combination to determine if a higher potency, or true synergy, could be achieved when, for example, testing two compounds together. The same methodology as that described above is applied, but the reader is referred to recent publications because interpretation of the data may not be simple.

Initial screening of compounds with potential virucidal activity for HIV

A simple and relatively rapid protocol for the initial screening of virucidal activity is described below. Given the dearth of highly effective clinical inhibitors of HIV, attention has moved to a more prosaic approach via destruction of virus particles or inhibition of virus attachment at the earliest stage of virus entry. Given that future infections with HIV will be mainly heterosexual, then such compounds must be applied to the vagina before or immediately after intercourse. Moreover, virucides could be applied for the disinfection of the birth canal as an approach to control mother-to-child HIV infection. Such a novel virucide should be colourless, odourless, with no toxicity and side effects, and most importantly be accepted by females. The non-ionic detergent nonoxynol-9 has been used as a spermicide but preliminary clinical trials have shown that over-use of the compound as a virucide could increase the incidence of HIV transmission by causing damage to the cells lining the reproductive tract and hence augmenting viral entry and enhancing infection. Hence an effective virucide should inactivate virus immediately on contact and have no concommitant effect on the membrane of mammalian cells. It is still not clear at present whether such compounds can be discovered. As described for the screening of anti HIV-1 activity, any compound to be screened for its potential virucidal activity should be prepared in a solution under sterile conditions. The concentration of the compound, its solubility, and its chemical composition should be recorded. An extra requirement is a preparation of infective HIV at high titre in excess of 10^7 $TCID_{50}$ ml^{-1}. In this way after the virucidal test *per se* the drug can be removed by simple dilution and residual virus detected by infectivity end-point titration in susceptible cells.

Preliminary cytotoxicity test for the virucide

1. Using a 96-well tissue culture plate, add 180 µl of H9 cells at a concentration of 2×10^5 cells ml^{-1} to each well.
2. Prepare the compound at the desired initial concentration in growth medium.
3. Add 20 µl of the compound, at the initial concentration, to the first 6 wells of the plate.
4. Make 10-fold dilutions across the plate and leaving the last row as a cell control by adding 20 µl of growth medium to each well in the last row.
5. Incubate the plate at 37°C for one week.
6. Count cells using the trypan blue method described above after the addition of the compound, 24 h, 3, 5, and 7 days later.
7. Determine the cytotoxicity of the compound.

Virucidal test

1. To a 96-well tissue culture plate add 180 µl of H9 cells at a concentration of 2×10^5 cells ml^{-1} to each well.
2. Prepare:
(A) 200 µl of virus at high titre + 200 µl

of compound Y (with potential virucidal activity).

(B) 200 μl of virus at high titre + 200 μl of complete growth medium as a control.

3. Incubate (A) and (B) for 10 min at 37°C.
4. Add 20 μl of (A) to each of the first six wells of the plate (from well A1 to A6) and 20 μl of (B) to each of the next 6 wells (from well A6 to A12), mix well, then make 10-fold dilutions using separate pipettes for each dilution moving down the plate and leaving the last row (H1–H12) as cell control. In this way an infectivity end-point can be determined for residual virus.
5. Incubate the plate at 37°C and 5% CO_2.
6. Record the cytopathic effects on days 3, 5, 7, and 11.
7. Compare the cytopathic effects, including syncytia formation, of the virus with and without Y, and hence determine whether any infective virus survived the contact with the drug.

Comments

1. The spermicidal detergent nonoxynol-9 can be used as a positive control. This compound has been shown to have detectable anti-HIV activity (Malkovsky et al 1988).
2. A different scale of time can be used and, for example, the virucidal effects can be recorded after only seconds contact with virus.
3. Different cell lines and PBMCs can be used to compare the cytotoxicity as well as virucidal activity of the compound being tested.

Virological screening of drug candidates against herpes simplex and influenza viruses

While new developments in HIV continue to dominate antiviral research, herpesviruses, in the widest sense, remain a very important target for the design and application of improved antiviral chemotherapy (Field 1994). Both HSV and influenza viruses have unique enzymes such as herpes DNA polymerase, nucleotide reductase, thymidine kinase, or influenza RNA replicase or neuraminidase which may be used in screening assays. However, in all these cases a vital assay is whether the new drug inhibits virus replication in cell culture. Furthermore, for both herpes and influenza there are well developed animal model systems for later evaluation of new drugs. In the case of influenza both the mouse pneumonia model and the classical ferret respiratory infection model are used (Oxford et al 1994). There are several well investigated animal models of herpesvirus such as the infection in the hairless mouse and genital infection of guinea-pigs. In essence the screening methods used for HSV and influenza are similar to those used for anti-HIV drugs. In practice the viruses are easier and faster to handle in a category II laboratory. However, scientific personnel must be well trained in avoidance of cross infection. For example, recently isolated strains of influenza, particularly those passaged briefly in mammalian cells, may be infectious and could in extreme cases trigger an epidemic. As with HIV, careful thought should be given to the virus to be used in the screening test. For influenza it is particularly important to discover drugs to inhibit both types A and B. For herpes, drugs are required to inhibit HSV type 1 and 2 as well as varicella-zoster virus (VZV).

Materials and reagents

24-well tissue culture plates.
Maintenance medium (MM): Eagle's Minimum Essential Medium (Sigma) containing 50 IU ml^{-1} Penicillin, 50 μg ml^{-1} Streptomycin and 2 mM L-Glutamine.
Trypsin/EDTA (Sigma).
Trypan blue 0.4% (Sigma).
Haemocytometer.
Gilson pipette (100 μl) and sterile tips.
5 and 10 ml pipettes.
Ordinary and inverted microscopes.
CO_2 incubator.
Different concentrations of the drug to be tested.
Falcon 96-well plates (herpes simplex).
25-cm^2 Falcon cell culture flasks (Influenza).
Phosphate buffered saline (PBS).
0.05% trypsin (Worthington) prepared in PBS.
Virus.
Drug test and drug positive control.
Eppendorf pipetter (0.5 and 2.5 ml).
Tubes for drug and virus dilution.
MTT (Sigma) 5 mg ml^{-1} in PBS.
10% SDS + 0.01 N HCl.
ELISA plate reader.

Toxicity assay for cells cultivated in monolayers

It must be clearly acknowledged that the cyto-toxicity assay can only give an approximate estimation of potential toxicity. For example, only one out of a thousand potential drugs selected in this way will later proceed to *in vivo* testing in animals. The remaining 999 drugs will be discarded because of unacceptable toxicity in other cells such as those in the gut, kidney, brain, skin, or the white blood progenitor cells. Yet more drugs will have unacceptable, surprising, and unpredictable toxicities in animals or patients.

1. Add 1 ml of cell suspension at a concentration of 2×10^5 cells ml^{-1} to a 24-well tissue culture plate.
2. Incubate at 37°C for 48 h.
3. Discard the growth medium and wash the cells using PBS.
4. Add a range of at least five different concentrations of the candidate antiviral agent to six wells per concentration, and leave six more wells with no drug as the cell control.
5. Incubate for three days at 37°C.
6. Daily, trypsinise two wells containing each concentration of the drug and two wells with no drug and count the viable cells using the trypan blue exclusion method described above.
7. Calculate the mean and then the percentage reduction of the viable cell count compared with the cell count in the drug free control cultures. The drug concentration required to reduce the viable cell count by 50% is called the CyD_{50} (Hu & Hsiung 1989).

Antiviral assays for herpes virus

Cytopathic end-point assay (low numbers of drugs to be screened)

1. Add 100 µl of a HEp-2 or Vero cell suspension at a concentration of 2×10^5 cells ml^{-1} to each well of a 96-well plate.
2. After 48 h at 37°C in an incubator with 5% CO_2 (when the monolayer is confluent), discard the growth medium and wash the cells using PBS.
3. Add 100 µl of each concentration of the drug to be tested to 4 wells. The drug should be diluted in MM. Keep 4 wells with no drug and add MM to the cells (virus control). Also keep two wells for each concentration of the drug with no virus.
4. Incubate for 60 min at 37°C for equilibration to be achieved of drugs and cells.
5. Add 10 µl of 100 $TCID_{50}$ of virus to all wells containing different concentrations of the drug and to the 4 wells of the virus control.
6. Incubate at 37°C in a 5% CO_2 incubator.
7. Observe daily, under the inverted microscope, until all the quadruplicate cultures in the virus control wells show CPE. The time required for visual observation of the culture obviously limits the number of drugs which can be tested simultaneously. The 50% effective dose (ED_{50}) of the antiviral agent is expressed as the concentration that inhibits CPE in half of the quadruplicate test cultures (Hu and Hsiung 1989). Acyclovir (ACV) is included as a positive control drug for HSV-1. Gancyclovir or Foscarnet may

be used as a positive control drug for Cytomegalovirus (CMV).

MTT assay (high number of drugs to be screened)

(Takeuchi et al 1991)

1. Add 100 µl of cells at concentration of 2×10^5 cells ml^{-1} to a 96-well plate. Suitable cells are L929 or MRC-5.
2. Incubate for 48 h at 37°C in a 5% CO_2 incubator.
3. Wash the cells using PBS.
4. Add 100 µl of MM with or without drug to be tested at the appropriate concentration.
5. Incubate for 60 min at 37°C.
6. Add 10 µl of 100 TCID$_{50}$ of virus to all wells containing different concentrations of the drug and to the control wells with no drug.
7. Incubate the plates for three days at 37°C in a 5% CO_2 incubator.
8. Add 10 µl of 5 mg ml^{-1} MTT in PBS to all wells.
9. Incubate for 4 h at 37°C in a 5% CO_2 incubator.
10. Add 100 µl of 10% SDS + 0.01 N HCl in distilled water.
11. Mix and incubate overnight.
12. Read the plates using ELISA reader at a wavelength of 540 nm.

Screening antiviral agents against influenza virus

Although influenza virus was first isolated in the embryonated hens egg, nowadays, at least for antiviral screening, the egg has been replaced by cell culture systems. Moreover, in many countries a specific animal license is now required before eggs, which have a developing embryo at midterm, can be inoculated and subsequently killed. Cultivating influenza virus in cell culture requires the addition of trypsin to the medium while evaluation of virus growth is performed most simply using the haemagglutination (HA) test to detect virus in the supernatant fluids. 96-well plates may be used in screening antiviral agents (Nagai et al 1990), but here we describe the assay using 25 cm^2 Falcon cell culture flasks which is applicable to investigation involving low number of compounds. The general principle is, however, the same for both methods. We should note that for high input screening a modification of the MTT method can be used.

1. Add 5 ml of MDCK cell suspension at a concentration of 2×10^5 cells ml^{-1} to each flask.
2. Incubate for 48 h at 37°C in an incubator containing 5% CO_2.
3. Discard the growth medium and wash the monolayer using PBS.
4. Add 5 ml of each of the different concentrations of the drug to be tested containing 2.5 μg ml^{-1} trypsin to two flasks per drug concentration.
5. Keep two flasks with only MM and trypsin and no drug (virus and trypsin control). Also keep one flask with only MM (cell control).
6. Incubate at 37°C for 60 min to allow cell-drug equilibration.
7. Add 500 μl of influenza virus diluted at 1:100 (concentration of the stock approximately equal to 128 HA units and 10^5 ID$_{50}$) to half of the flasks containing the different concentrations of the drug and to the virus control. After 1 h at 37°C, wash to remove excess virus, add further drugs and reincubate the cultures.
8. Incubate at 37°C for 5 days.
9. Include amantadine hydrochloride (25 μg ml^{-1}) as a positive control drug for influenza A virus and Ribavirin for influenza A and B viruses.
10. Take out daily aliquots of 50 μl of medium and measure the quantity of virus by the HA test.
11. Compare the HA titres in the drug treated and untreated flasks. A difference of 4-fold or more between the HA titre of the treated and untreated cultures is considered as significant inhibition.

Haemagglutination (HA) assay

Materials

V bottomed 96 well plates
Turkey RBC at 0.5% v/v in PBS
Sterile PBS

Method

1. Add 50 μl of PBS into each well of the plate.
2. Make serial two fold dilutions of the samples.

3. Add 50 μl of 0.5% washed RBC into each well.
4. Incubate the plate at room temperature for 1 h and read the agglutination patterns and hence calculate the HA titre.

Comments

1. For each virus-cell system described above, the Therapeutic Index is expressed as the ratio:

$$\text{Therapeutic index (TI)} = CyD_{50}/ED_{50}$$

where CyD_{50} is the maximum drug concentration which causes cytotoxic effects in 50% of the cultured cells and ED_{50} is the minimum drug concentration which is effective to inhibit virus induced cytopathic changes by 50%.

2. All procedures described here are general methods to screen new drugs and they are useful to select candidates for their potential antiviral activity. After the initial selection, other methods can be used to study the mechanism of action of the active compounds.

3. Importantly XTT is a more soluble compound and can substitute MTT in this assay (Weislow et al 1989).

4. The Therapeutic Index calculated using the cell culture data is an *in vitro* parameter and obviously can not be correlated to the index *in vivo* or in the patients. Although it is reassuring to have a high TI at the commencement, drugs with a low *in vitro* TI, should not be discarded since, like the tortoise in the 'Tortoise and the Hare' tale, although starting with disadvantages, they may yet win the race and become effective antivirals in humans.

References

Field H (1994) Int Antiv News 2: 81.

Holmes HC, Mahmood N, Karpas A, Petrik J, Kinchington D, O'Conner T, Jeffries DJ, Desmyter J, De Clercq E, Pauwels R, Hay A (1990) Antiviral Chem & Chemother 2 (5): 287–293.

Hu JM, Hsiung GD (1989) Antiviral Res 11: 217–232.

Johnson VA (1991) Techniques in HIV Research. Stockton Press, USA pp 223–237.

Malkovsky M, Newell A, Dalgleish AG (1988) Lancet 1: 645.

Mossman T (1983) J Immunol Methods 65: 55–63.

Nagai T, Miyaichi Y, Tomimori T, Suzuki Y, Yamada H (1990) Chem Pham Bull 38: 1329–1332.

Oxford JS, Zuckerman MA, Race E, Dourmashkin R, Broadhurst K, Sutton PM (1994). Antiviral Chem & Chemother 5 (3): 176–181.

Pauwels R, Balzarini J, Baba M, Snoeck R, Scholes D, Herdewijin P, Desyter J, De Clercq E (1988) J Virol Meth 20: 309–321.

Schwartz O, Henin Y, Marechal V, Montagnier L (1988) AIDS Res Human Retrov 4 (6): 441–448.

Takeuchi M, Babo M, Shigeta S (1991) J Virol Meth 33: 61–71.

Weislow O, Kiser R, Fine DL, Bader J, Shoemaker RH, Boyd MR (1989) J Natl Cancer Inst 81: 577–586.

Detection of virus and viral antigens

15

S. Specter
D. Jeffries

The ability of the physician to manage a variety of viral infections either through chemotherapy or other manipulation of the patient has made rapid viral diagnosis a necessity. The development of sophisticated technology to detect viruses or viral antigens in specimens obtained from patients has made rapid viral diagnosis a reality in most types of infections. Rapid viral diagnosis is here defined as the ability to identify a virus in a clinical sample within 48 hours and in some cases within 1 hour. The key to effective viral diagnosis is properly collecting a specimen(s) from an appropriate site(s), transporting the specimen under the proper handling conditions, and using appropriate methods to process and detect the virus. It is important to note that the majority of false negative samples result from errors in handling of the specimen before it reaches the laboratory. Thus, it is vital for health care professionals to understand appropriate methods for the handling of specimens to be tested for detection of viruses. These methods are outlined in this chapter. However, it is important to recognize that different institutions have procedures that may vary from general recommendations and that over time recommendations are likely to change. Therefore, those unfamiliar with the procedures of the particular laboratory to which they will be submitting specimens should communicate with the laboratory on a regular basis to insure the highest quality of the specimens they are submitting, until such time as they are familiar with the appropriate procedures to follow.

Virology Methods Manual
ISBN 0–12–465330–8

Specimen collection

Correct specimen collection requires selection of the best body sites for obtaining virus, begins with the use of sterile implements, is enhanced by collecting the specimen as early in the course of infection as is practical, and is completed by transporting the specimen to the laboratory as rapidly as possible. Remember also that generally, the greater the number of cells collected in a specimen the higher the probability that a virus can be isolated and/or identified.

Specimen selection

The selection of appropriate specimens is based on both the clinical presentation and suspected virus(es) associated with the disease. Although several viruses may cause the same disease signs and symptoms the specimens required for their detection usually are the same. Occasionally infections may, however, require specimens from different sites for different viruses causing similar symptoms (e.g. central nervous system [CNS] infections).

Timing of collection

It is best to collect specimens for viral detection as early as possible in the acute stages of infection. While virus may be detected in specimens sometimes for weeks after onset of disease, the duration of viral shedding varies greatly depending on the virus, the host and the course of infection. Respiratory viruses may be shed for only a few days during upper respiratory tract infection but may be present for a month or longer if the lower respiratory tract becomes infected. Virus from vesicular lesions is readily obtained while there is fluid in the lesion but becomes more difficult to detect once the lesion dries out. Thus, it is often important to collect specimens for viral detection very early in infection and store them

if viruses are low on the differential diagnosis. Specimens should be stored at 4°C (refrigerated) for up to five days in most cases, thereafter storage should be at −70°C. Certain viruses are labile, e.g. RSV, and when they are suspected, specimens should be frozen (−70°C) immediately after collection. Specimen storage is discussed further on page 316. It is far easier to discard an unneeded specimen than to try to detect virus later in infection when the viral titer might be significantly reduced.

Viruses may be shed from individuals for long periods of time under certain circumstances. Adenovirus, cytomegalovirus (CMV), enteroviruses and rubella may be shed for months or years in asymptomatic individuals. Individuals with chronic diseases due to viruses like hepatitis B virus (HBV), hepatitis C virus (HCV), and human immunodeficiency virus (HIV) also may shed virus for long periods of time. Additionally, those with reactivated latent viruses such as herpes simplex virus (HSV) or varicella-zoster virus (VZV) may shed virus sporadically throughout their lifetime. Thus, it is vitally important in these cases to associate virus shedding with onset of disease symptoms in order to make an etiologic association of virus and disease. By contrast, immunocompromised individuals may shed viruses as a result of their immune system's failure to control infection. In these cases it becomes important to determine if the virus is the cause of symptoms or the result of progressing disease that has induced their replication. Thus, the fact that a particular virus has been isolated from a patient is not nearly so important to the interpretation of etiology as are the circumstances of infection, regarding disease progression, specimen source, etc.

Types of specimens

Throat and nasopharynx

Washings or aspirates of the throat and naso-pharynx are usually more useful than swabs of these areas for performing virus isolation in cell cultures. For respiratory syncytial virus (RSV) especially, nasopharyngeal aspirates generally yield better diagnosis (Ahluwalia et al 1987). By contrast, it is often easier to collect a nasal swab because the patient accepts this method more readily and it is more conveni-ent for medical personnel that are responsible for collection of the specimen. In addition, direct detection of virus using fluorescent anti-body is preferred using swabs. The nasal wash is discouraged for direct detection of most respiratory viruses, since it often contains deb-ris, mucus, red or white blood cells, or squa-mous cells (Blumenfeld et al 1984; Kim et al 1983).

In young children however, Frayha et al (1989) reported that nasopharyngeal aspi-rates and swabs were equally effective for the diagnosis of respiratory viruses. When swabs are collected, it is best to collect one nasopharyngeal and one throat swab. When comparing yield from swabs of different loca-tions, nasopharyngeal swabs are more likely to yield a positive specimen for influenza viruses, parainfluenza viruses and RSV, while throat swabs are better for recovering adenoviruses, enteroviruses and HSV (Wiedbrauk and John-ston 1993). Nasal swabs or washes are best for recovering rhinoviruses.

Sputum

The value of sputum as a source for viral infections of the lower respiratory tract is unclear. Also, one must be wary of contamina-tion by organisms in the throat. Thus, sputum is not usually a preferred specimen for diag-nosis of viral infections. However, Kimball et al (1983) reported that 20% of patients with radi-ologically proven pneumonias yielded virus when isolation was performed. In this study both influenza A virus and RSV were isolated from sputum in association with disease, lead-ing the authors to conclude that this is a useful specimen for diagnosis of viral infection of the lower respiratory tract. Unfortunately, this study did not compare sputum to other meth-ods of specimen collection, such as throat washings or bronchoalveolar lavage (BAL). Nevertheless, BAL samples are generally con-sidered to be superior to sputum for lower respiratory tract infections.

Bronchoalveolar lavage

Bronchoalveolar lavage is a preferred alterna-tive to open lung biopsy for the collection of specimens for rapid viral diagnosis. Martin and Smith (1986) have shown this to be especially useful for CMV infections. Using a broncho-scope it is possible to identify localized lesions in the lower respiratory tract and to wash the involved area with saline to retrieve infected cells. Specimens can be examined for direct detection or placed into cell culture. The value of this procedure is noted in a study at the Mayo Clinic, where 71 of 80 specimens yielded CMV, while parainfluenza, influenza, and enterovirus also were detected in a few specimens (Smith 1992).

Stool and rectal swab

Stools or rectal swabs can be especially useful when submitted for diagnosis of infections due to enteroviruses. This specimen is especially useful when submitted in addition to cere-brospinal fluid (CSF) for the diagnosis of CNS disease. In fact, it is often easier to isolate virus from the gastrointestinal tract than the CSF in cases of aseptic meningitis, which is caused most frequently by enteroviruses. However, recovery of an enterovirus from the stool is not always proof that it is the etiologic agent of the current infection, since these viruses are frequently isolated from the gut of healthy individuals.

The use of fecal material for diagnosis of cases of viral gastroenteritis is limited by the fact that many of the viruses (rotavirus, enteric adenoviruses, Norwalk agent, other small round viruses) that are responsible for this are not readily cultured. However, stool specimens can be useful for detection of gastrointestinal viruses if electron microscopy is to be performed. Another problem is that enteroviruses and reoviruses are as often isolated from fecal material of healthy individuals as they are from patients with gastrointestinal disorders. The use of stool specimens is preferred over rectal swabs, since more fecal material can be obtained, when testing for viral gastroenteritis is performed (Mintz and Drew 1980). However, it should be noted that during acute disease patients may have difficulty producing a stool. In these situations it is reasonable to collect a fecal sample as soon as possible, rather that awaiting a stool sample, as long as the swab contains fecal material. Nucleic acid probes for the detection of enteroviruses (Romero and Rotbart 1993), enteric adenoviruses (Krajden et al 1990) and perhaps others may make detection of viruses from fecal material more useful in the near future.

CMV can be recovered in stool and is especially important to detect in the G.I. tract in immunocompromised individuals, usually using direct detection (Drew 1988). By contrast, enveloped viruses are not easily isolated in cell cultures from fecal material.

Urine

Recovery of viruses from urine is relatively common. This is accomplished during clinically apparent infections by adenovirus, CMV and mumps and many other viruses are present in urine during their incubation period. The best time to collect specimens for detection of virus is from the first morning urine sample, since materials are more concentrated at this time. Recovery of CMV from urine of perinatally infected infants and mumps virus from urine of individuals with

encephalitis are especially important since they may be the only sites yielding virus at times. In the case of CMV, the virus is in relatively low titer and may be directly inoculated into standard cell culture; however, for enhanced detection in shell vials low speed centrifugation is often helpful (Lee and Balfour 1977; Lipson et al 1990). The detection of CMV by nucleic acid probes requires centrifugation in order to concentrate the virus (Landini et al 1990). It must be noted that CMV can be isolated from multiple sites, with urine usually being the best. However, at times urine might be negative when throat swabs/washes are positive and vaginal secretions may be positive when urine is negative in pregnant women. Thus, obtaining specimens from several sites for routine CMV detection is recommended.

Blood

Blood is a useful specimen for certain infections that are in the acute phase or in chronic diseases. Enteroviruses are generally cell free in blood, whereas CMV, Epstein-Barr virus (EBV), HIV, human herpes viruses 6 (HHV-6) and 7 (HHV-7), HSV, measles, rubella and VZV are mostly cell associated. Specific separation of leukocytes by differential centrifugation is recommended as compared to the use of a buffy coat for the isolation of CMV or VZV (Paya et al 1988). Detection of CMV antigen in blood is one of the earliest predictors of active infection, which is so important to detect early in immunocompromised patients. Cell-free CMV may also be detected in plasma or serum but this is frequently defective virus, so direct detection is superior to virus isolation in such cases. The clinical significance of this cell-free CMV is not yet clear.

Cerebrospinal fluid and other sterile body fluids

Cerebrospinal fluid is a useful specimen for detection of viruses in association with

meningitis but is less so in patients with encephalopathies. Most commonly non-polio enteroviruses (67–80% of samples in which virus is detected) are detected in CSF but HSV 2 may be detected in cases of meningitis (Rubin 1983). The overall rate of virus positive CSF specimens associated with clinical disease is about 4% (Wilden and Chonmaitree 1987). While these viruses can be isolated from CSF, more recent attempts using nucleic acid hybridization have proven useful (Romero and Rotbart 1993; Rowley et al 1990) and the polymerase chain reaction (PCR) has been used to detect HSV DNA (Rowley et al 1990). Other less common isolates from CSF in CNS infections include adenovirus, CMV and VZV in immunocompromised hosts. Although togaviruses, flaviviruses and a variety of other arboviruses are associated with CNS disease they are not readily detected from CSF and generally require serology for detection.

Other sterile body fluids, e.g. pericardial, pleural, synovial, may also be tested for the presence of viruses. Like CSF, virus is usually present in low concentration in these fluids and should not be diluted before inoculation into tissue culture.

Ocular

The majority of positive specimens from eyes exhibiting keratoconjunctivitis yield HSV or adenoviruses, with the former present about twice as often (Chastel et al 1988; Claoué et al 1988; Smith 1984). In addition, enteroviruses can be isolated in cases of hemorrhagic conjunctivitis (Pal et al 1983) or pharyngoconjunctivitis. More recently, CMV has been detected in cases of retinitis in immunocompromised hosts, especially in AIDS patients (Henderly et al 1987). In neonates, ocular infections may be seen in the context of generalized disease and accompany dermatologic manifestations due to rubella, VZV or HPV (Lambert et al 1989; Naghashfar et al 1986). *Chlamydia trachomatis* (bacteria that are frequently detected in virology labs) must also be considered in conjunctivitis in newborns. Usually, a swab is obtained from the palpebral conjunctiva but corneal scrapings may be required when there is keratoconjunctivitis. The latter should be collected by an ophthalmologist or other well trained personnel.

Dermal lesions

The agents most commonly recovered from dermal lesions include the viruses that cause vesicular lesions, HSV and VZV (Smith 1992). Coxsackieviruses type A and other enteroviruses are also obtained but to a much lesser extent. When lesions are in the form of unopened vesicles or pustules virus is recovered nearly 90% of the time; however, when lesions become crusty or dry out this is reduced to about 25% success (Moseby et al 1981). Direct examination of these specimens by histologic or immunologic staining techniques also reveals that materials from closed vesicles yield cells in which viral antigens or inclusions are more easily observed.

Tissues containing human papillomaviruses (HPV) also can be used to detect virus but this generally requires nucleic acid hybridization.

Solid tissue

Autopsy or biopsy specimens are useful in the diagnosis of a variety of viral infections. Autopsy specimens are complicated by decline in viral titers after death and the increase in the levels of bacteria. Thus, postmortem specimens should be collected quickly after death. The most useful specimens for isolation of virus from solid tissues are lung, respiratory tract tissue and brain. Infrequently, liver or spleen may yield CMV or HSV. The recovery rate of viruses from tissue in one study was about 4% (Smith 1983) and even in the best of circumstances (CMV isolated from open lung biopsy of immunocompromised individuals) is generally below 10%. Isolation of viruses from tissue is hampered by the release of viral inhibitors from tissue upon homogenization. Shope et al (1972) demonstrated that isolation can be improved if enzymatic digestion is used instead of homogenization. More recently, the use of sectioning formaldehyde fixed, paraffin embedded tissue, *in situ* hybridization or the PCR and nucleic acid probes have resulted in the detection of HPV, adenovirus and others in a variety of tissues (Jiwa et al 1989; Shibata et al 1988; Telenti et al 1990).

Specimen transport

A serious problem in the isolation of viruses is the loss of infectivity suffered from the time the specimen is collected until it reaches the laboratory. Viral titers are negatively affected by time in transit, temperature, pH, the type of protein in the sample, the amount of virus present and how much the sample is disturbed (shaken) in transit. It is therefore critical to understand the appropriate conditions for transporting the specimens to the laboratory.

Virus stability

Naked (non-enveloped) virus, such as adeno-viruses and enteroviruses are generally very stable and are readily transported to the laboratory without much loss of infectivity. By contrast enveloped viruses, such as herpes-viruses, influenza viruses and paramyxo-viruses and rubella, are labile and quickly lose infectivity if not properly protected. Since it is not possible to determine which virus a specimen will contain when it is collected, all specimens for virologic examination must be treated as if they contain labile virus. Thus, specimens should be rapidly transported to the laboratory in a sterile container placed in wet ice and stored at 4°C until inoculated into cell culture. For transport to a remote labora-tory, specimens can be held at 4°C for up to 48 h without much loss of infectivity (Levin et al 1984). It is not advisable to freeze speci-mens for transport to the laboratory; CMV is especially labile if frozen at −20°C. If speci-mens must be transported for longer than 48 h, then freezing at −70°C and shipping in dry ice is advised. RSV is a particularly labile virus and inoculation into tissue culture is recommended as soon as possible. In several institutions respiratory specimens are inocu-lated into cell culture directly from the patient at the bedside. While this is perhaps extreme, it underscores the concern for the lability of this virus.

Transport materials

Swabs

The most common specimen submitted to the virus laboratory for isolation or direct detection is the swab. Smith and Wold (1991) report that nearly two-thirds of submitted specimens in one year were swabs. These can be collected from nasopharynx, throat, rectum, skin lesions and conjunctiva. Swab tips used for collection may be comprised of cotton, dacron, rayon or polyester but *not calcium alginate*, as it is toxic to HSV (Wiedbrauk and Johnston 1993). An aluminum shafted swab should be used as materials used to treat the wood in some swabs may be toxic to viruses and *Chlamydia*.

Other specimens

Sterile, leak-proof containers should be used for the submission of body fluids. Specimens should be submitted as collected and not diluted in transport medium. Blood or bone marrow should be collected in tubes contain-ing an anti-coagulant (preservative free heparin or EDTA), transported to the labora-tory at room temperature and processed as soon as possible (within 8 h).

Media

The use of appropriate transport medium will greatly facilitate the ability of the laboratory to isolate virus from clinical specimens. Such media are comprised of balanced salt solu-tion, D-glucose and often a small amount of protein (bovine serum albumin, serum, gelatin or lactalbumin hydrolysate) to help stabilize the virus, they also contain antibiotics and a buffer to maintain neutral pH. More common media

Detection of virus and viral antigens

for viral transport include Stuart's medium, Hanks' balanced salt solution, Leibovitz-Emory medium and sucrose–phosphate–glutamate, used with or without added protein. Comparative studies of the different media are limited and have not provided conclusive results as to which medium is most effective at maintaining virus titer (Smith 1992).

Transport media commonly used for diagnostic virology

Hanks' balanced salt solution with gelatin

Hank's balanced salt solution (100 ml)
Gelatin (0.5 g)
Autoclave at 15 lb pressure for 15 min. Before use add antibiotics to desired concentration and dispense in aliquots in screw-capped containers (2–3 ml). Store at 4°C.

Veal infusion broth with gelatin

Veal infusion broth (25 g)
Phenol red (0.5%) (0.4 ml)
Distilled water (100.0 ml)
Autoclave as above. After cooling add 0.5 g bovine serum albumin and filter to sterilize (0.45 μM filter). Before use add antibiotics to desired concentration, aliquot and store as above.

Buffered tryptose phosphate broth with gelatin

Tryptose phosphate broth (2.95 g)
$NaH_2PO_4H_2O$ (0.08 g)
$Na_2HPO_47H_2O$ (2.06 g)
Gelatin (0.5 g)
Phenol red (0.5%) (0.4 ml)
Distilled water (100.0 ml)
Autoclave, add antibiotics, aliquot and store as above.

Transport systems

The earliest transport systems for submitting specimens to the virology laboratory were systems originally designed for submission of samples for bacteriologic studies. The Culturette (Becton Dickinson Microbiology Systems, Cockeysville, MD) has been used by virus labs for more than 20 years. This consists of a sterile rayon tipped swab in a plastic tube containing an ampule of modified Stuart's transport medium. More recent systems include the Virocult (Medical Wire and Equipment Co., Cleveland, OH), Microtest M4 TM (Microtest, Inc., Snellville, GA) and Amplicor TM (Roche Diagnostics, NJ), which was designed for samples submitted for PCR assays. M4 is an example of a universal transport medium that is useful for maintenance of specimens submitted for isolation of viruses, *Chlamydia*, and other microorganisms. In a recent study it was also shown to be highly effective for samples submitted for PCR assay (Salmon et al 1994).

Specimen storage

Storage of viruses for short periods of time, up to 5 days, should be at 4°C, as there is less loss of infectivity at this temperature compared to room temperature or freezing. HSV has been shown to retain 90% of titer for up to 30 days at this temperature, whereas even one freeze–thaw cycle reduced titer by 2 log_{10}. Thus, for short term storage 4°C is recommended (Gleaves et al 1994). By contrast, storage for stable viruses (adenoviruses, enteroviruses, HSV) for long periods of time should be at −70°C using a stabilizing medium (Johnson 1990) and labile viruses, such as RSV or VZV, are better maintained if freeze dried in stabilizing medium (Gallo et al 1989; Gleaves et al 1994; Tannock et al 1982).

Specimen processing

Inoculation

Standard tissue culture

A variety of cell lines may be used for diagnosis of viral infections, the particular cell lines used for any sample is determined by the specimen source and the types of virus(es) suspected (Specter and Lancz 1992; Wiedbrauk and Johnston 1993) (also see Chapters 1 & 2). Regardless, a normal inoculum of 0.2–0.3 ml is generally used. Prior to inoculation maintenance medium is removed from the cells and then the inoculum is added for a period of 1–2 h to allow the virus particles to adsorb to the cells. The cells are then washed free of any non-absorbed material and placed in fresh medium for daily examination for evidence of infection. When the inoculum is a body fluid, such as urine, it can be added directly to cells. However, in some instances the fluid may contain toxic substances which require dilution of the fluid prior to inoculation. In addition, some fluids, as well as fecal material and homogenized tissues suspended in balanced salt solution, will require low speed centrifugation (2000–3000 g) to remove debris. For inoculation of cell culture with specimens suspected of containing RSV, direct inoculation at the bedside has enhanced isolation rates. Hall and Douglas (1975) report that this could increase viral titers by 500-fold compared to transport to the laboratory (average time held at 4°C was 3 h). By contrast, another study showed no significant difference in isolation rate between bedside and laboratory inoculation (Bromberg et al 1984).

The choice of whether or not the laboratory should produce their own tubes of cells or purchase them commercially is a personal one. It is dependent on the technician time available, the number of specimens tested by the laboratory and the commercial availability of consistently good quality cell cultures.

Shell vials

Enhanced cell culture can be performed in dram vials (shell vials) containing a coverslip, as first described by Gleaves et al (1984) for the detection of CMV. By this method cells from which medium has been removed are inoculated with 0.2 ml of sample and then the vial is spun in a centrifuge at 700 g for 1 h, medium is added back and vials are incubated for 16–48 h depending on the virus. At this time cells may be treated with antibodies, specific for the suspected virus(es), that are labeled with an enzyme or fluorescein tag. This method often has resulted in viral detection many days sooner than standard cell culture. Shell vials are used in the detection of CMV, HSV, influenza virus, RSV, adenovirus and an expanding number of other viruses. The main limitation to the variety of viruses to be tested in this manner is the availability of reagents to detect viruses that are present. The spectrum of viruses to be detected in this manner is likely to be expanded as newer monoclonal antibodies and nucleic acid probes are developed. Shell vial culture should be supplemented with standard culture when low virus titers are suspected or other viruses for which shell vial culture is not effective may be present in the specimen.

Hen's eggs

The use of eggs for detection of viruses has been replaced for the most part by cell culture. Chicken eggs are useful for growing influenza and mumps viruses in the amniotic sac and the chorioallantoic membrane can be used to culture HSV and poxviruses (Hsiung 1994); however, use of eggs is mainly limited to production of vaccines since cell culture is routinely used to detect these viruses.

Animals

Inoculation of suckling mice for the detection of coxsackievirus types A and B and for togaviruses in suspected CNS infections is currently the only routine use of animals in diagnostic virology (Hsiung 1994). This approach is hardly used any more as most of these viruses can be cultured in tissue culture (Landry et al 1987; Schmidt et al 1975; Shope and Sather 1979). Use of animal inoculation should be limited to laboratories with personnel experienced in this technique.

Direct antigen detection

The direct detection of viral antigens in clinical specimens allows for rapid diagnosis of infection, sometimes resulting in detection within minutes of specimen collection. Most frequently this is accomplished using fluorescein isothiocyanate labeled antibodies but can be accomplished using enzyme labeled antibody, radiolabeled antibody or using antibodies labeled in another manner (Fig. 15.1). In addition to antigen detection, virus can be detected in specimens using nucleic acid hybridization, electron microscopy, or by cytopathologic examination of cells for inclusion bodies, which are described elsewhere in this volume. Selection of the method to use is often a matter of preference of the laboratory but can be influenced by the availability of reagents to perform the test.

The key to effective antigen detection is the acquisition of a good specimen containing intact cells. This is because the detection of virus is dependent upon both the presence of reactive material and its distribution within the cells. Furthermore the assays must be performed by experienced technologists to assure quality results.

In addition to the classical laboratory techniques there are newer methods by which rapid diagnosis of viral infections using viral antigens is accomplished. Using ELISA technology commercial concerns have developed kits for rapid detection in which the antibody is

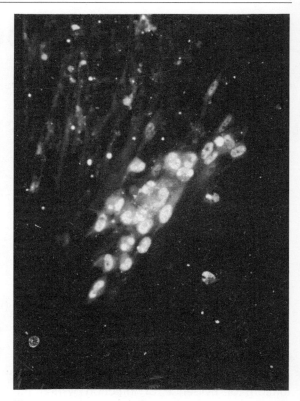

Figure 15.1. Immunofluorescence. The example shown is a focus of varicella zoster virus replicating in human embryo fibroblasts; stained with fluorescein-labelled monoclonal antibody using a fluorescence microscope.

bound to a solid state in a pattern to denote the presence of virus. The Becton Dickinson Directigen kits can be used to detect either Influenza A or RSV in this way. A negative test yields a small purple dot to denote that the test was properly performed, whereas a positive specimen yields a purple triangle. A specimen (e.g. a nasal wash) is appropriately diluted, poured through the self-contained reagent and membrane filter, and this is followed by the stepwise addition of several reagents and wash buffers which ultimately yield the colorimetric reaction that is readily observed. The Abbott Test-Pack is another example of this technology with the exception that the test yields a (−) line for a negative and a (+) plus sign for a positive result. These tests can be performed within a period of 30 min or less. Other viruses that can be detected using these types of membrane immunoassays include HSV and rotavirus (Smith 1992).

More sophisticated technology, such as the Biomerieux Vitek Vidas system, is based on fluorescence technology and is available for detection of adenovirus, CMV, HSV and other antigens. The specimen is placed into the machine with the appropriate reagents and the other steps are performed automatically with results available within a few hours.

The latter tests described here have the advantage of simplicity and/or automation and therefore require less training of technologists, and performance requires less technician time. However, for specimens for which there is not a clear cut result, care must be taken to have specimens examined further by skilled personnel.

Method to detect respiratory syncytial virus by immunofluorescence in nasopharyngeal aspirates

1. Add 20 ml phosphate buffered saline (PBS) to the specimen.
2. Mix thoroughly to disperse any mucus.
3. Centrifuge 1000–1200 rpm for 10 min (Chilspin 2 MSE centrifuge).

4. Discard the supernatant and resuspend pellet in 1–2 drops PBS.
5. Add 15–20 µl of cell suspension to required number of spots on a microscope slide.
6. Air dry (36°C).
7. Fix in acetone for 10 min.
8. Add 7–10 µl of fluorescein labeled RSV monoclonal antibody.
9. Incubate in a moist chamber (36°C) for 15 min.
10. Remove monoclonal antibody with PBS using a wash bottle.
11. Wash in fresh PBS for 5 min.
12. Air dry.
13. Add a few drops of mounting fluid.
14. Place coverslip on slide.
15. Examine using a UV microscope.

Examination of specimens

Cytopathic examination (CPE)

The examination of cell cultures using microscopy is necessary to determine the extent of the changes in cells induced by virus infection (Figs. 15.2 and 15.3). Generally, standard cell

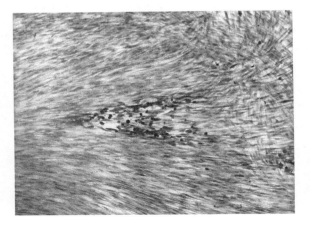

Figure 15.2. The cytopathic effect of cytomegalovirus in human embryo fibroblasts.

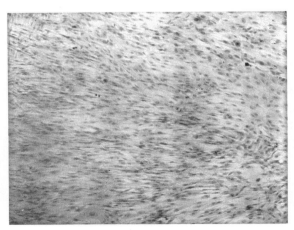

Figure 15.3. The uninfected control cells.

Detection of virus and viral antigens

cultures are examined using an inverted phase contrast microscope, with the 10× to 40× objective used to observe distinctive CPE. Since this is not always a reliable way to identify the infecting virus the use of labeled antibodies to tag the infected cells has become popular. Thus, more rapid diagnosis can be accomplished by combining the techniques of cell culture and antigen detection.

In addition to observation of CPE, cells may be used in a variety of other detection techniques including hemadsorption (Fig. 15.4), neutralization and interference assays (Hughes 1993; Specter and Lancz 1992) (see p. 33).

Antigen detection

The utilization of shell vials and centrifugation to enhance infection of cell cultures has speeded up detection of virus by combining infection and detection of virus using labeled antibodies (Gleaves et al 1994). Shell vials are now routinely used for detection of CMV, HSV, adenovirus, influenza and some additional viruses. Most antibodies are enzyme- or FITC-labeled for use in this assay. Detection of virus in most cases occurs in 1–2 days, often well before cytopathogenic effects can be seen. Thus this method has led to more rapid diagnosis in most cases, as compared to standard cell culture.

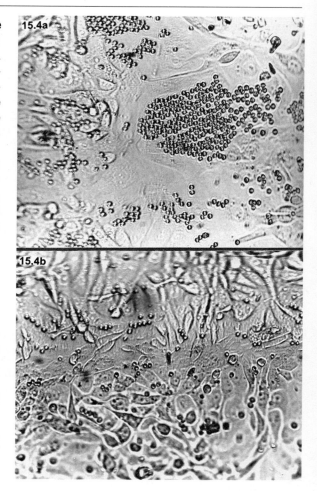

Figure 15.4. Hemadsorption. (a) shows hemadsorption in primary monkey cells infected with parainfluenza virus type 1. Guinea pig blood cells are firmly adherent to the infected tissue culture cells. (b) shows an uninfected culture with non-adherent red blood cells.

Summary

The rapid and effective diagnosis of virus infections has evolved as a most useful tool in the management of many virally induced diseases. This success is dependent upon the acquisition of appropriate specimens, their proper transport to the laboratory and continually evolving technology. The key to using these resources effectively is the establishment of excellent communications channels between health care professionals and the laboratory.

References

Ahluwalia G, Embree J, McNicol P, Law B, Hammond GW (1987) J Clin Microbiol 25: 763–767.

Blumenfeld W, Wager E, Hadley WK (1984) Am J Clin Pathol 81: 1–5.

Bromberg K, Daidone B, Clarke L, Sierra M (1984) J Clin Microbiol 20: 123–124.

Chastel C, Adrian T, Demazure M, Legrand-Quillien MC, Lejune B, Colin J, Wigand R (1988) J Med Virol 24: 199–204.

Claoué CMP, Ménage MJ, Easty DL (1988) Brit J Ophthalmol 72: 530–533.

Drew L (1988) J Infect Dis 158: 449–456.

Frayha H, Castriciano S, Mahony J, Chernesky M (1989) J Clin Microbiol 27: 1387–1389.

Gallo D, Klimpton JS, Johnson PJ (1989) J Clin Microbiol 27: 88–90.

Gleaves CA, Hodinka RL, Johnston SLG, Swierkosz EM (1994) Cumitech 15A Baron EJ (Coordinating Ed.) Am Soc Microbiol, Washington D.C.

Gleaves CA, Smith TF, Shuster EA, Pearson GR (1984) J Clin Microbiol 19: 917–919.

Hall CB, Douglas RG Jr (1975) J Infect Dis 131: 1–5.

Henderley DE, Freeman WR, Smith RE, Causey D, Rao NA (1987) Am J Ophthalmol 103: 316–320.

Hsiung GD (1994) Diagnostic Virology, 3rd Ed. Yale University Press, New Haven.

Hughes JH (1993) Clin Microbiol Rev 6: 150–175.

Jiwa NM, Raap AK, van de Rijke FM, Mulder A, Weening JJ, Zwaan FE, The TH, van der Ploeg M (1989) J Clin Pathol 42: 749–754.

Johnson FB (1990) Clin Microbiol Rev 3: 120–131.

Kim HW, Wyatt RG, Fernie BF, Brandt CD, Arrobio JO, Jeffries BC, Parrott RH (1983) J Clin Microbiol 18: 1399–1404.

Kimball AM, Foy HM, Cooney MK, Allan ID, Mattock M, Plorde JJ (1983) J Infect Dis 147: 181–184.

Krajden M, Brown M, Petrasek A, Middleton PJ (1990) Pediatr Infect Dis 9: 636–641.

Lambert SR, Taylor D, Kriss A, Holzel H, Heard S (1989) Am J Ophthalmol 107: 52–56.

Landini MP, Trevisani B, Guan MX, Ripalti A, Lazzarotto T, La Placa M (1990) J Clin Lab Anal 4: 161–164.

Landry ML, Fong CKY, Neddermann K, Solomon L, Hsiung GD (1987) Am J Med 83: 555–559.

Lee MS, Balfour HH Jr (1977) Transplantation 24: 228–230.

Levin MJ, Leventhal S, Master HA (1984) J Clin Microbiol 19: 880–883.

Lipson SM, Costello P, Forlenza S, Agins B, Szabo K (1990) Curr Microbiol 20: 39–42.

Martin WJ II, Smith TF (1986) J Clin Microbiol 23: 1006–1008.

Mintz L, Drew WL (1980) Am J Clin Pathol 74: 324–326.

Moseby RC, Corey L, Benjamin D, Winters C, Remington MI (1981) J Clin Microbiol 13: 913–918.

Naghashfar Z, McDonnell PJ, McDonnell JM, Green WR, Shah KV (1986) Arch Ophthalmol 104: 1814–1815.

Pal SR, Szucs GY, Melnick JL (1983) Intervirology 20: 19–22.

Paya CV, Wold AD, Smith TF (1988) J Clin Microbiol 26: 2031–2033.

Romero JR, Rotbart HA (1993) In: Diagnostic Molecular Microbiology: Principles and Applications, Persing DH, Smith TF, Tenover FC, White TJ, (Eds) ASM Press, Washington D.C. pp 401–406.

Rowley AH, Whiteley RJ, Lakeman FD, Wolinsky SM (1990) Lancet 1: 440–441.

Rubin SJ (1983) Am J Med 75: 124–128.

Salmon VC, Kenyon BR, Overall JC Jr, Anderson R (1994) Abstr 10th Ann Clin Virol Symp p 33.

Schmidt NH, Ho HH, Lennette EH (1975) J Clin Microbiol 2: 183–185.

Shibata DK, Arnheim N, Martin WJ (1988) J Exp Med 167: 225–230.

Shope RE, Sather GE (1979) Arboviruses. In: Diagnostic Procedures for Viral, Rickettsial and Chlamydial Infections. Lennette EH, Schmidt NH (Eds) Am Public Health Assoc, Washington D.C.

Shope TC, Klein-Robbenhaar J, Miller G (1972) J Infect Dis 125: 542–544.

Smith TF (1983) Med Clin North Am 67: 935–951.

Smith TF (1984) Postgrad Med 75: 215–223.

Smith TF (1992) Specimen requirements: selection, collection, transport and processing.: Clinical Virology Manual 2nd Edition, Specter S, Lancz G (Eds) Elsevier Science Publishers, New York, pp 19–41.

Smith TF, Wold AD (1991) Changing trends of diagnostic virology in a tertiary care medical center. In: Medical Virology X. de la Maza LM, Peterson EM (Eds) Elsevier Science Publishers, New York, pp 1–16.

Specter S, Lancz G (Eds) (1992) Clinical Virology Manual, Elsevier Science Publishers, New York.

Tannock GA, Hierholzer JC, Bryce DA, Chee C-F, Paul JA (1982) J Clin Microbiol 25: 1769–1771.

Telenti A, Aksamit AJ Jr, Proper J, Smith TF (1990) J Infect Dis 162: 858–861.

Wiedbrauk DL, Johnston SLG (1993) Manual of Clinical Virology, Raven Press, New York, 273 pp.

Wilden S, Chonmaitree T (1987) Am J Dis Child 141: 454–457.

Chapter 15

Detection of viral nucleic acids in clinical material

16

J. B. Mahony

Techniques for the detection of viral nucleic acid have evolved from techniques developed by bacterial geneticists almost three decades ago. The principles of nucleic acid hybridization are based on the biochemical properties of DNA and RNA in physiological solutions and were first elucidated by biochemists studying the reassociation kinetics of double stranded DNA using liquid hybridization and *Cot* curves. The major parameters affecting the kinetics and fidelity of hybridization are salt concentration, solvent, temperature, complexity of nucleic acid, probe concentration and post-hybridization stringency washing. Few virologists using DNA hybridization today realize that commonly used hybridization conditions are based on the following rule – the hybridization of a nick translation labeled double stranded DNA probe should be allowed to proceed for a time sufficient to enable the probe in solution to achieve $3 \times Cot_{\frac{1}{2}}$ at which time most of the probe will be present in hybrid or duplex form where the $Cot_{\frac{1}{2}}$ (half-renaturation) is determined by the volume of the reaction volume, the base sequence complexity of the probe and the concentration of probe. Other important points include the following: (1) the use of single stranded cDNA probes shortens the hybridization time since the lack of a competing DNA strand in solution favours hybridization of the probe DNA to the target DNA, and (2) dextran sulphate is used to accelerate the rate of reassociation of nucleic acids by excluding nucleic acids from the volume of the solution occupied by the polymer and effectively increasing the concentration of the probe and the rate of reassociation by up to 10-fold. Hybridization fidelity is generally provided by using stringent washing conditions usually achieved by a combination of high temperature (5°C below the melting temperature [Tm] of the hybrid) together with low salt concentration. The temperature and salt conditions can be determined empirically, although this is rarely done any more. The Tm of oligonucleotide probes or PCR primers can be approximated using the formula:

$$Tm = (A + T) + 2 \times (G + C).$$

Virology Methods Manual
ISBN 0–12–465330–8

Specimens

Viral nucleic acids can be detected in a wide range of clinical specimens using a variety of hybridization and amplification techniques. Blood, CSF, urine, bronchoalveolar lavage (BAL) and other body fluids can be tested by filter paper hybridization with viral probes after nucleic acids have been extracted and purified. These specimens also lend themselves to *in situ* hybridization using cytocentrifugation. Solid tissues usually obtained at biopsy or post mortem can be processed for either filter paper hybridization by extracting nucleic acids or by *in situ* hybridization by cutting sections of fresh frozen tissue on a cryostat or paraffin preserved tissue on a microtome. Clinical specimens may be also examined for specific viral nucleic acids using amplification techniques including polymerase chain reaction (PCR), ligase chain reaction (LCR), or other methods such as Q-beta replicase, or transcription-based amplification systems. PCR and LCR can also be performed *in situ* on cells or tissue sections on microscope slides.

Materials and reagents

TE Buffer

10 mM Tris-Cl, pH 7.4, 0.1 mM EDTA.

Chaos Buffer

For 100 ml combine the following: 50 g GuSCN (4.2 M), 2.5 ml 20% Sarkosyl, 1.25 ml 2 M Tris HCl pH 8.0, dH$_2$O to 99.7 ml and filter these 0.45 μ, Millipore filter then add 0.7 ml beta mecaptoethanol per 100 ml just prior to use.

T4 Polynucleotide Kinase Buffer

0.5 M Tris-Cl, pH 7.5, 0.1 M MgCl$_2$, 50 mM DTT, 0.5 mg ml^{-1} BSA.

SSC Buffer (20×)

3 M sodium chloride, 300 mM sodium citrate, pH 7.0.

SSPE (20×)

Dissolve 174 g of NaCl, 27.6 g of NaH$_2$PO$_4$H$_2$O, and 7.4 g of EDTA in 800 ml of H$_2$O. Adjust pH to 7.4 with NaOH and adjust volume to 1 liter.

Denhardt's Solution (100×)

Add 10 g polyvinylpyrrolidone (PVP), 10 g bovine serum albumin (BSA), and 10 g Ficoll 400 to 470 ml water. Dissolve sterile filter, and store at −20°C in 50 ml aliquots.

PCR Master Mix

Glass-distilled sterile H$_2$O (2310 μl)
10X PCR Reaction Buffer (300 μl)
dNTP Mix, 12.5 mM each (48 μl)
Primer 1 200 μM (15 μl)
Primer 2 200 μM (15 μl)
Cetus Ampli Taq (5 U μl^{-1}) (12 μl)
Total volume 2700 μl.

PCR Reaction Buffer (10x)

500 mM KCl, 100 mM Tris-Cl pH 8.3 (RT), 25 mM MgCl$_2$, 0.1% (w/v) gelatin.

In situ PCR Reaction Mix

PCR Buffer (500 mM KCl, 100 mM Tris HCl, pH 8.3) (2.5 μl)
MgCl$_2$ (25 mM) (4.5 μl)
dNTPs (final concentration 200 μM) (4.0 μl)
BSA (2% w/v) (1.0 μl)
DIG-11-dUTP (100 μM) (0.4 μl)
Primers 1 and 2 (each, 20 μM) (1.0 μl)
H$_2$O (11.0 μl)
Taq Polymerase (4 U μl^{-1}) (0.6 μl)
Total volume 25.0 μl.

LCR Reaction Mix

50 mM Hepes, pH 7.8, 10 mM MgCl$_2$, 10 mM NH$_4$Cl, 100 mM KCl, 1 mM DTT, 10 ug ml^{-1} BSA, 0.1 mM NAD, 50 μM dCTP or appropriate dNTP for G-LCR, thermostable DNA ligase from *Thermus thermophilus* (2 U/50 μl) from Molecular Biological Resources (Milwalkee), 10^{11} · molecules of each of 4 primers.

SDA Master Mix

For each reaction add the following reagents in sequence: 1.37 μl of H$_2$O, 1 μl of the amplification control, 1 μl of primer solution, 3.63 μl of 0.5 M K$_2$HPO, pH 7.6, 1 μl dNTP solution, 10 μl 55% (v/v) glycerol, 1 μl BSA solution and 1 μl 0.35 M MgCl$_2$. Mix by vortexing.

Nick Translation Buffer (10×)

0.5 M Tris-HCl, pH 7.4, 0.1 M MgCl$_2$, 1 mM DTT, 0.5 mg ml^{-1} BSA.

Random Priming Buffer Mix

Buffer Mix (BRL): 0.67 M Hepes, 0.17 M Tris-Cl, 17 mM MgCl$_2$, 33 mM

Detection of viral nucleic acids in clinical material

2-mercaptoethanol, 1.3 mg ml^{-1} BSA, 18 OD$_{260}$ units ml^{-1} of random hexamer primers. Adjust pH to 6.8, and store at −20°C.

Tailing Buffer (5×)

0.5 M potassium cacodylate, pH 7.2, 5 mM CoCl$_2$, 5 mM DTT.

Methods

Extraction of nucleic acids

DNA extraction

1. For isolation of DNA from mammalian cells, pellet approximately 10^4–10^6 cells in a 1.5 ml microfuge tube. For tissue samples, homogenize approximately 100 mg of tissue, transfer to a 1.5 ml microfuge tube and pellet. For urine samples or specimens collected in transport media, pellet approximately 100 µl of sample in a microfuge tube. Retain the pellet for cell-associated pathogens, the supernatant for lytic pathogens.
2. Discard the supernatant and process the pellets by adding a 100 µl volume of freshly prepared lysis buffer containing 50 mm KCl, 10 mm Tris-Cl, pH 8.3, 2.5 mm $MgCl_2$, 0.01% gelatin, 1% Tween 20 and 200 µg ml^{-1} Proteinase K.
3. Incubate the specimens at 55°C for 1 h or overnight at room temperature.
4. Heat inactivate proteinase K by heating samples at 94°C for 10 min.
5. Briefly spin the tubes in a microfuge to pellet the condensation.
6. Add an equal volume (200 µl) of phenol/$CHCl_3$/isoamyl alcohol (50:48:2) to the lysate and mix by inversion.
7. Centrifuge 5 min at 12,000 rpm to separate the phases.
8. Transfer the top aqueous phase to a fresh microfuge tube and add an equal volume (approximately 200 µl) of $CHCl_3$/isoamyl alcohol (98:2 v/v).
9. Mix well and centrifuge as above.
10. Transfer the aqueous phase to a fresh microfuge tube and add 3 m sodium acetate, pH 5.2 to a final concentration of 0.25 m.
11. Add 2 volumes of 95% ETOH (400 µl) and precipitate the DNA at −70°C for 30 min or at −20°C overnight.
12. Centrifuge the samples at 12,000 rpm at 4°C for 30 min.
13. Wash the pellet once with 70% ETOH and centrifuge at 12,000 rpm for 10 min at 4°C.
14. Air dry the pellet and resuspend in dH_2O or TE buffer.

Extracting DNA from paraffin sections

1. Cut 5–10 3 µ sections from each block and collect in 1.5 ml microcentrifuge tubes (packed volume should be about 300–400 µl).
2. Dewax by adding 1 ml of xylene, vortexing, and centrifuging for 5 min at 10,000 g. Discard the supernatant, and repeat the extraction.
3. Wash the pellet twice with 1 ml ethanol, vortex, and centrifuge as above.
4. Dry in a 37°C incubator for 2 h.
5. Resuspend in 300 µl of 50 mm Tris, 5 mm EDTA, 300 µg ml^{-1} proteinase K, pH 8. Larger volumes may be required, depending on the amount of tissues sectioned.
6. Incubate for 1–2 days at room temperature or until most of the tissue has disintegrated. Vortexing or brief sonication during this step will help in breaking down larger tissue pieces.

7. Spin the digests 10 min at 10,000 *g* to remove remaining unsolubilized tissue.
8. Aliquots can be tested by filter paper hybridization or PCR. If necessary, these preparations can be further purified by phenol-chloroform extraction and ethanol precipitation. Extracts can be stored at $-20°C$.

10. Mix well by inversion. Store at $-20°C$ for at least 1 h.
11. Centrifuge for 30 min at 4°C, at 14,000 rpm.
12. Wash pellet once with 75% EtOH.
13. Dry pellet and dissolve in 10–30 µl of dH_2O.

Labeling of probes

RNA extraction

All solutions must be RNase free and should be prepared with double filtered deionized water using disposable plastic pipettes and diethylpyrocarbonate (DEPC) treated glassware. DEPC-treated water should be used throughout to prevent degradation of RNA. Include negative and positive patient specimens as controls for the extraction procedure.

1. Transfer 100 µl of serum, 100 mg of homogenized tissue, or $10^4–10^6$ mammalian cells to a 1.5 ml microfuge tube. Resuspend tissue and cells in 100 µl of dH_2O or TE buffer.
2. Add 600 µl of chaos buffer (with mercaptoethanol added).
3. Incubate for 30 min at room temperature.
4. Add 700 µl of Phenol/$CHCl_3$/isoamyl alcohol and mix well by inversion.
5. Centrifuge for 10 min at 14,000 rpm.
6. Transfer the aqueous phase to a fresh 1.5 ml microfuge tube and add 700 µl of $CHCl_3$/isoamyl alcohol.
7. Mix well by inversion and centrifuge as above.
8. Transfer the upper aqueous phase to a fresh 1.5 ml microfuge tube.
9. Add 3 M NaOAc pH 5.2 to a final concentration of 0.25 M and add 1 volume of Isopropanol.

Nick translation

This method (see Chapter 10) can be used to label double stranded (ds) DNA with nucleotide triphosphates tagged with ^{32}P or non-radioactive ligands such as biotin, fluorescein or digoxigenin. Incorporation of 70% or better can be expected with probe specific activities of $1–2 \times 10^9$ cpm $µg^{-1}$. Commercial kits are available from Amersham (N5000) and BRL. Following the labeling, a 2 µl aliquot, of the reaction mixture is counted in scintillation fluid and (a) the specific activity and (b) percent incorporation for the labeled DNA is calculated:

a) $\dfrac{\text{cpm incorporated}}{\text{µg input DNA}} \times 125 = \text{cpm µg}^{-1}$

b)
$\dfrac{\text{cpm incorporated}}{\text{total cpm added}} \times 125 \times 100\% = \text{\% incorporation.}$

Note

The factor 125 is used to convert the counts from a 2 µl aliquot back to the 250 µl total reaction volume.
Biotin-labeled probes can be checked by dotting serial dilutions onto nitrocellulose and detecting with an enzyme-labeled streptavidin conjugate and substrate. Unincorporated bases can be removed

by precipitation or in a Sephadex G-50 spun column:

1. Pipette into a 1 ml plastic syringe, plugged with siliconized glass wool, Sephadex G-50 swollen in 50 mM Tris-HCl, pH 7.5, 1 mM EDTA, 0.1% SDS, until the syringe is filled to about 1.2 ml.
2. Place the syringe in a 15 ml plastic conical centrifuge tube with a pad of paper towel or tissue in the bottom, so that the syringe is suspended from the top of the centrifuge tube.
3. Spin in a bench top centrifuge at low speed for 3–4 min to form a packed bed in the syringe with a volume between 0.85 and 0.90 ml.
4. Remove the syringe and insert an eppendorf tube with the top flap removed and place into the bottom of the conical centrifuge tube.
5. Reinsert the syringe so that the tip is over the open eppendorf.
6. Pipette the nick translation reaction mixture onto the top of the Sephadex column.
7. Centrifuge 3–4 mm at low speed.
8. The liquid collected in the eppendorf contains the DNA probe free of unincorporated nucleotides, in a volume equal to or slightly less than that applied (50 µl). The unincorporated nucleotide is retained in the column. The volume of the sample is adjusted to give a final concentration of 20 µg ml^{-1} (1 µg 50 µl^{-1}).

Note

The elution of the probe may be tracked by the addition of 0.5% blue dextran to the reaction mixture prior to the fractionation on the Sephadex column. This will aid in the identification of those fractions containing the DNA fragments, as both are eluted in the void volume. Commercial products are now available from several companies (Amicon, Biorad or Pharmacia) to remove unincorporated nucleotides.

Random priming

This method (see Chapter 10) can be used to label linear DNA with a variety of reporter molecules. Between 10 ng and 3 µg of linear DNA can be labeled per standard reaction and larger amounts can be labeled by scaling up of all components and volumes.

5' Terminal labeling

T4 polynucleotide kinase catalyses the transfer of a γ^{32}P phosphate to the 5' OH and of either single or double stranded DNA or dsRNA. The method is the method of choice for labeling short single stranded oligonucleotide probes.

1. To a 1.5 ml microfuge tube add the following:
   1–50 pmol dephosphorylated DNA, 5' ends
   3 µl 10 × T4 polynucleotide kinase buffer
   20 µl [α^{32}P]-ATP (3000 Ci mmol)
   2 µl T4 Polynucleotide kinase (10 U µl^{-1})
   dH$_2$O to 30 µl final volume.
2. Incubate for 1 h at 37°C.
3. Stop the reaction by adding 2 µl of 0.5 M EDTA.
4. Adjust volume to 100 µl with 70 µl dH$_2$O and extract once with phenol/CHCl$_3$.
5. Mix well by inversion and centrifuge for 5 min at 12,000 rpm.
6. Transfer the top aqueous phase to a fresh microfuge tube.
7. Separate the labeled DNA from unincorporated labeled nucleotides by filtration with a spin column or commercially available products such

as a Bio Rad Bio Spin 6 columns or Pharmacia Micro Spin S200 HR or S300 HR columns.

3′ Terminal labeling

This method may be used to tag an oligo-nucleotide probe with ^{32}P, fluorescein, digoxigenin or other reporter molecules for dot blot hybridization or fluorescent *in situ* hybridization. Terminal deoxynucleotidyl transferase catalyzes the addition of dNTPs to the 3′ hydroxyl termini of single stranded DNA. Commercial products are now available from Amersham (ECL 3′-biolabeling and detection system).

1. To a 1.5 ml microfuge tube on ice add the following:
   oligonucleotide (10 ng of 30-mer) (5 μl)
   Fluorescein-11-dUTP (1 mM) (1.5 μl)
   Or α-^{32}P-dATP (3,000 Ci/mmol, 10 μCi μl^{-1})
   5× Tailing buffer pH 7.2 (4 μl)
   Terminal transferase (50 U μl^{-1}) (1 μl)
   Sterile dH$_2$O (3.5 μl)
2. Mix by pipetting up and down.
3. Incubate 60–90 min at 37°C.
4. If necessary, the labeled probe may be purified by affinity chromatography using glass particles.
5. Store at −20°C in the dark.

Membrane hybridization

Dot/slot blot hybridization

1. Pre-wet Nitrocellulose (NC) paper for 5–10 min in dH$_2$O and again in 1 M sodium acetate, pH 7.0.
2. Spot 5–10 μl of sample DNA onto nitrocellulose using BRL Hybri-slot TM Manifold.

3. Remove the filter and air dry for 60 min at room temperature.
4. Place the filter in denaturing alkali (1 M Sodium acetate, 0.1 N NaOH) for 20 min.
5. Rinse the filter with neutralizing buffer (0.1 M Tris-HCl pH 7.4, 1 M NaCl).
6. Place the filter in 2 × SSC on orbital shaker for 20 min.
7. Dry and fix DNA to membrane under vacuum for 2 h at 80°C.
8. Place nitrocellulose into plastic bag and add prehybridization mixture; 2 × Denhardt's, 6 × SSC, 0.5% SDS, 0.1 mg ml^{-1} heat denatured herring sperm DNA. Seal bag with heat sealer.
9. Prehybridize at 65°C in shaking water bath for 2 h.
10. Pour off the prehybridization mixture and add hybridization mixture: 3 × Denhardt's, 0.4 × SSC, 0.5 SDS, 10% Dextran Sulphate, 0.1 mg ml^{-1} heat denatured herring sperm DNA and heat denatured probe (95°C 10 min) (200 ng ml^{-1} for biotin labeled probe or 10^9 cpm for dCTP labeled probe). Reseal the bag.
11. Incubate in shaking water bath at 65°C overnight.
12. Wash using stringent conditions at 65°C: 3 times (20 min each) in 1 × Denhardt's, 6 × SSC and 0.5% SDS, 3 times (10 min each) in 1 × Denhardt's, 1 × SSC, and 0.5% SDS, 3 times (10 min each) in 0.1 × SSC and 0.5 SDS.
13. For detection of biotin-labeled probe wash the NC in solution I (0.1 M Tris HCl, pH 7.5, 0.1 M NaCl, 2 mM MgCl$_2$, 0.05% Triton x-100) then inoculate with 2 ug ml^{-1} streptavidin in the same buffer for 10 min with gentle agitation.
14. Wash three times (3 min each) with solution I.
15. Add 3 ml of 1 ug ml^{-1} biotinylated polymer of alkaline phosphatase (poly AP, BRL) in Solution I and

incubate for 10 min with gentle agitation.

16. Wash twice (3 min each) with Solution I, twice (3 min each) with Solution II (0.1 M Tris-HCl, pH 9.5, 0.1 M NaCl, 50 mM MgCl$_2$).

17. Just prior to use prepare NBT/BCIP substrate solution by adding 18 μl NTB (75 mg ml^{-1} in dimethyl formamide) and 13 μl of BCIP (50 mg ml^{-1} in dimethly formamide) to 4 ml of Solution II.

18. Incubate the NC in the substrate in a sealed bag or petri dish for up to 4 h and cover with aluminium foil.

19. Wash NC in 20 mM Tris-HCl, pH 7.5, 5 mM EDTA to stop color reaction, air dry and store dried filter – protected from light.

Comment

Hybridizations are commonly performed in either aqueous buffer such as 5 × SSC at 60–65°C or in 50% formamide at 40–42°C. Biotin-labeled probes are sometimes difficult to read and have been gradually replaced by digoxigenin- or FITC-labeled probes. Several companies (Boehringer Mannheim, Amersham, and others) now supply probe labeling and detection kits which perform well. The use of alkaline phosphatase conjugated antibodies to digoxigenin or fluorescein and substrates, such as lumiphos 530^{TM} allows for the chemiluminescent detection of bound probe and imaging on x-ray film. Nylon membranes offer some advantages over NC but, because backgrounds vary for different membranes, it is always best to use the membrane recommended by the supplier of the kit.

Southern hybridization

Southern blotting is a membrane hybridization assay in which DNA fragments generated by restriction endonuclease digestion are first separated by agarose gel electrophoresis, transblotted to a membrane either electrophoretically or by capillary action then reacted with a DNA probe. Southern blotting is often used to determine whether viral DNA such as EBV or HPV is integrated into the host chromosome or remains as an episome in the cell. Southern blotting is also regularly used to verify the specificity of a PCR amplification. In this case 10 μl of a PCR product is electrophoresed in 2% agarose gels and the DNA transblotted to a membrane then probed with an internal oligonucleotide. We use the BioRad transblotter for the Mini Protean electrophoresis apparatus but other companies also supply similar transblotters.

Immerse the gel in 2–3 gel volumes of solution A (300 ml of 5 M NaCl, 50 ml 10 M NaOH in 1 liter with H$_2$O) at room temperature for 30–45 min with occasional agitation to denature the DNA. Decant solution A, add 2–3 volumes solution B (200 ml of 10 M ammonium acetate, 3 ml 10 M NaOH in 1 liter with H$_2$O) and incubate for 30–45 min with occasional agitation. Add 500 ml solution B to a large dish. Soak a large piece of Whatman 3MM paper with solution B and lay over a support with both ends contacting the buffer in the dish, to serve as a wick for buffer during the transfer. Smooth the wick to remove any bubbles. Carefully lift the gel and slide onto the buffer-soaked wick. Squeeze out any bubbles trapped between the gel and the wick. Pre-wet two sheets of Whatman 3MM paper cut to the size of the gel and place over the gel. Pre-wet two sheets of Whatman 3MM paper cut to the size of the gel in solution B and place over the nitrocellulose. Place a stack of paper towels, 2–4 inches, cut to fit the size of the gel on top of the Whatman 3MM paper. Place a glass plate on top of the blotting paper stack, and place a light weight on top of the plate. Transfer for 4 h to overnight. After transfer, mark the position of the sample wells on the membrane with pinholes and indicate the right and left side. Air dry the membrane for a few minutes and bake in an 80°C vacuum oven for 30 min to 2 h. The membrane can be stored between sheets of Whatman 3MM paper in a dry place at room temperature prior to hybridization.

Northern hybridization

Northern blotting is used for the analysis of RNA and follows a similar procedure to Southern blotting. Total RNA from cell cultures infected with virus or from clinical specimens, such as blood, serum, stool or CSF, is extracted and purified, usually with 5M guanidine isothiocyanate (to inactivate RNase in the specimen) followed by cesium chloride ultracentrifugation to remove traces of DNA and protein. The purified RNA is then electrophoresed, transferred to NC or nylon and probed using either radioactive or non-radioactive probes. Northern blots are used to detect viral genomes or determine the size or presence of viral transcripts. Care must be taken during the extraction step to ensure that RNA is not degraded. The use of DEPC-treated water and scrupulous rinsing of all glassware with DEPC is imperative. The use of commercially available RNase inhibitors such as RNasin from Promega or vanadyl-riboside complex from Gibco BRL is highly recommended.

In situ hybridization

In situ hybridization can be performed on any type of fixed specimen but is most often performed on paraffin-embedded tissue. After removal of paraffin wax, tissues are hydrated and permeabilized by limited proteolysis. The conditions for proteolysis vary according to tissue type and the reader is advised to refer to the comprehensive literature on this topic.

Specimens containing single cells such as peripheral blood mononuclear cells (PBMC), bronchoalveolar lavage (BAL) and urine sediments can be centrifuged onto a microscope slide using a Shandon Cytocentrifuge. Although ^{32}P-labeled DNA probes were originally used other reporter molecules such as biotin, FITC and digoxigenin are gaining in popularity. A number of different labeling techniques including nick translation, random priming, 3'-terminal labeling, 5'-terminal labeling, and PCR can be used for *in situ* hybridization. The following procedure can be used for most types of tissue and all single cell specimens.

1. Paraffin sections should be fixed onto microscope slides treated with either poly-L-lysine or Silane (Sigma). (Cells in suspension can be deposited onto treated slides using a cytocentrifuge and fixed in 10% buffered formalin for 2 h.)
2. Tissue sections are deparaffinized by immersion in xylol twice for 10 min each followed by absolute ethanol for 3 min then progressively rehydrated (95% ethanol for 3 min, 70% ethanol for 3 min, dH$_2$O for 3 min).
3. Tissue is permeabilized by limited proteolysis with 2 mg ml^{-1} trypsin or pepsin at room temperature for 10–90 min depending on the length of time in formalin.
4. Inactivate the enzyme by treating for 1 min with DEPC-treated water then 1 min with absolute ethanol. Air dry the slide.
5. Cover the slide with hybridization solution and prehybridize for 10 min with 5 × SSC or 50% formamide in 1 × SSPE.
6. Pour off the prehybridization solution and cover the tissue with hybridization solution containing probe. Cover with a glass coverslip and seal edges with silicone or rubber cement.
7. Place the slide on heat block at 94°C for 3 min to denature DNA, then place

at room temperature and hybridize for 30 min.

8. Remove the coverslip and wash with wash solution for 10 min at room temperature.

9. For the detection of biotin-labeled probes, apply 3–4 drops of avidin-horse radish peroxidase conjugate and incubate for 30 min at room temperature. Rinse the slide with wash buffer then add aminoethyl carbazole/hydrogen peroxide substrate and incubate for 10 min. Rinse and counterstain the cytoplasm with fast green or the nucleus with methyl green for 1–2 min then rinse with dH$_2$O. Mount with water or glycerin jelly and observe under a light microscope for reddish brown stain deposits over cells.

Comment

Kits for the detection of several viruses using biotinylated probes are available from Enzo Biochem, New York. *In situ* hybridization lends itself to short oligonucleotide probes of 18–30 mer length as well as PCR labeled probes in the 200–400 bp range. These can be tagged with either digoxigenin-11-dUTP and detected with alkaline phosphatase conjugated antibody and NBT/BCIP substrate. FITC-11-dUTP labeled probes can be detected by fluorescence microscopy or by flow cytometric analysis when a single cell suspension such as peripheral blood mononuclear cells are examined.

Nucleic acid amplification

Polymerase chain reaction

Conventional PCR

1. Prepare sufficient PCR master mix for 30 × 100 µl reactions.

2. Aliquot 90 µl of the master mix into 0.5 ml microfuge tubes and cover with 75 µl light mineral oil.

3. Add 10 µl of DNA or processed specimen. Include positive and negative controls. It is useful to include a sensitivity panel consisting of dilutions of control DNA ranging from 1 fg to 1 pg. Interspersing negative controls in a large run is a useful way of detecting carryover contamination if uracil-N-glycosylase is not used.

4. Amplify for 35–40 cycles as follows using a Cetus Perkin Elmer thermocycler model 4800 (or equivalent): 1 min at 94°C (denaturation), 1 min at 55°C (annealing), 2 min at 72°C (extension). The last cycle should be followed by an extension at 72°C for 8 min. (If a 9600 thermocycler is used, the cycles can be shortened to 30 s, 30 s, 60 s).

5. Analyze amplification products by electrophoresizing 10 µl on a 2% agarose gel for 2 h at 75 V.

Reverse transcriptase-PCR

RT-PCR can be used to detect either viral genomic RNA or RNA transcripts and involves first the synthesis of a single stranded complimentary DNA using reverse transcriptase followed by amplification using a thermostable DNA polymerase (*Thermus aquaticus, Thermus thermophilus, Bacillus steareothermophilus*). Nested PCR using first an outer set of primers with 10 cycles of amplification followed by a second amplification (20 cycles) using an inner set of primers located within the first amplicon has been used to improve the sensitivity of RT-PCR. The use of a new recombinant DNA polymerase from *Thermus thermophilus* (rTth, Cetus Perkin Elmer) that contains both reverse transcriptase and DNA polymerase activity has simplified the procedure and helped reduce contamination by eliminating the need to open the tubes between the reverse transcriptase and PCR setup.

The following protocol describes a nested RT-PCR using AMV reverse transcriptase and Taq polymerase for the detection of Hepatitis C virus (Shindo et al 1991).

1. Prepare the following master mix (enough for 10 × 45 µl reactions).
   Glass-distilled sterile dH$_2$O (382 µl)
   10× PCR Reaction Buffer (50 µl)
   dNTP Mix, 12.5 mM (8 µl)
   Outer primers 1 and 2 (3 µl)
   Cetus Ampli-Taq (5 U µl^{-1}) (2 µl)
   AMV reverse transcriptase:
      (Promega 10 U ml^{-1} (2 µl)
   Total volume 450 µl.
2. Aliquot 45 µl of the master mix into 0.5 ml microfuge tubes.
3. Add 5 µl of specimen. Set up appropriate positive and negative controls.
4. Programme the Cetus Perkin Elmer 9600 thermocycler as follows:
   20 min at 42°C, 35 cycles of 30 s at 94°C, 30 s at 50°C, 45 s at 72°C, and 8 min at 72°C.
5. Prepare the second PCR master mix as in Step 1 *except* increase the volume of dH$_2$O to 380 µl, use 5 µl of the inner nested Primers 3 and 4 (instead of 1 and 2), and do not add the reverse transcriptase.
6. Aliquot 48 µl of this master mix to each tube and lightly cap tubes.
7. In a separate area away from the specimen preparation area, set up the nested PCR by opening one tube at a time from the first amplification and transferring 2 µl to a fresh tube. Ensure that each tube from the first amplification is closed after transfer of an aliquot. (Take extra care as nested PCRs are especially prone to carryover contamination.)
8. Repeat the amplification cycles as in Step 6 omitting the RT step.
9. Analyze 10 µl of the second amplification product on a 2% agarose gel with ethidium bromide staining.

Multiplex PCR

Multiplex PCR can be used to simultaneously co-amplify two targets in a single reaction tube. Successful co-amplification is dependent upon compatible primer sets that have similar melting temperatures (Tm) and MgCl$_2$ requirements so that they will both anneal to their target at the same temperature. It is absolutely essential that there is no sequence homology between any of the primers to prevent the formation of primer dimers. Multiplex PCR is particularly suited to the detection of viruses in stool specimens or respiratory tract specimens where several different viruses may be present. Multiplex assays can also be developed for the simultaneous detection of both DNA and RNA viruses. In the future, multiplex PCR will be developed for the detection of both genomic DNA or RNA and RNA transcripts that may be useful in assessing latency or studying pathophysiological mechanisms.

We have used the following protocol to detect *C. trachomatis* and *N. gonorrhoeae* in first void urine specimens (Mahony et al 1995) using primers for the *C. trachomatis* plasmid (Mahony et al 1993a) and *N. gonorrhoeae* plasmid (Ho et al 1992).

1. Prepare the following master mix enough for 30 × 100 µl reactions:
   Glass-distilled sterile H$_2$O (2280 µl)
   10 × PCR Reaction Buffer (300 µl)
   dNTP Mix 12.5 mM each (48 µl)
   C. trachomatis primers KL1, KL2 200 µM (15 µl each)
   N. gonorrhoeae primers HO1, HO3 200 µM (15 µl)
   Cetus Ampli Taq (5U µl^{-1}) (12 µl)
   Total volume 2700 µl.
2. Aliquot 90 µl of the master mix into 0.5 ml microfuge tubes and cover with 75 µl of light mineral oil.
3. Add 10 µl of processed specimen (urine, endocervical or urethral swab). Set up appropriate positive and negative controls.

4. Program the Cetus Perkin Elmer thermocycler model 4800 for 40 cycles of 1 min at 94°C (denaturation), 1 min at 55°C (annealing), and 2 min at 72°C (extension) followed by 8 min at 72°C (hold at 15°C overnight if necessary).

5. Analyze 10 μl of the amplified products by agarose gel electrophoresis and Southern blot hybridization using specific probes for each product.

In situ PCR

PCR can be used to detect specific viral DNA or RNA sequences in formalin fixed paraffin imbedded tissue by performing the amplification *in situ*. The methods for DNA and RNA detection are similar, RNA being detected by overnight digestion with DNase followed by RT-PCR. Complete DNase treatment of the tissue is essential to eliminate the non-specific amplification of DNA that is inherent with RT-PCR. The detection part of the protocol can be streamlined by direct incorporation of digoxigenin 11-dUTP into the PCR product with detection by alkaline phosphate-conjugated anti-digoxigenin antibody and NBT/BCIP substrate. For detection of RNA, non-specific amplification can be prevented by digesting with protease and DNase prior to reverse transcription (Nuovo et al 1993). It is absolutely essential to use both a negative control (to assess removal of DNA) and a positive control (to assess tissue permeabilization) together with the test section, preferably together on one slide.

1. Tissue must be fixed with a cross-linked fixative such as formalin to inhibit diffusion of PCR product from the cell. Fixation should be in 10% neutral buffered formalin for 2–24 h.

2. Place three tissue sections (3–5 μm) or two cytospin preparations on a silane coated slide.

3. Deparaffinize the sections twice with xylol followed by alcohol.

4. Hydrate the sections with buffer then digest with trypsin or pepsin (2 mg ml^{-1}) at room temperature for 10–90 min. (If the tissue was fixed in 10% formalin for 4 h perform a 10 min digestion. If fixation was for 24 h, digest for 90 min.)

5. Inactivate the enzyme by washing for 1 min in diethylpyro carbonate-treated (DEPC) water and for 1 min in 100% ethanol. Air dry the sections.

6. For RT-PCR treat with RNase-free DNase (10 U ml^{-1}) in DEPC-water overnight at 37°C.

7. Wash for 1 min in DEPC-water and for 1 min in 100% ethanol and air dry.

8. Add reverse transcriptase and buffer to one section and cover with coverslip. Anchor the coverslip with nail polish or silicon. Place the slide in an 'aluminium boat' on the block of a thermal cycler and cover with mineral oil. Incubate for 30 min at 42°C.

9. Remove the coverslip and wash the slide in xylene for 5 min followed by 100% ethanol for 5 min, then air dry.

10. Prepare sufficient *in situ* PCR reaction mix for each slide.

11. Add the mixture to each slide, cover with a large coverslip, seal as before and place on the thermal cycler block.

12. Ramp to 80°C, add mineral oil and heat to 94°C for 3 min.

13. Cycle at 55°C for 2 min and 94°C for 1 min for 20 cycles.

14. Remove the coverslip and wash with xylene and ethanol as above.

15. Detect incorporated digoxigenin-11-dUTP with alkaline phosphatase-conjugated anti digioxigenin antibody (diluted 1:50, 30 min) and NBT/BCIP (5–10 min).

Interpretation

It is imperative that the negative and positive controls are run on the same slide as the actual test. This is crucial because one must demonstrate with the negative control section (addition of DNase but no reverse transcriptase) that the native DNA repair and mispriming pathways have been eliminated, and with the positive control (no DNase pretreatment) that the protease conditions are optimal for amplification of DNA inside the cell. Using these controls, a meaningful result is obtained when: no signal is evident with the negative control and at least 50% of the cells on the positive control section show an intense signal. If both criteria are not satisfied the most likely problem was inadequate protease digestion. Both of these criteria must be met before the test is valid.

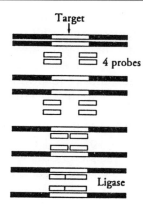

Figure 16.1. LCR amplification of DNA. After heat denaturation of DNA at 94°C, oligonucleotide probes anneal at 55°C and are ligated together by DNA ligase resulting in a doubling of the number of target molecules for each cycle of amplification.

second reporter molecule at the distal end of the other primer.

Ligase chain reaction

LCR utilizes four oligonucleotide primers (instead of two used in PCR), a thermobile DNA ligase to ligate the contiguous primers and a thermal cycler to cycle the reaction between the denaturation temperature (94°C) and the ligation (72°C) temperature. A variation of LCR called gapped LCR employs Taq polymerase to fill in one nucleotide prior to the ligation of adjacent primers. LCR has been used to detect HPV DNA in cell lines established from cervical carcinomas and clinical specimens (Hampl et al 1991), *C. trachomatis* and *N. gonorrhoeae* in genito-urinary specimens (Birkenmeyer et al 1992). Abbott Diagnostics is developing LCR and have used a microparticle EIA to detect specific LCR products with the automated IMx instrument (Dille et al 1993). Briefly, ligated product is captured by antibody immobilized onto the surface of microparticles via a ligand attached to the end of one primer then detected by an enzyme conjugated antibody directed at a

1. First void urine specimens (1 ml of first 20 ml urine) are centrifuged 14,000 *g* for 10 min and the pellet resuspended in buffer. Boil specimens by heating to 95–100°C for 15 min to release DNA.
2. Prepare sufficient LCR reaction mixture for the desired number of specimens and controls (50 μl for each specimen).
3. When specimens have cooled to ambient temperature, add 50–100 μl of sample to a tube containing 100 μl LCR reaction mixture.
4. Place tubes in thermal cycler and program for 40 cycles of 10 s at 94°C, 10 s 55°C, 60 s at 62°C (the times and temperatures will vary for LCR or G-LCR and Tms of primers).
5. Ligated product can be detected by gel electrophoresis and autoradiography or by chemiluminescence following capture of amplified product onto microparticles using immobilized antibodies directed against one of the haptens (Dille et al 1993; Chernesky et al 1993). The other end of the LCR

product containing a second hapten is recognized by a second antibody conjugated to a reported enzyme such as alkaline phosphatase. Only ligated product with both haptens covalently attached will generate a chemiluminescent signal. Abbott Diagnostics uses microparticles EIA to detect LCR products on the LCx™ analyzer: 100 μl of the LCR reaction is pipetted into the reaction wedge of the LCx and the wedges are placed in the IMx carousel. Results are expressed as counts per second per second and positives are defined using run calibrators that establish the cutoff.

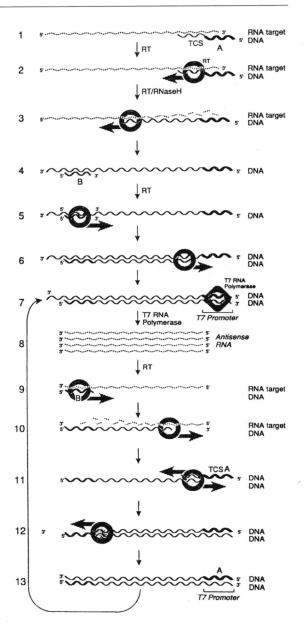

Nucleic acid sequence-based amplification

Nucleic acid sequence-based amplification (NASBA) is an isothermal amplification technique in which specific RNA sequences are amplified in an isothermal reaction using three enzymes: reverse transcriptase (RT), T7 RNA polymerase and RNase H (Kievits et al 1991). In the first non-cyclical phase of the reaction a downstream primer containing a tail-sequence of the T7 promotor sequence anneals to a single stranded target sequence. A cDNA is made by the RT and RNase H then digests away the target RNA from the DNA–RNA hybrid leaving a single strand of DNA to which the upstream primer can anneal. The RT (through its DNA function) then synthesizes the complimenting strand producing a dsDNA intermediate which. has a transcriptionally active promoter sequence. T7 RNA polymerase then produces up to a thousand ssRNA copies that serve as a template in cyclical phase producing a potential amplification of up to 10^9 copies in a 1.5–2 h reaction.

Figure 16.2. NASBA amplification of RNA by continuous cycles of reverse transcriptase and RNA transcription. Oligonucleotides A and B prime DNA synthesis forming a double-stranded cDNA containing a T7 promoter sequence (steps 2–6). T7 polymerase produces multiple copies of antisence RNA transcripts (step 7) which act as templates for cDNA synthesis and the synthesis of sense strand RNA transcripts (steps 9–13).

1. Prepare a reaction mixture consisting of a 0.2 μM of primer 1 and primer 2, 40 mM Tris-HCl, pH 8.5, 12 mM MgCl₂, 40 mM KCl, 5 mM DTT, 15% DMSO, 1 mM of four dNTPs, 2 mM of each NTP, 12 U RNA Guard (Pharmacia).
2. Pipitte 21 μl of reaction mix into a microfuge tube and add 2 μl of nucleic acid solution to be tested.
3. Heat the reaction to 65°C for 5 min.
4. Add 2 μl enzyme mix containing 20 U T7 RNA polymerase (Pharmacia), 4 U AMV reverse transcriptase (Seikagaku, Japan), 0.2 U RNase H (Pharmacia) and 0.1 ug ml⁻¹ BSA.
5. Incubate at 41°C for 90 min.
6. Analyze 10 μl of the product by gel electrophoresis and hybridization with a ³²P-labeled internal oligonucleotide probe.

Strand displacement amplification (SDA)

SDA is an isothermal method of amplifying target that can produce a 10⁸-fold amplification during a single 2 h incubation at 41°C. SDA requires two enzymes, a DNA polymerase and a restriction enzyme (Walker et al 1992). In the first step, a primer bearing a *Hinc* II restriction site (⁵′GTTGAC) binds to a complementary target nucleic acid and the primer and target are extended by the exo⁻ Klenow fragment of DNA polymerase in the presence of dGTP, dCTP, dUTP and dATP containing an alpha-thiol group (dATPαS) forming a double stranded *Hinc* II recognition site, one strand of which contains phosphorothioate linkages located 5′ to each dA. *Hinc* II nicks the hemiphosphorothioate recognition site between the T and G in the sequence ⁵′GTT↓GAC, without cutting the complementary thiolated strand (⁵′GUCₛAₛAC). *Hinc* II then dissociates from the nicked site and Klenow fills in the new downstream DNA strand. The extension/displacement step regenerates

an unnicked *Hinc* II site. The nicking and strand displacement steps cycle continuously. Since SDA works with target DNA fragments with defined 5′- and 3′-ends, a target generation step is included that uses two additional primers to generate target fragments with defined 5′- and 3′-ends. During target

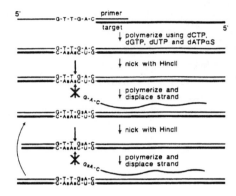

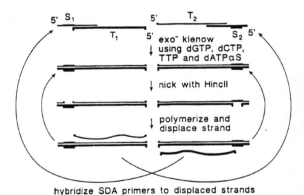

hybridize SDA primers to displaced strands

Figure 16.3. SDA amplification of DNA. A primer containing a *Hinc* II restriction site anneals to the target sequence and is extended by an exonuclease deficient Klenow fragment of DNA polymerase incorporating alpha-throl group derivatized dATP in place of dATP. *Hinc* II nicks on strand at the restriction site between T and G without cutting the complementary thiolated strand. The Klenow fragment then initiates another round of DNA synthesis at the nick displacing the downstream strand as the new strand is made. The displacement strand regenerates the *Hinc* II site and the nicking and strand displacement steps cycle continuously. The amplification becomes experimental while both sense and antisense primers containing *Hinc* II sites are used (bottom half of figure).

generation, the sample is heat denatured in the presence of four primers and Klenow simultaneously extends all four primers and initiates a cascade of extension and displacement steps. The end result is a number of target fragments with hemi-phosphorothioate *Hinc* II sites at one or both ends that enter the amplification cycle upon nicking by *Hinc* II. The inability of SDA to efficiently amplify long (>200 nucleotides) target sequences may restrict its use in the research laboratory but should not limit its use in clinical diagnostic laboratories where the length of the amplified product is generally not important. The SDA product can be analyzed by hibridization and chemiluminescent detection (Spargo et al 1993).

1. Treat the specimen to release DNA (e.g. boiling for 5 min).
2. Prepare an SDA master mix sufficient for the number of SDA reactions to be performed.
3. Add 20 µl of master mix to 25 µl processed clinical sample and mix by vortexing.
4. Heat sample for 2.5 min in a boiling water bath. Cool for 2 min in a 41°C water bath.
5. Dilute exo⁻ Klenow (United States Biochemical, Cleveland OH) 1:5 in 50 mM K_2HPO, pH 7.0, 1 mM dithiothreitol (DTT), 50% (v/v) glycerol to a concentration of 3 units μl^{-1}.
6. Prepare enough SDA 'enzyme mix' for the number of SDA reactions. The enzyme mix for a single SDA reaction consists of 2 µl H_2O, 2 µl of 75 units μl^{-1} *Hinc* II and 1 µl of 3 units μl^{-1} exo-Klenow.
7. Add 5 µl of enzyme mix to each SDA reaction and mix.
8. Incubate for 2 h at 41°C, followed by 1 min at 95°C.
9. Amplification products can be detected by hybridization with specific capture and detection probes using 96-well microtitre plate luminometer.

Applications

Amplification methods are rapidly replacing membrane hybridization for the detection of viral nucleic acids in clinical specimens. An impressive literature has developed over the last five years with examples of the detection of most if not all clinically relevant viruses by PCR. Amplification techniques are particularly well suited for the detection of non-cultivable viruses and PCR in particular has been a god-send to clinical laboratories working on Hepatitis C virus, Parvovirus B19, JC and BK Papovavirus and more recently Hantavirus. We have used PCR for the antenatal detection of Parvovirus B19 in fetal serum obtained by cordocentesis in cases of hydrops fetalis (Barrett et al 1994). JC virus can be detected by PCR in CSF from about 75% of patients with progressive multifocal leukoencephalopathy (Fong et al 1995). In addition to detecting these fastidious viruses PCR and NASBA have been extremely useful for detecting conventional viruses in 'difficult' clinical specimens such as stool, CSF or biopsied tissue. Detection of HSV in CSF from patients from encephalitis has been reported by a number of laboratories and may obviate the need for physicians to perform brain biopsy. RT-PCR and NASBA are now being used for the routine detection of HIV and Hepatitis C virus in blood and recently quantitative assays have been used for monitoring response to antiviral drug therapy. Quantitation of HIV viral load by either PCR or NASBA has been shown to correlate with p24 antigen levels, β_2-microglobulin and neopterin and is now used routinely in clinical trials for monitoring anti retroviral drug therapy (Verhofstede et al 1994). PCR amplification together with gene sequencing has facilitated virus strain typing or genotyping and in the case of HCV has led to the identification of six major genotypes and up to 12 subtypes (Simmonds et al 1994). This is useful clinically since type II (1b) has been associated with higher levels of virus in the blood and poorer response to interferon alpha therapy (Nousbaum et al 1994). A variation of PCR called 3'-mismatch PCR has been used to detect base mutations and codon substitutions in the reverse transcriptase of HIV that confer resistance to Azidothymidine (Larder et al 1993). We have expanded this approach using 3'-mismatch PCR to detect mutant codons in the UL97 protein kinase gene of CMV that confer resistance to Ganciclovir (Mahony et al 1995).

Pitfalls

Although PCR is rapidly becoming a 'routine' test in the clinical laboratory there are some pitfalls to be aware of. The first is the need for verification of a positive PCR test result. This usually involves specific oligonucleotide probe hybridization performed either in solution or on a solid phase. Hybridization remains the best way to confirm the specificity of a PCR reaction. Alternatively a second PCR using a separate and distinct target can be used to confirm positives. This approach has been used to confirm *C. trachomatis* PCR and LCR positives; the second target being a chromosomal gene either MOMP or 16S rRNA with the first target being a plasmid gene (Mahony et al 1994). The second concern with amplification assays is the presence of inhibitors of Taq polymerase and DNA ligase that can result in false negative amplification results. These inhibitors have been poorly characterized and may be present at different rates in various types of clinical material. To rule out the possibility of a false negative result due to the presence of inhibitors clinical specimens should be tested in duplicate with and without exogenously added DNA that can be amplified with the same or different primers.

References

Barrett J, Ryan G, Morrow R, Farine D, Kelly E, Mahony J (1994) J Soc Obst Gyn Can 16: 1253–1258.

Brikenmeyer L, Armstrong AS (1992) J Clin Microbiol 30: 3083–3094.

Chernesky MA, Jang D, Lee H, Burczak JO, Hu H, Sellors J, Tomazic-Allen SJ, Mahony JB (1993) J Clin Microbiol 32: 2682–2685.

Dille BJ, Butzen CC, Birkenmeyer LG (1993) J Clin Microbiol 31: 729–731.

Fong IW, Britton CB, Luinstra KE, Toma E, Mahony JB (1995) J Clin Microbiol 33: 484–486.

Hampl H, Marshall RA, Perko T, Soloman N (1991) In: PCR topics. Rolfs A, Schumacher HC, Marx P (Eds) Springer-Verlag, Berlin, pp 22–25.

Ho BSW, Feng WG, Wong BKC, Egglestone SI (1992) J Clin Pathol 45: 439–442.

Kievits T, van Gemen B, van Strijp D, Schuukkink R, Dircks M, Adriannse H, Malek L, Sooknanan R, Lens P (1991) J Virol Methods 35: 273–286.

Larder BA, Boucher CAB (1993) In Pershing DH, Smith TF, Tenover FC, White TJ (Eds) Diagnostic Molecular Microbiology, Principles and Applications pp 527–533.

Mahony J, Luinstra K, Sellors J, Chernesky M (1993a) J Clin Microbiol 7: 1753–1758.

Mahony J, Luinstra K, Tyndall M, Sellors J, Krepel J, Chernesky M (1995) J Clin Microbiol 33: 3049–3053.

Mahony JB, Luinstra KE, Sellors JW, Pickard L, Chong S, Jang D, Chernesky MA (1994) J Clin Microbiol 32: 2490–2493.

Mahony J, Luinstra K, Lipson M (1995) 95th American Society for Microbiology General Meeting Abstract, Washington D.C.

Nousbaum JB, Pol S, Nalpas B, Landais P, Berthelot P, Brechot C et al (1994) Ann Intern Med 122: 161–168.

Nuovo GJ, Gallery F, Hom R, MacConnell P, Block W (1993) PCR Methods Applic 3: 305–312.

Shindo M, DiBisceglic AM, Cheung L, Shik WK, Cristiano K, Feinstone SM, Hoofnagle JH (1991) Ann Intern Med 115: 700–704.

Simmonds P, Smith DB, McOmish F, Yap PL, Kolberg J, Urdea MS, Holmes EC (1994) J Gen Virol 75: 1053–1061.

Spargo CA, Haaland PD, Jurgensen SR, Shank DD, Walker GT (1993) Mol Cell Prob 7: 395–404.

Verhofstede C, Reniers S, Van Wanzeele FV, Plum J (1994) AIDS 8 (10): 1421–1427.

Walker GT, Fraiser MS, Schram JL, Little MC, Nadeau JG, Malinowoski DP (1992) Nucl Acids Res 20: 1691–1696.

Serological diagnosis

17

S. Specter
D. Jeffries

The introduction of rapid diagnostic techniques to detect viruses or viral antigens has vastly improved the isolation and/or identification of etiologic agents in viral diseases; however, there are still many instances for which serologic diagnosis is necessary. Agents that do not replicate well in cell culture or for which there are as yet no good reagents for direct detection of virus are routinely diagnosed using measurement of antibody. Routine testing for ARBOviruses, Epstein-Barr virus (EBV), hepatitis B virus (HBV), hepatitis C virus (HCV), human immunodeficiency virus (HIV), human T lymphotropic viruses (HTLV) and in some circumstances cytomegalovirus (CMV), herpes simplex virus (HSV), varicella-zoster virus (VZV), measles and rubella is performed by serologic techniques.

Serologic testing is performed both for screening of susceptible populations and for the diagnosis of acute or chronic diseases. The use of serologic testing in these circumstances is delineated in this chapter.

Principles for serologic diagnosis and for screening

The detection of antibodies as a measure of infection by a particular virus may be used in one of several ways for diagnosis. One may measure the presence of antibody as: (1) an indication of immune status, following natural infection or vaccination; (2) seroconversion (i.e. appearance of antibody) or an increase in titer as an indicator of recent infection; (3) a particular class of immunoglobulin to determine the nature of the infection; (4) responses to various antigens associated with the same virus to indicate disease progression; (5) a combination of antibody and antigen levels also to monitor disease state or progression, and (6) levels in different body fluids, such as serum versus CSF, to determine involvement of possible site of infection, such as CNS.

Qualitative assessment of immune status

The qualitative measurement of antibody presence or absence is a useful measure of immune status relative to a particular virus. This can confirm either exposure to a natural infection or successful vaccination of an individual. Immune status is extremely important in circumstances for which secondary exposure to a virus may have very different consequences than primary exposure. For a pregnant female, evidence of prior CMV infection may have devastating consequences for the fetus, whereas a reactivated latent infection is less likely to have pathologic consequences for the fetus. Similarly, screening tests for antibodies to rubella virus in pregnant women indicate that the mother will not likely get rubella if she is antibody positive and thus the fetus is also protected. In rare instances, reinfection with rubella has been recorded but this is an insignificant problem.

Virology Methods Manual
ISBN 0–12–465330–8

Screening tests are also important for a variety of other medical circumstances. Transplant donors and recipients must be screened for CMV immune status, and organs from CMV positive donors should not be used in CMV negative recipients, if this can be avoided, as there is a high likelihood of transmitting infection. Blood products are routinely screened for several viruses that are blood borne pathogens, including CMV, HBV, HCV, HIV and HTLV. This practice has severely reduced the incidence of disease caused by these viruses that is attributed to transfusion.

It must be noted here that qualitative assessment of antibody is of limited value, merely indicating exposure to a particular virus. Although in many cases the presence of antibody can be equated with protective immunity, diagnosis of acute infection requires a quantitative analysis of antibody.

Quantitative analysis of antibody

The detection of antibodies in serum is not always diagnostic for an acute infection, because it is not possible to determine qualitatively whether these antibodies are due to a current, recent or past infection. Since several viruses can cause similar symptoms the presence of antibody in conjunction with clinical evidence of disease still is not sufficient for diagnosis. Thus, it is necessary to measure virus-specific antibody titers in acute and convalescent sera to determine the cause of an acute infection. Acute sera should be collected as soon as possible after onset of infection and convalescent serum should be collected 2–3 weeks later. A two tube (usually four-fold using two-fold dilutions) rise in titer is indicative of a significant change in antibody titer denoting a current infection. The disadvantage to this method is that it takes a considerable amount of time for antibodies to rise and hence for a meaningful result to be obtained; thus utility for diagnosing and, if necessary, treating an acute infection is severely hampered. An alternative to using the titer rise is

to examine an acute serum for indicators of acute infection.

Immunoglobulin class assessment

IgM determination

The determination of immunoglobulin (Ig) M levels in a serum is often useful for rapid identification of acute, primary infection. Numerous methods have been devised to detect IgM and these are well described (Hermann and Erdman 1992) (see chapter 7). More importantly the limitations of this approach must be noted. Considerable care must be taken in measuring IgM levels to a particular virus to be certain that the results are not confused by the presence of rheumatoid factor in the serum (Ziola et al 1979). A variety of strategies have been devised to avoid this problem and are also described by Herrmann and Erdman (1992) (see chapter 7).

While IgM generally is diagnostic of primary infection this is not always so. With certain herpesviruses, particularly CMV and HSV, IgM levels may rise with reactivation of infection (Pass et al 1983; Lopez et al 1993). Thus, detection of IgM is not necessarily indicative of primary infection with these viruses and is only useful in this regard when IgM can be measured in the absence of significant amounts of IgG.

Immunoglobulin A

IgA is important as an antibody in fluids associated with mucosal surfaces, since it is more stable than other Ig as secretory IgA in secretions such as saliva, nasal secretions, gastrointestinal secretions, etc. (Cremer 1985). Thus, measurement of IgA levels in such secretions may be an important and useful measurement of protective immunity against respiratory and enteric viral infections. It also is important in the assessment of generation of protective immunity on mucosal surfaces. By contrast

IgA is less important in systemic immunity since it is usually minimal compared to IgM and IgG responses. In fact, measurement of IgA in serum can often be obscured by high affinity IgG (Cremer 1985). Thus, IgA is not routinely measured in the diagnostic laboratory but is used only in special circumstances.

One such circumstance is the measurement of IgA antibodies against the viral capsid antigen (IgA-VCA) of EBV. IgA is considered diagnostic for nasopharyngeal carcinoma (NPC) that is EBV induced (Lennette 1985). In such cases, IgA-VCA titers can be used prognostically in following the tumor burden due to NPC and to monitor the effectiveness of treatment.

Assessment of antibodies to different antigens

The onset of antibody production to various antigens of a particular virus can occur sequentially and quantitative testing for these different antibodies using one serum specimen can be diagnostic of the state of infection (Fig. 17.1). For infectious mononucleosis due to EBV, antibody responses are first detected against the VCA, followed by the early antigen (EA) then the Epstein-Barr nuclear antigen (EBNA) (Paar and Strauss 1992). Thus, high VCA and EA titers in the absence of EBNA would be indicative of a current acute infection, whereas a high EBNA titer along with high VCA but low EA would suggest a past EBV infection. When combined with comparing IgM-VCA (higher early in infection) to IgG-VCA (higher later in infection) titers more specific information can be gained as to how early in infection the sample was collected.

It should be noted that while these titers provide some very specific information about EBV infection, there is a very simple test for infectious mononucleosis. This test involves detection of the Paul-Bunnell heterophile antibody. This antibody is a common anti-red blood cell antibody that is induced in humans by EBV infection (Lennette 1985). When properly controlled, this test is a far less expensive way of diagnosing EBV induced infectious mononuclesosis than the specific anti-EBV antibody tests. Heterophile testing that gives a negative result may be indicative of CMV

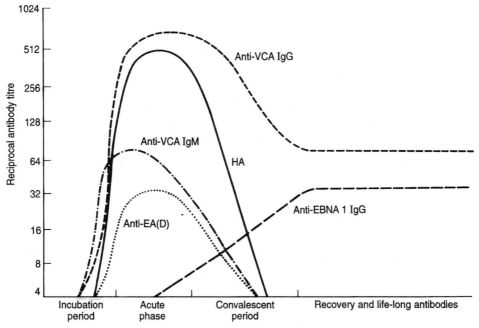

Figure 17.1. Antibody responses following primary Epstein-Barr virus infection.

induced mononucleosis or may be a false negative. This can be confirmed by specific testing for antibodies to CMV or EBV.

For the diagnosis of mumps infection the combination of antibodies to S and V antigens can be used in a similar manner to indicate current versus past infection with this virus (Kleiman 1985). Anti-S antibody rises first and persists for only 2–3 months, whereas anti-V rises later and persists for a significantly longer time period.

tion is prognostic for disease progression. The presence of HBeAg indicates that a patient has infectious virus in their blood and is associated with a poor prognosis, while the presence of anti-HBe suggests that a patient is recovering. The conversion from HBsAg positive to anti-HBs positive along with anti-HBe denotes complete recovery from HBV infection. Thus, by using these various markers one can diagnose HBV infection and can ascertain a prognosis for the disease.

Assessment of antibody and antigen combinations

Hepatitis B virus diagnosis is dependent upon the detection of a combination of viral antigens and anti-viral antibodies in serum (Fig. 17.2). Three antigens of HBV, the surface (s) antigen, core (c) antigen and e antigen are used for this testing as are the antibodies to these antigens (Escobar 1992). The presence of hepatitis B surface (HBsAg) is indicative of active infection and is used to screen for HBV. The detection of anti-HBs is indicative of recovery from HBV infection, while presence of HBc in the absence of either HBsAg or anti-HBs (the core 'window') indicates a late acute infection. The use of HBeAg and anti-HBe detec-

Detection of antibody in fluids other than serum

Cerebrospinal fluid

The measurement of antibodies in the CSF may be useful in the diagnosis of CNS disease. Antibodies may be present in high levels in the CSF as a result of CNS infection and an active immune response or because of leakage of serum into the CSF due to breakdown of the blood–brain barrier (BBB). The two situations can be distinguished by calculating CSF/serum ratios of albumin and IgG (Cremer 1985). The normal levels for albumin and IgG are 200-fold and 500-fold lower, respectively in

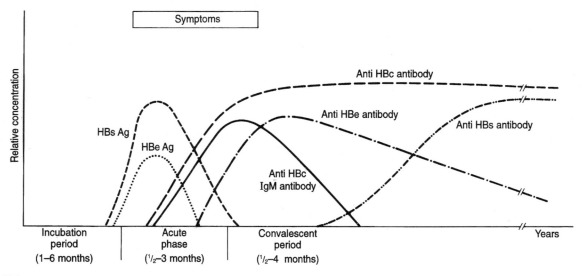

Figure 17.2. Antigen and antibody responses in hepatitis B infection.

CSF. If there is antibody synthesis in the CSF, then only the IgG ratio changes but if there is BBB damage then both the IgG and albumin ratios between CSF and serum will change.

The presence of increased levels of Ig in the CSF is indicative of local antibody synthesis and therefore local viral infection. For the most part this is an IgG response; however, in HSV encephalitis and chronic measles leading to subacute sclerosing panencephalitis IgM class antibody may also be detected (Doerr et al 1976). Additionally, one may compare ratios of antibody in serum versus CSF, such that low ratios, e.g. 8–32, are of diagnostic importance for CNS infection.

Saliva

The detection of antibodies in saliva is not a common laboratory practice. Nevertheless this source of antibody is being examined in circumstances where drawing blood for serum is impractical for reasons of both convenience and cost. There is currently a test kit that is commercially available for testing HIV antibodies in saliva and is based on a similar test that has been reported for testing anti simian immunodefiency virus antibodies in monkeys (Israel et al 1993). While this is marketed in the United States for convenience use, the approach may be very useful in developing nations, where AIDS has become a severe problem and serum collection and testing is far too expensive for the large numbers of people that require testing. The reliability of such testing remains to be verified using large numbers of samples.

Confirmatory testing

The need for confirmatory testing of serum antibodies is most notable for HIV. This is necessitated by the nature of the infection and the primary test used to detect antibody. Because there is a desire to eliminate false negative results, the HIV test is performed so that sensitivity is very high at the cost of decreased specificity. This results in a relatively high false positive rate, necessitating a confirmatory test. In the case of HIV, the primary test is most often performed using ELISA technology. Early tests had a false positive rate as high as 10% (Veronese et al 1992), although later generation tests have reduced this significantly (<1% and for some tests below 0.1%). The most common confirmatory tests are performed using immunoblotting (Western blotting, Chapters 7 & 12) (Veronese et al 1992). The advantages of this latter test is that it is highly specific since a pattern of bands denoting HIV antigens is detected, indicating antibodies to several antigens. Alternative to the Western blot, confirmation may be performed using ELISA or immune fluorescence systems based on different principles than the initial testing. For example, viral lysates, recombinant antigens or peptide antigens can be used for confirmation of positivity. Other testing that requires confirmation generally results from the use of high sensitivity, lowered specificity testing.

Antigen testing

The detection of viral antigen in serum may be used for blood-borne diseases in which there is a substantial period of infection of the blood, to monitor the presence of infection and the progress of that infection, and for the evaluation of drug therapy of such infections. Viruses for which this can be readily performed include HBV, HIV, and HTLV. Antigen testing of blood specimens is not particularly useful for viral infections in which there is a transient viremia, since virus is usually eliminated from the blood prior to the onset of overt disease.

Monitoring infection

Routine testing of serum for viral antigens is limited mainly to HBV and HIV infections. We have discussed above (page 346) the monitoring of HBV infection by antigen detection in concert with detection of the antibody to those antigens. The detection of the HBV antigens has been used more extensively than any other serum antigen detection.

More recently, the detection of HIV p24 antigen has been used to monitor the progression of HIV from clinical latency through the development of overt AIDS (Fig. 17.3). While the detection of this antigen per se is not an indicator of the stage of development of HIV, when used in conjunction with other markers it can be used prognostically (Phillips et al 1991; Henrard et al 1992). Generally, in latent infection, there is little p24 present in blood. When virus replication increases and immune deficiency begins to appear p24 levels increase. This is usually associated with a decline in the number of CD4+ lymphocytes in circulation and these two indicators are prognostic for progressing disease. Additionally, the presence of p24 in a newborn from an HIV infected mother is diagnostic for HIV infection during pregnancy (Amirhessami-Aghili and Spector 1991). It must be noted that a significant proportion of HIV infected individuals may be p24 antigenemia negative during much of their infection, with negative results observed in 30% or more of HIV infected individuals in developed nations and higher percentages of negative samples seen from blood of African patients.

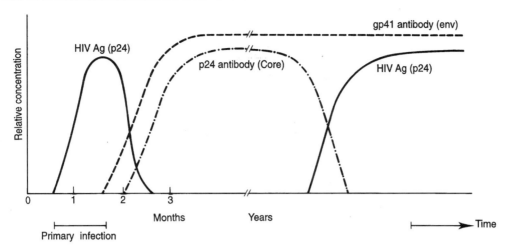

Figure 17.3. Antigen and antibody responses during the course of HIV infection.

Evaluation of drug therapy

The detection of viral antigen to monitor drug therapy is again mainly limited to HBV, HCV and HIV. In the case of the hepatitis viruses the levels of HBsAg and HBeAg are measured following treatment of chronic HBV with interferon alpha (Davis and Hoofnagle 1986). These antigens are usually tested along with the antibodies to the same antigens, as well as liver enzyme levels and HBV DNA polymerase levels. For HCV testing, measurement of antibodies or, more sensitively, the presence of virus genome by PCR, is used to follow the efficacy of interferon therapy for chronic infection (Davis 1994).

Therapy of HIV with azidothymidine (AZT) or other drugs is followed by the monitoring of p24 levels in conjunction with measuring the number of CD4+ lymphocytes in peripheral blood (Japour et al 1993). This method has been very useful for documenting efficacy of therapy. It must be noted that technology such as the development of quantitative PCR has diminished some testing for antigen since the former provides a more precise assessment of the amount of virus present (Persing et al 1993). This is especially true with techniques that can assess quantitatively the amounts of cell associated versus cell free virus in blood.

Use of commercial kits

The serologic assessment of antibodies and antigens using commercially prepared and marketed kits is commonplace. These kits are available for most of the common viruses and are highly reputable for the most part. They use ELISA, radioimmunoassay, immunofluorescence, immunoblotting, latex agglutination, hemagglutination and a variety of other methods for detection. The quality of such kits has improved over the past decade due to the availability of monoclonal antibodies, recombinant technologies and the automation of some testing procedures.

The use of these kits in lieu of reagents developed in-house is encouraged because it adds to the standardization of testing and results in reduced time technologists are required to put in developing and testing reagents. With this in mind however, it is essential for the laboratory to have a thorough quality assurance/quality control program to insure that reagents are of the highest quality and are properly used.

The list of available tests is extensive and constantly changing so it is of little value to list them here. Linscott's Directory provides information on available reagents and tests (Linscott 1992).

Summary

The use of serology to detect viruses remains a vital adjunct to virus isolation and direct detection of virus for the diagnosis of infections. The wide variety of immunoassays is delineated in Chapter 7. This chapter has not dealt with the issue of which assay is best for each virus, since this is often a matter of preference and changes as new assays are introduced. The use of serology requires excellent quality assurance and control and when combined with other viral detection techniques provides the laboratory with the ability to assist the physician in the identification of etiologic agents and to monitor the progression of infection and the success of therapeutic intervention.

References

Amirhessami-Aghili N, Spector SA (1991) J Virol 65: 2231–2236.

Cremer NE (1985) In: Laboratory Diagnosis of Viral Infections, Lennette EH (Ed.) Marcel Dekker, New York, pp. 73–85.

Davis GL (1994) Am J Med 96: 41S–46S.

Davis GL, Hoofnagle JH (1986) Hepatology 6: 1038–1041.

Doerr HW, Gross G, Schmitz H (1976) Med Microbiol Immunol 162: 183–192.

Escobar MR (1992) In: Clinical Virology Manual 2nd Ed. Specter S, Lancz G (Eds.) Elsevier Science, New York, pp. 397–424.

Henrard DR, Mehaffey WF, Allain J-P (1992) AIDS Res Human Retroviruses 8: 47–52.

Herrmann KL, Erdman DD (1992) In: Clinical Virology Manual 2nd Ed. Specter S, Lancz G (Eds.) Elsevier Science, New York, pp. 263–273.

Israel ZR, Dean GA, Maul DH, O'Neil SP, Dreitz MJ, Mullins JI, Fultz PN, Hoover EA (1993) AIDS Res Human Retroviruses 9: 277–286.

Japour AJ, Mayers DL, Johnson VA, Kuritzkes DR, Beckett LA, Arduino J-M, Lane J, Black RJ, Reichelderfer PS, D'Aquila RT, Crumpacker CS, The RV-43 Study Group and The AIDS Trials Clinical Group Virology Committee Resistance Working Group (1993) Antimicrob Agents Chemother 37: 1095–1101.

Kleiman MB (1985) In: Laboratory Diagnosis of Viral Infections, Lennette EH (Ed.) Marcel Dekker, New York, pp. 369–384.

Lennette ET (1985) In: Laboratory Diagnosis of Viral Infections, Lennette EH (Ed.) Marcel Dekker, New York, pp. 257–271.

Lincott's Directory of Immunological and Biological Reagents, 7th Ed. 1992. Santa Rosa, CA p. 237.

Lopez C, Arvin AM, Ashley R (1993) In: The Human Herpesvirus, Roizman B, Whitley RJ, Lopez C (Eds.) Raven Press, New York, pp. 397–425.

Paar D, Straus SE (1992) In: Clinical Virology Manual 2nd Ed. Specter S, Lancz G (Eds.) Elsevier Science, New York, pp. 501–526.

Pass RF, Griffiths PD, August AM (1983) J Infect Dis 147: 40–46.

Persing DH, Smith TF, Tenover FC, White TJ (Eds.) (1993) Diagnostic Molecular Microbiology: Principles and Applications. ASM Press, Washington, DC, p. 641.

Phillips AN, Lee CA, Elford J et al (1991) AIDS 5: 1217–1222.

Veronese F.diM, Lusso F, Schüpbach J, Gallo RC (1992) In: Clinical Virology Manual 2nd Ed. Specter S, Lancz G (Eds.) Elsevier Science, New York, pp. 585–625.

Ziola B, Salmi A, Panelius M, Halonen P (1979) Clin Immunol Immunopathol 13: 462–474.

Disinfection

18

S. Specter
D. Jeffries

Virucidal agents may inactivate viruses either because of their physical or chemical properties. These agents generally are effective on viruses outside of their host cells. The ability of these agents to inactivate virus is very closely associated with the conditions under which they are used. Depending on the agent, this may include temperature, pH, moisture content of the sample, concentration and composition of the virus, concentration of the agent, and time of exposure. Thus, viruses kept at room temperature will become inactivated more rapidly than those held at 4°C. Likewise some viruses maintained at neutral pH may be inactivated less rapidly than at either lower or higher pH (Lancz 1976), other viruses such as enteroviruses may be stable at highly acidic pH. Some viruses are also known to lose infectivity as the sample in which they are collected dries (Parker et al 1944). Thus, virus maintained in mucus containing secretions on an environmental surface is likely to retain infectivity longer than the same amount of virus in saliva, since the latter will dry more quickly (Dunham 1977).

An important factor in the effectiveness of disinfection is the virus titer present at the outset of addition of the disinfectant. The loss of infectivity over time is such that if a sample that is treated with a virucidal agent is held for 15 min it may lose 50% of its infectivity, after 30 min 90% is lost, and by 60 min there is a 99% loss. If a sample contains 1000 infectious particles per milliliter at outset, after 15 min 0.1 ml will contain approximately 5 infectious units, whereas after 60 min 0.1 ml has a 10% chance of containing infectious material. By contrast, if the original concentration of virus is 10^6 particles per milliliter, then even a 99% inactivation after 1 h may leave sufficient infectious material to cause infection; i.e. 1000 infectious units will be present in 0.1 ml.

The ability of various agents to inactivate viruses is also dependent on the composition of the virus. Many viruses contain a lipid envelope that is sensitive to lipid solvents such as ether, chloroform or detergents, whereas naked (non-enveloped) viruses are resistant to such agents (Dunham 1977). Finally, the nature of the disinfection agents can determine the extent of inactivation. This will depend upon whether the agent is physical or chemical and if it is organic or inorganic. It should be noted that other organic material in solutions containing viruses may inhibit the virucidal effects of many disinfectants. Wiedbrauk and Johnston (1993) have delineated which compounds are particularly useful for viruses that are commonly encountered both in the laboratory and on environmental surfaces. Inactivation of commonly used disinfectants is shown in Table 18.1.

The methods for testing virucidal agents are well delineated (Koski and Chen 1977).

Inorganic chemical agents

The most commonly used inorganic disinfectants are halophilic compounds, including

Virology Methods Manual
ISBN 0–12–465330–8

Table 18.1. Inactivation of commonly used disinfectants

	Protein	Hard Water	Detergents
Hypochlorites	++++	+	C
Phenolics	+	+	C
Alcohols*	+	+	–
Formaldehyde	+	+	–
Glutaraldehyde	+	+	–

* Alcohols are extremely poor in penetrating proteinaceous material and are, therefore, of very limited use as disinfectants.
C, Cationic detergents

chlorine and bromine (Brown et al 1963; Clarke and Kabler 1964; Lund 1964). The most readily available antiviral for use is common household bleach (sodium hypochlorite), which usually can be used as a 10% solution (the solution must contain 10,000 ppm available chlorine), to inactivate many enveloped and naked viruses. The bleach is capable of destroying nucleic acids, making it a universally effective disinfectant for viruses. Thus, it is the recommended disinfectant for routine use in the clinical laboratory, the physician's office, and any setting where concerns about viral contamination exist. Its ability to inactivate nucleic acids makes household bleach an ideal agent for decontamination of a laboratory where polymerase chain reactions are performed, and carry over of nucleic acids is a concern (Prince and Andrews 1992). Chlorine and bromine are useful for the inactivation of viruses in swimming pools when used at about 0.5 parts per million. Iodine also can be used as a disinfectant of contaminated water supplies (Dunham and MacNeal 1944; Kabler 1962).

Ozone is considered to be safer and more effective than chlorine for the disinfection of water, but is not practical for widespread use due to cost (Sliter 1974). Similarly, hydrogen peroxide can be used to inactivate viruses. However, the presence of other organic materials in fluids will compete with the viruses and block the effects of the H_2O_2. Acid solutions, such as 1 N HCl, and alkaline compounds, such as 2% NaOH are also useful disinfectants for inactivation of viruses.

Metals and metal salts also have antiviral properties. Copper salts, mercury, potassium permanganate and silver nitrate have been used as virucidal agents (Dunham 1977).

Organic chemical agents

The list of organic compounds with virucidal activity is quite long, and includes quaternary ammonium compounds, alcohols, aldehydes, ether, glycerol, beta-propiolactone, ethylene oxide, digestive enzymes and a preparation known as liquor antisepticus.

Benzalkonium chloride (Zephiran) has been demonstrated to be useful for the disinfection of skin. It is the preparation of choice for cleansing animal bites, due to its ability to inactivate rabiesvirus when used at a 1:1000 dilution. By contrast this compound is not highly effective against naked viruses. O-phenylphenol is likewise active against enveloped but not naked viruses (Klein and Deforest 1963). Diethyl ether is also an effective agent for inactivating lipid containing viruses, showing virucidal activity at concentrations of 3–10% for these viruses. However, ether is not effective against poliovirus (a non-enveloped virus), even at 95% concentration.

Seventy percent ethanol is an effective disinfectant for naked and enveloped viruses, but can be decreased in activity by substances that precipitate alcohol. This can be overcome by the addition of 0.005 N NaOH to the alcohol solution. While lower concentrations of ethanol may be effectively virucidal, the higher concentration is more effective, with most virus destroyed within a few minutes by 70%. Methanol also may be used to inactivate virus, but is considerably less effective than ethanol (Cox et al 1947). However, alcohols penetrate organic matter rather poorly and are not effective for disinfection of such materials. Furthermore, the inactivation of HIV and other viruses by alcohols is slow and the alcohol is likely to evaporate, if used for surface decontamination, before the virus is inactivated (Hanson et al 1989). Liquor antisepticus is a compound described in the National Formulary that can be used as a mouthwash (National Formulary 1965). Its principal ingredient is ethyl alcohol (28.5% by volume).

Formaldehyde is an excellent virucidal agent, and can be used to inactivate viruses as a 0.3% solution (Dunham 1977; Wiedbrauk and Johnston 1993). Similarly gluteraldehyde is very useful for cold sterilization and a 2% solution will inactivate most virus in 10 min when buffered with sodium bicarbonate at pH 7.5–8.5.

Beta-propiolactone is an effective virucidal agent, even when virus is in plasma, that has low toxicity in mammalian systems. It has been used in the preparation of vaccines, such as the Merieux rabies vaccine.

Physical agents

Elevated temperature has a distinct antiviral effect, increasing the rate of virus inactivation. The inactivation rate due to high temperature varies for different viruses and can be changed greatly by the pH of a solution. The presence of a protein stabilizer such as serum decreases the ability of heat to inactivate virus in a suspension. Most viruses lose some infectivity when heated at 56°C for 30 min. All viruses are destroyed by appropriate autoclaving, 121°C under 15 psi pressure for 15 min.

Ultraviolet radiation is also a highly effective virucidal physical agent, as long as it is of suitable wavelength and intensity. Wavelengths of approximately 250 nm have been demonstrated to be effective against influenza virus (Dunham 1977). The effectiveness is significantly diminished when the virus suspension is moved away from the source of radiation. In addition, ultraviolet rays are more effective through air than water, and particulate matter (dust particles or salt crystals) can further decrease effectiveness.

Ionizing radiation, including X-rays, gamma rays, high energy electrons, deuterons and alpha particles, is capable of inactivating viruses. This is effected by the damaging of viral nucleic acids. However, radical scavengers are able to inhibit the effects of ionizing radiation. Viruses have different levels of resistance to ultraviolet and gamma radiation, depending on the target size of the nucleic acid. Many of the doses necessary for inactivation of mammalian viruses are listed by McCrea (1960). Ionizing radiation has been used for many years for sterilization of disposable medical supplies, and has become more popular of late for more common consumable items including food.

Filters may also be used for the sterilization of liquids or air. While most common filters that are used to remove bacteria from solutions do not remove viruses, small pore filters can be used to hold back viruses. This practice is most commonly used for filtering air in biological safety cabinets or 'clean rooms' using hepa-filters. The use of such filters is generally reserved for areas where tissue culture is performed, to provide sterile air, or in Biosafety level 3 and 4 rooms, to remove the risk of contamination of the environment when pathogenic viruses are studied.

Summary

There are a wide variety of methods that can be used for sterilization, disinfection and antisepsis. When possible, the recommended method for sterilization is steam heating using an autoclave. An alternative effective method of limiting contamination is to use disposable sterile items (needles, syringes, pipettes, tubes, flasks, etc.) that come in a sealed sterile container. Such items, if not autoclavable, can be sterilized using γ-irradiation or ethylene oxide gas after packaging, to achieve sterilization. The recommended disinfectants for decontamination of surfaces or solutions containing viruses are bleach or gluteraldehyde. Instruments that are reused should be cleaned with detergents that will remove organic matter, prior to disinfection with these substances, as such material promotes survival of viruses.

References

Brown JR, McLean DM, Nixon MC (1963) Can J Pub Hlth 54: 267–270.

Clarke NA, Kabler PW (1954) Am J Hyg 59: 119–127.

Cox HR, van der Scheer J, Aiston S, Bohnel E (1947) J Immunol 56: 149–166.

Dunham WB (1977) In: Disinfection, Sterilization and Preservation, 2nd Edn, Block SS (Ed.) Lea and Febiger, Philadelphia, pp. 426–441.

Dunham WB, MacNeal WJ (1944) J Immunol 49: 123–128.

Hanson PJV, Gor D, Jeffries DJ, Collins JV (1989) Brit Med J 298: 862–864.

Kabler PW (1962) Ann Rev Microbiol 16: 127–140.

Klein, M Deforest A (1963) Soap Chem Spec 39: 70–72.

Koski TA, Chen JHS (1977) In: Disinfection, Sterilization and Preservation 2nd Edn, Block SS (Ed.) Lea and Febiger, Philadelphia, pp. 116–134.

Lancz GJ (1976) Virology 75: 488–491.

Lund E (1964) Am J Hyg 80: 1–10.

McCrea JF (1960) Ann NY Acad Sci 83: 692–705.

National Formulary, 12th Ed. (NF XII) (1965) American Pharmaceutical Assoc, Washington, pp. 36–37.

Parker ER, Dunham WB, MacNeal WJ (1944) J Lab Clin Med 29: 37–42.

Prince AM, Andrus L (1992) BioTechniques 12: 358–360.

Sliter JT (1974) J Water Pollut Control Fed 46: 4–6.

Wiedbrauk DL, Johnston SLG (1993) Manual of Clinical Virology, Raven Press, New York, 273 pp.

Chapter 18

Appendix A: Biosafety in the virology laboratory

Working with viruses which are infectious to humans poses a considerable risk of laboratory-acquired infection. This was demonstrated on numerous occasions in the past, and led to the establishment of a classification of viruses and other infectious agents into four groups depending upon the hazards to the laboratory worker. A full description of the historical development and current guidelines for biosafety can be found in *Biosafety in Microbiological and Biomedical Laboratories* edited by JW Richmond and RW McKinney, third edition, May 1993. Published by the US Department of Health and Human Services, Publication number (CDC) 93-8395.

Here we reprint from that publication the summary description of recommended safety practices at each of the four levels (Table 1).

Biosafety level 4 (maximum containment) laboratories are expensive to maintain and exist only in Australia, Canada, France, Germany, Russia, South Africa, the UK and the USA.

For human blood-borne pathogens, biosafety precautions have been issued to health care and clinical laboratory workers under the term 'Universal Precautions' and these need to be observed for all work involving contact with potentially infectious blood and body fluids in addition to utilization of the appropriate biosafety level laboratory. A full description of universal precautions has been published. (*Occupational Exposure to Bloodborne Pathogens, Final Rule, US Federal Register 56,* 64175–64182, 1991).

Since the eradication of smallpox, routine vaccination with vaccinia virus has ceased throughout the world. However work with vaccinia virus continues in many virology laboratories because of its value as a gene vector, e.g. in various vaccinia-based expression systems. In persons vaccinated within the previous ten years, work with vaccinia virus poses no special risk, and the US policy is that such work can be conducted at Biosafety Level 2 by appropriately vaccinated persons in a laboratory area with appropriate warning signs to prevent entry of unvaccinated persons. However, vaccination itself can be associated with significant adverse reactions, and in the UK and other European countries vaccination of laboratory workers is not advised (and is illegal in some countries, e.g. Germany). The danger to unvaccinated laboratory workers who use vaccinia virus is that they could become infected at an inappropriate site (e.g. the eye), with the possibility of a serious adverse reaction. The laboratory director may wish, therefore, to raise work with vaccinia virus to Biosafety Level 3, where such unvaccinated persons are involved.

The following classification of vertebrate viruses potentially infectious for humans indicates the appropriate biosafety level (2, 3 or 4) at which work should be performed. Note that some viruses appear twice, depending upon the type of work being undertaken. In general, work involving virus concentration to high titre, production of aerosols, or virus infection of an animal host may require a higher biosafety level than that needed for other types of work. The laboratory director is responsible for appropriate risk assessment, and on occasion may decide to select a biosafety level higher than that recommended in the following classification.

Virology Methods Manual
ISBN 0–12–465330–8

Level Two

Aabahoyo
Abras
Abu Hammad
Acado
Acara
Adeno-associated virus
Adenoviruses
Aguacate
Alfuy
Almpiwar
Amapari
Ananindeua
Anhanga
Anhembi
Anopheles A
Anopheles B
Apeu
Apoi
Aride
Arkonam
Aroa
Aruac
Arumowot
Astrovirus
Aura
Avalon
B19
Bagaza
Bahig
Bakau
Baku
Bandia
Bangoran
Bangui
Banzi
Barmah Forest
Barur
Batai
Batama
Bauline
Bebaru
Belmont
Benevides
Benfica
Betioga
Bimiti
Birao
Bluetongue
Boraceia

Botambi
Boteke
Bouboui
Buffalopox
Bujaru
Bunyamwera
Bunyip
Burg E Arab
Bushbush
Bussuquara
Buttonwillow
Bwamba
Cacao
Cache valley
California encephalitis
Calmito
Calovo
Candiru
Cape Wrath
Capim
Caraparu
Carey Island
Catu
Chaco
Chagres
Chandipura
Changuinola
Charleville
Chenuda
Chikungunya (vs 131/25)*
Chilibre
Chobar Gorge
Clo Mor
Colorado tick fever
Coronavirus
Corriparta
Cotia
Cowbone Ridge
Cowpox
Coxsackie
Csiro Village
Cuiaba
Cytomegalovirus
D'Aguilar
Dakar Bat
Dengue 1[†]
Dengue 2[†]
Dengue 3[†]
Dengue 4[†]
Dera Ghazi Khan

Eastern equine encephalitis[†]
Edge Hill
Entebbe bat
Enteroviruses
Epizootic haemorrhagic
    disease (of deer)
Epstein-Barr
Erve
Eubenangee
Eyach
Flanders
Fort Morgan
Frijoles
Gamboa
Gan Gan
Gomoka
Gossas
Grand Arbaud
Great Island
Guajara
Guama
Gumbo Limbo
Hart Park
Hazara
Hepatitis A
Hepatitis B
Hepatitis C
Hepatitis D
Hepatitis E
Hepatitis F
Hepatitis G
Highlands J
Huacho
Hughes
Human herpesvirus
Human papillomaviruses
Icoaraci
Ieri
Ilesha
Ilheus
Influenza A
Influenza B
Influenza C
Ingwavuma
Inkoo
Ippy
Irituia
Isfahan
Itaporanga
Itaqui

Jamestown Canyon
Japanaut
Jerry Slough
Johnstone Atoll
Joinjakaka
Juan Diaz
Jugra
Junin (vs Candid #1)
Jurona
Jutiapa
Kadam
Kaeng Khoi
Kaikalur
Kaisodi
Kamese
Kammavan pettai
Kannaman galam
Kao Shuan
Karimabad
Karshi
Kasba
Kemerovo
Kern Canyon
Ketapang
Keterah
Keuraliba
Keystone
Kismayo
Klamath
Kokobera
Kolongo
Koongol
Kotonkan
Kowanyama
Kunjin
Kununurra
Kwatta
La Crosse
La Joya
Lagos bat
Landjia
Langat
Lanjan
Las Maloyas
Latino
Le Dantec
Lebombo
Lednice
Lipovnik
Lokern

Lone Star
Lukuni
Lymphocytic choriomeningitis
M'poko
Madrid
Maguari
Mahogany Hammock
Main Drain
Malakal
Manawa
Manzanilla
Mapputta
Maprik
Marco
Marituba
Marrakai
Matariya
Matruh
Matucare
Measles
Melao
Mermet
Milkers nodule
Minatitlan
Minnal
Mirim
Mitchell River
Modoc
Moju
Molluscum contagiosum
Mono Lake
Montana myotis
    leukoencephalitis
Moriche
Mosqueiro
Mossuril
Mount Elgon bat
Mumps
Murutucu
Mykines
Navarro
Nepuyo
Ngaingan
Nique
Nkolbisson
Nola
Norwalk
Ntaya
Nugget
Nyamanini

Nyando
O'nyong nyong
Okhotskiy
Okola
Olifantsvlei
Oliveros
Orf
Oriboca
Ossa
Pacora
Pacui
Pahayokee
Palyam
Parainfluenza
Parana
Pata
Pathum Thani
Patois
Phnom-Penh bat
Pichinde
Pixuna
Point
Poliovirus
Pongola
Ponteves
Precarious
Pretoria
Prospect Hill
Puchong
Punta Salinas
Punta Toro
Qalyub
Quaranfil
Rabies virus
Reoviruses
Respiratory syncytial
Restan
Retroviruses, including human
    and simian immunodeficiency
    viruses (HIV-1, HIV-2, and SIV)
Rhinoviruses
Rift Valley fever (vs MP-12)
Rio Bravo
Rio Grande
Ross River
Rotaviruses
Royal farm
Rubella
Sabo
Saboya

Saint Floris
Sakhalin
Salehabad
San Angelo
Sandfly fever (Sicilian)
Sandfly fever (Naples)
Sandjimba
Sango
Sathuperi
Sawgrass
Sebokele
Seletar
Sembalam
Serra do Navio
Shamonda
Shark River
Shuni
Silverwater
Simbu
Simian hemorrhagic fever
Sindbis
Sixgun City
Snow Mountain
Snowshoe Hare
Sokuluk
Soldado
Sororoca
Spumavirus
Stratford
Sunday Canyon
Tacaiuma
Tacaribe
Taggert
Tahyna
Tamiami
Tanapox
Tanga
Tanjong Rabok
Tataguine
Tehran
Tembe
Tembusu
Tensaw
Tete
Tettnang
Thimiri
Thottapalayam
Tibrogargan
Timbo
Timboteua

Tindholmur
Torovirus
Toscana
Toure
Transmissible spongiform
    encephalopathies[†]
    (Creutzfeldt-Jakob, kuru,
    scrapie and related agents)
Tribec
Triniti
Trivittatus
Trubanaman
Tsuruse
Turlock
Tyuleniy
Uganda S
Umatilla
Umbre
Una
Upolu
Urucuri
Usutu
Uukuniemi
Vaccinia (vaccinated persons)
Varicella-zoster
Vellore
Venezuelan equine encephalo-
    myelitis (vs TC-83)*[†]
Venkatapuram
Vesicular stomatitis – Indiana
Vesicular stomatitis – New
    Jersey
Vinces
Virgin River
Wad Medani
Walla
Wanowrie
Warrego
Western equine encephalitis
Whataroa
Witwatersrand
Wonga
Wongorr
Wyeomyia
Yabapox
Yaquinea Head
Yatapox*
Yellow fever (vs 17-D)
Yogue
Zaliv Terpeniya

Zegla
Zika
Zingilamo
Zirqa

Level Three
Adelaide River
Agua Preta
Aino
Akabane
Alenquer
Almeirim
Altamira
Andasibe
Antequera
Araguari
Aransas Bay
Arbia
Arboledas
Babanki
Batken
Belem
Berrimah
Bhanja
Bimbo
Black Creek Canal
Bobaya
Bobia
Bozo
Buenaventura
Cabassue
Cacipacore
Calchaqui
Cananeia
Caninde
Chikungunya
Chim
Coastal Plains
Cocal
Connecticut
Corfu
Dabakala
Dhori[†]
Dobrava-Belgrade
Douglas
Dugbe
Enseada
Estero Real
Everglades
Flexal

Fomede
Forecariah
Fort Sherman
Gabek Forest
Gadgets Gully
Garba
Germiston
Getah
Gordil
Hantaan
Herpesvirus simiae (B virus)
Human polyomaviruses (JC,
   BK)
Iaco
Ibaraki
Ife
Ingangapi
Inini
Israel Turkey meningitis
Issyk-kul
Itaituba
Itimirim
Itupiranga
Jacareacanga
Jamanxi
Japanese encephalitis
Jari
Junin
Kairi
Kedougou
Khasan
Kimberley
Kindia
Koutango
Kyzylagach
Lake Clarendon
Llano Seco
Louping III
Lymphocytic choriomeningitis
   (infected animals)
Macaua
Mapuera
Mayaro
Mboke
Meaban
Middleburg
Mobala
Mojui Dos Compos
Monte Dourado
Mopeia

Mucambo
Munguba
Murray Valley encephalitis
Nairobi sheep disease
Naranjal
Nariva
Nasoule
Ndelle
Ndumu
Negishi
New Minto
Ngari
Ngoupe
Nodamura
Northway
Odrenisrou
Omo
Oriximina
Oropouche
Orungo
Ouango
Oubangui
Oubi
Ourem
Palestina
Para
Paramushir
Paroo River
Peaton
Perinet
Pery
Petevo
Picola
Piry
Playas
Powassan
Pueblo Viejo
Purus
Puumala[†]
Radi
Razdan
Resistencia
Rift Valley fever
Rochambeau
Rocio
Sagiyama
Sal Vieja
Salanga
San Perlita
San Juan

Santa Rosa
Santarem
Saraca
Saumarez Reef
Sedlec
Semliki Forest[†]
Sena Madureira
Seoul
Sepik
Shokwe
Sin Nombre
Slovakia
Somone
Spipur
Spondweni
St Louis encephalitis
Tai
Tamdy
Telok Forest
Termeil
Thiafora
Thogoto
Tilligerry
Tinaroo
Tlacotalpan
Tocio
Tonate
Ttinga
Turuna
Venezuelan equine
   encephalitis
Vesicular stomatitis (infected
   animals)
Wesselbron
West Nile
Xiburema
Yacaaba
Yaounde
Yellow fever
Yoka
Yug Bogkanovac

Level Four
Absettarov[†]
Black Creek Canal (infected
   animals)
Congo-Crimean hemorrhagic
   fever
Ebola
Guanarito

Hanzalova	Machupo	Russian Spring-Summer
Hypr	Marburg	encephalitis
Junin	Omsk hemorrhagic fever	Sabià
Kumlinge	Rift Valley Fever (infected	Sin Nombre (infected animals)
Kyasanur Forest disease	animals)	Tick-borne encephalitis
Lassa		

* Vaccine Strain

† Viruses marked with this dagger are classified in Europe either one level above (for Level Two) or below (for Level Three) the US levels.

Table 1 Summary of recommended biosafety levels for infectious agents

Biosafety Level	Agents	Practices	Safety Equipment (Primary barriers)	Facilities (Secondary Barriers)
1	Not known to cause disease in healthy adults	Standard Microbiological Practices	None required	BSL-1 plus: autoclave available
2	Associated with human disease, hazard=auto-inoculation, ingestion, mucous membrane	BCL-1 practice plus: • Limited access • Biohazard warning signs • Biosafety manual defining any needed waste decontamination or medical surveillance policies	Primary barriers= Class I or II BSCs or other physical containment devices used for all manipulations of agents that cause splashes or aerosols of infectious materials; PPEs; laboratory coats; gloves; face protection as needed	BSL-1 plus: autoclave available
3	Indigenous or exotic agents with potential for aerosol transmission; disease may have serious or lethal consequences	BSL-2 practice plus: • Controlled access • Decontamination of all waste • Decontamination of lab clothing before laundering • Baseline serum	Primary barriers= Class I or II BSCs or other physical containment devices used for all manipulations of agents; PPEs: protective lab clothing; gloves; respiratory protection as needed	BSL-2 plus: • Physical separation from access corridors • Self-closing, double door access • Exhausted air not recirculated • Negative airflow into laboratory
4	Dangerous/exotic agents which pose high risk of life-threatening disease, aerosol-transmitted lab infections; or related agents with unknown risk of transmission	BSL-3 practices plus: • Clothing change before entering • Shower on exit • All material decontaminated on exit from facility	Primary barriers=All procedures conducted in Class III BSCs or Class I or II BSCs *in combination with* full-body, air-supplied, positive pressure personnel suit	BSL-3 plus: • Separate building or isolated zone • Dedicated supply/ exhaust, vacuum, and decon systems • Other requirements as outlined in the recommended text

Based on '*Biosafety in Microbiological and Biomedical Laboratories*' with kind permission of the Editor, JW Richmond

Appendix B: Metabolic inhibitors used in virology

Most inhibitors are highly toxic, and it is essential that they are used strictly in accordance with all relevant safety instructions and procedures.

Inhibitor	Molecular mass	Effect	Typical concentration for use
Cycloheximide (3-[2-{3,5-dimethyl-2-oxocyclohexyl}-2-hydroxyethyl]glutarimide	281.4	Inhibitor of eukaryotic protein synthesis at translational level; used to induce high levels of mRNA prior to removal	100–360 μM
Puromycin (3'-[α-amino-p-methoxycinnamamido]-3'-deoxy-N,N-dimethyladenosine	544.4	Protein synthesis inhibitor, Disrupts polyribosomes	200 μM
Castanospermine (8$\alpha\beta$-indolizidine-1α,6β,7α,8β-tetrol)	189.2	Inhibits processing of high-mannose oligosccharides to complex-type	530–1320 μM
1-Deoxymannojirimycin (1,5-dideoxy-1,5-imino-D-mannitol)	199.6	Inhibits processing of high-mannose oligosaccharides to complex-type	1000–4000 μM
1-Deoxynojirimycin (1,5-dideoxy-1,5-imino-D-glucitol)	163.2	Inhibits formation of high-mannose oligosaccharides	1000–5000 μM
Monensin	692.9	Monovalent ionophore: Multiple effects on glycosylation due to disruption of passage through the Golgi	1.0–1.5 μM
Swainosine (8α,β-indolizidine-1α,2α,8β-triol)	173.2	Inhibits processing of high-mannose oligosaccharides	0.1–29 μM
Tunicamycin	840 approximately; very variable, multiple isomers	Prevents N-linked glycosylation	1.0–6 μM
Actinomycin D	1255.4	Irreversible inhibitor of transcription from double-standard DNA (RNA synthesis is inhibited at lower concentrations than is DNA synthesis)	0.4–8 μM

Virology Methods Manual
ISBN 0–12–465330–8

Inhibitor	Molecular mass	Effect	Typical concentration for use
Aphidicolin	338.5	Reversible inhibitor of eukaryotic DNA polymerases α and β and some viral DNA polymerases. May be used to synchronize cell growth	3–20 μM
Phosphonoacetic acid	140.0	Inhibits some viral DNA polymerases (notably in herpesviruses, where it is used to assay DNA synthesis-dependent protein synthesis)	2140 μM
α-Amanitin	919.0	Inhibits RNA polymerases II (mRNA) and III (tRNA)	0.001–0.01 μM (polymerase II) 10–100 μM (polymerase III)
Cordycepin (3'-deoxyadenosine)	251.2	Inhibits RNA synthesis and mRNA polyadenylation	200 μM

This table is derived from *Virology Labfax*, D.R. Harper (Ed.), 1993, Bios Scientific Publishers, and is presented here with permission of the publishers.

Appendix C: Virus taxonomy

Viruses are classified on the basis of:

Morphology

Size, capsid structure (icosahedral symmetry, helical symmetry, complex symmetry) and appearance in the electron microscope, presence of envelope, other structural features (presence of cellular structures or unusual viral structures, e.g. ribosomes in *Arenaviridae*, tegument in *Herpesviridae*).

Genome

Type of nucleic acid (RNA or DNA), number of strands (single or double) and relationship to messenger RNA if single stranded (termed 'positive sense' if of the same base sequence as mRNA, 'negative sense' if of complementary sequence) or segments present, sequence homology and similarities of genetic organization to other viruses.

Physical and biochemical properties

Buoyant density (in cesium chloride) and sedimentation constant, pH stability, number and size of proteins present, presence of lipid (usually as an envelope).

Serology

Presence of antigens cross-reactive with other viruses.

Pathology

Nature of disease caused, mechanisms involved.

A novel virus will be assigned to a family (ending -*viridae*) and genus (ending -*virus*), and possibly to other taxonomical subdivisions, on the basis of these properties. The heirarchy of classification is:

Classification	Suffix	Example	Notes
Order	-virales	*Mononegavirales*	Only one order defined to date.
Family	-viridae	*Paramyxoviridae*	Always defined.
Subfamily	-virinae	*Pneumovirinae*	Not always defined.
Genus	-virus	*Pneumovirus*	Always defined.
Species	None	Respiratory syncytial virus	Always defined.

The size of individual virus families varies enormously, for example:

Filoviridae: Two members, Marburg and Ebola viruses

Picornaviridae: Over two hundred members, including poliovirus, rhinoviruses (common cold), hepatitis A virus.

As an example of the processes involved in virus classification:

Human herpes virus 6 was assigned to the family *Herpesviridae* on the basis of its morphology (enveloped, with a 100–110 nm icosahedral nucleocapsid and visible tegument between the nucleocapsid and the envelope) and the presence of a large double-stranded DNA genome, and noted to be related to Epstein-Barr virus (human herpes virus 5, subfamily *Gammaherpesvirinae*) on the basis of its behaviour in cell culture, has since been reclassified as closer to cytomegalovirus (human herpes virus 4, subfamily *Betaherpesvirinae*) on the basis of its genomic structure and sequence.

While the nature of the disease caused by a virus has little effect on its placement in taxonomy, it may influence the name used for the virus itself. For example: The human hepatitis

Virology Methods Manual
ISBN 0–12–465330–8

viruses A to E are only very distantly related, and belong to four different virus families (A, *Picornaviridae*; B, *Hepadnaviridae*; C, *Flaviviridae*; E, *Caliciviridae*), while Hepatitis D 'virus' is a sub-viral infectious agent related to the viroids of plants. Despite this, they have very similar names, based on their role in hepatitis.

A virus is usually named, often from the disease caused, before it is assigned a place in the taxonomical structure, and it may take a great deal of time before a final classification is agreed by the International Committee on the Taxonomy of Viruses (ICTV), the responsible body in these matters, and even this may change when new evidence becomes available. For the current classification of most known viruses, readers are directed to the latest report of the International Committee on Taxonomy of Viruses, whose details are as follows:

Virus Taxonomy. Sixth report of the International Committee on Taxonomy of Viruses ed. FA Murphy, CM Fauquet, DHL Bishop, SA Ghabriel, AW Jarvis, GP Martelli, MA Mayo, MD Summers. Archives of Virology, Supp. 10, Vienna: Springer Verlag, 1995.

Index

Index

Index